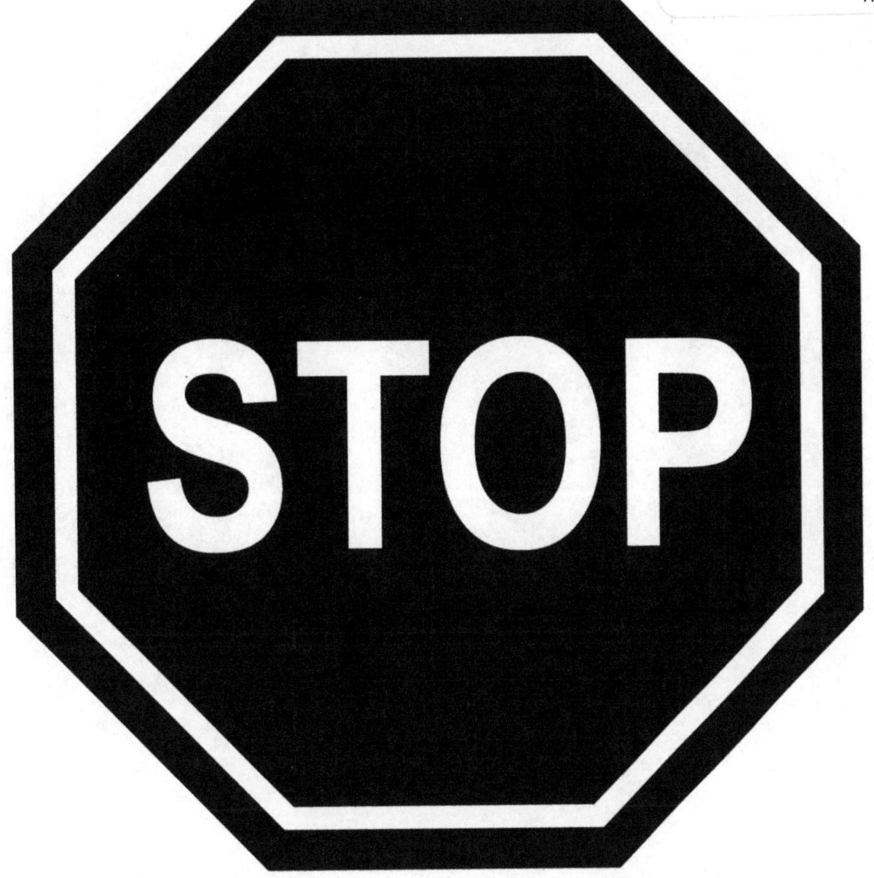

FREE Test Taking Tips DVD Offer

To help us better serve you, we have developed a Test Taking Tips DVD that we would like to give you for FREE. **This DVD covers world-class test taking tips that you can use to be even more successful when you are taking your test.**

All that we ask is that you email us your feedback about your study guide. Please let us know what you thought about it – whether that is good, bad or indifferent.

To get your **FREE Test Taking Tips DVD**, email freedvd@studyguideteam.com with "FREE DVD" in the subject line and the following information in the body of the email:

a. The title of your study guide.

b. Your product rating on a scale of 1-5, with 5 being the highest rating.

c. Your feedback about the study guide. What did you think of it?

d. Your full name and shipping address to send your free DVD.

If you have any questions or concerns, please don't hesitate to contact us at freedvd@studyguideteam.com.

Thanks again!

PCAT Prep Book 2020-2021

PCAT Study Guide & Practice Test Questions for the Pharmacy College Admissions Test [2nd Edition]

Test Prep Books

Written and edited by Test Prep Books.

ISBN 13: 9781628458480
ISBN 10: 1628458488

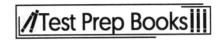

Table of Contents

Quick Overview

As you draw closer to taking your exam, effective preparation becomes more and more important. Thankfully, you have this study guide to help you get ready. Use this guide to help keep your studying on track and refer to it often.

This study guide contains several key sections that will help you be successful on your exam. The guide contains tips for what you should do the night before and the day of the test. Also included are test-taking tips. Knowing the right information is not always enough. Many well-prepared test takers struggle with exams. These tips will help equip you to accurately read, assess, and answer test questions.

A large part of the guide is devoted to showing you what content to expect on the exam and to helping you better understand that content. In this guide are practice test questions so that you can see how well you have grasped the content. Then, answer explanations are provided so that you can understand why you missed certain questions.

Don't try to cram the night before you take your exam. This is not a wise strategy for a few reasons. First, your retention of the information will be low. Your time would be better used by reviewing information you already know rather than trying to learn a lot of new information. Second, you will likely become stressed as you try to gain a large amount of knowledge in a short amount of time. Third, you will be depriving yourself of sleep. So be sure to go to bed at a reasonable time the night before. Being well-rested helps you focus and remain calm.

Be sure to eat a substantial breakfast the morning of the exam. If you are taking the exam in the afternoon, be sure to have a good lunch as well. Being hungry is distracting and can make it difficult to focus. You have hopefully spent lots of time preparing for the exam. Don't let an empty stomach get in the way of success!

When travelling to the testing center, leave earlier than needed. That way, you have a buffer in case you experience any delays. This will help you remain calm and will keep you from missing your appointment time at the testing center.

Be sure to pace yourself during the exam. Don't try to rush through the exam. There is no need to risk performing poorly on the exam just so you can leave the testing center early. Allow yourself to use all of the allotted time if needed.

Remain positive while taking the exam even if you feel like you are performing poorly. Thinking about the content you should have mastered will not help you perform better on the exam.

Once the exam is complete, take some time to relax. Even if you feel that you need to take the exam again, you will be well served by some down time before you begin studying again. It's often easier to convince yourself to study if you know that it will come with a reward!

Test-Taking Strategies

1. Predicting the Answer

When you feel confident in your preparation for a multiple-choice test, try predicting the answer before reading the answer choices. This is especially useful on questions that test objective factual knowledge. By predicting the answer before reading the available choices, you eliminate the possibility that you will be distracted or led astray by an incorrect answer choice. You will feel more confident in your selection if you read the question, predict the answer, and then find your prediction among the answer choices. After using this strategy, be sure to still read all of the answer choices carefully and completely. If you feel unprepared, you should not attempt to predict the answers. This would be a waste of time and an opportunity for your mind to wander in the wrong direction.

2. Reading the Whole Question

Too often, test takers scan a multiple-choice question, recognize a few familiar words, and immediately jump to the answer choices. Test authors are aware of this common impatience, and they will sometimes prey upon it. For instance, a test author might subtly turn the question into a negative, or he or she might redirect the focus of the question right at the end. The only way to avoid falling into these traps is to read the entirety of the question carefully before reading the answer choices.

3. Looking for Wrong Answers

Long and complicated multiple-choice questions can be intimidating. One way to simplify a difficult multiple-choice question is to eliminate all of the answer choices that are clearly wrong. In most sets of answers, there will be at least one selection that can be dismissed right away. If the test is administered on paper, the test taker could draw a line through it to indicate that it may be ignored; otherwise, the test taker will have to perform this operation mentally or on scratch paper. In either case, once the obviously incorrect answers have been eliminated, the remaining choices may be considered. Sometimes identifying the clearly wrong answers will give the test taker some information about the correct answer. For instance, if one of the remaining answer choices is a direct opposite of one of the eliminated answer choices, it may well be the correct answer. The opposite of obviously wrong is obviously right! Of course, this is not always the case. Some answers are obviously incorrect simply because they are irrelevant to the question being asked. Still, identifying and eliminating some incorrect answer choices is a good way to simplify a multiple-choice question.

4. Don't Overanalyze

Anxious test takers often overanalyze questions. When you are nervous, your brain will often run wild, causing you to make associations and discover clues that don't actually exist. If you feel that this may be a problem for you, do whatever you can to slow down during the test. Try taking a deep breath or counting to ten. As you read and consider the question, restrict yourself to the particular words used by the author. Avoid thought tangents about what the author *really* meant, or what he or she was *trying* to say. The only things that matter on a multiple-choice test are the words that are actually in the question. You must avoid reading too much into a multiple-choice question, or supposing that the writer meant something other than what he or she wrote.

5. No Need for Panic

It is wise to learn as many strategies as possible before taking a multiple-choice test, but it is likely that you will come across a few questions for which you simply don't know the answer. In this situation, avoid panicking. Because most multiple-choice tests include dozens of questions, the relative value of a single wrong answer is small. As much as possible, you should compartmentalize each question on a multiple-choice test. In other words, you should not allow your feelings about one question to affect your success on the others. When you find a question that you either don't understand or don't know how to answer, just take a deep breath and do your best. Read the entire question slowly and carefully. Try rephrasing the question a couple of different ways. Then, read all of the answer choices carefully. After eliminating obviously wrong answers, make a selection and move on to the next question.

6. Confusing Answer Choices

When working on a difficult multiple-choice question, there may be a tendency to focus on the answer choices that are the easiest to understand. Many people, whether consciously or not, gravitate to the answer choices that require the least concentration, knowledge, and memory. This is a mistake. When you come across an answer choice that is confusing, you should give it extra attention. A question might be confusing because you do not know the subject matter to which it refers. If this is the case, don't eliminate the answer before you have affirmatively settled on another. When you come across an answer choice of this type, set it aside as you look at the remaining choices. If you can confidently assert that one of the other choices is correct, you can leave the confusing answer aside. Otherwise, you will need to take a moment to try to better understand the confusing answer choice. Rephrasing is one way to tease out the sense of a confusing answer choice.

7. Your First Instinct

Many people struggle with multiple-choice tests because they overthink the questions. If you have studied sufficiently for the test, you should be prepared to trust your first instinct once you have carefully and completely read the question and all of the answer choices. There is a great deal of research suggesting that the mind can come to the correct conclusion very quickly once it has obtained all of the relevant information. At times, it may seem to you as if your intuition is working faster even than your reasoning mind. This may in fact be true. The knowledge you obtain while studying may be retrieved from your subconscious before you have a chance to work out the associations that support it. Verify your instinct by working out the reasons that it should be trusted.

8. Key Words

Many test takers struggle with multiple-choice questions because they have poor reading comprehension skills. Quickly reading and understanding a multiple-choice question requires a mixture of skill and experience. To help with this, try jotting down a few key words and phrases on a piece of scrap paper. Doing this concentrates the process of reading and forces the mind to weigh the relative importance of the question's parts. In selecting words and phrases to write down, the test taker thinks about the question more deeply and carefully. This is especially true for multiple-choice questions that are preceded by a long prompt.

9. Subtle Negatives

One of the oldest tricks in the multiple-choice test writer's book is to subtly reverse the meaning of a question with a word like *not* or *except*. If you are not paying attention to each word in the question, you can easily be led astray by this trick. For instance, a common question format is, "Which of the following is...?" Obviously, if the question instead is, "Which of the following is not...?," then the answer will be quite different. Even worse, the test makers are aware of the potential for this mistake and will include one answer choice that would be correct if the question were not negated or reversed. A test taker who misses the reversal will find what he or she believes to be a correct answer and will be so confident that he or she will fail to reread the question and discover the original error. The only way to avoid this is to practice a wide variety of multiple-choice questions and to pay close attention to each and every word.

10. Reading Every Answer Choice

It may seem obvious, but you should always read every one of the answer choices! Too many test takers fall into the habit of scanning the question and assuming that they understand the question because they recognize a few key words. From there, they pick the first answer choice that answers the question they believe they have read. Test takers who read all of the answer choices might discover that one of the latter answer choices is actually *more* correct. Moreover, reading all of the answer choices can remind you of facts related to the question that can help you arrive at the correct answer. Sometimes, a misstatement or incorrect detail in one of the latter answer choices will trigger your memory of the subject and will enable you to find the right answer. Failing to read all of the answer choices is like not reading all of the items on a restaurant menu: you might miss out on the perfect choice.

11. Spot the Hedges

One of the keys to success on multiple-choice tests is paying close attention to every word. This is never truer than with words like almost, most, some, and sometimes. These words are called "hedges" because they indicate that a statement is not totally true or not true in every place and time. An absolute statement will contain no hedges, but in many subjects, the answers are not always straightforward or absolute. There are always exceptions to the rules in these subjects. For this reason, you should favor those multiple-choice questions that contain hedging language. The presence of qualifying words indicates that the author is taking special care with his or her words, which is certainly important when composing the right answer. After all, there are many ways to be wrong, but there is only one way to be right! For this reason, it is wise to avoid answers that are absolute when taking a multiple-choice test. An absolute answer is one that says things are either all one way or all another. They often include words like *every*, *always*, *best*, and *never*. If you are taking a multiple-choice test in a subject that doesn't lend itself to absolute answers, be on your guard if you see any of these words.

12. Long Answers

In many subject areas, the answers are not simple. As already mentioned, the right answer often requires hedges. Another common feature of the answers to a complex or subjective question are qualifying clauses, which are groups of words that subtly modify the meaning of the sentence. If the question or answer choice describes a rule to which there are exceptions or the subject matter is complicated, ambiguous, or confusing, the correct answer will require many words in order to be expressed clearly and accurately. In essence, you should not be deterred by answer choices that seem excessively long. Oftentimes, the author of the text will not be able to write the correct answer without offering some qualifications and modifications. Your job is to read the answer choices thoroughly and completely and to select the one that most accurately and precisely answers the question.

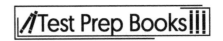

13. Restating to Understand

Sometimes, a question on a multiple-choice test is difficult not because of what it asks but because of how it is written. If this is the case, restate the question or answer choice in different words. This process serves a couple of important purposes. First, it forces you to concentrate on the core of the question. In order to rephrase the question accurately, you have to understand it well. Rephrasing the question will concentrate your mind on the key words and ideas. Second, it will present the information to your mind in a fresh way. This process may trigger your memory and render some useful scrap of information picked up while studying.

14. True Statements

Sometimes an answer choice will be true in itself, but it does not answer the question. This is one of the main reasons why it is essential to read the question carefully and completely before proceeding to the answer choices. Too often, test takers skip ahead to the answer choices and look for true statements. Having found one of these, they are content to select it without reference to the question above. Obviously, this provides an easy way for test makers to play tricks. The savvy test taker will always read the entire question before turning to the answer choices. Then, having settled on a correct answer choice, he or she will refer to the original question and ensure that the selected answer is relevant. The mistake of choosing a correct-but-irrelevant answer choice is especially common on questions related to specific pieces of objective knowledge. A prepared test taker will have a wealth of factual knowledge at his or her disposal, and should not be careless in its application.

15. No Patterns

One of the more dangerous ideas that circulates about multiple-choice tests is that the correct answers tend to fall into patterns. These erroneous ideas range from a belief that B and C are the most common right answers, to the idea that an unprepared test-taker should answer "A-B-A-C-A-D-A-B-A." It cannot be emphasized enough that pattern-seeking of this type is exactly the WRONG way to approach a multiple-choice test. To begin with, it is highly unlikely that the test maker will plot the correct answers according to some predetermined pattern. The questions are scrambled and delivered in a random order. Furthermore, even if the test maker was following a pattern in the assignation of correct answers, there is no reason why the test taker would know which pattern he or she was using. Any attempt to discern a pattern in the answer choices is a waste of time and a distraction from the real work of taking the test. A test taker would be much better served by extra preparation before the test than by reliance on a pattern in the answers.

FREE DVD OFFER

Don't forget that doing well on your exam includes both understanding the test content and understanding how to use what you know to do well on the test. We offer a completely FREE Test Taking Tips DVD that covers world class test taking tips that you can use to be even more successful when you are taking your test.

All that we ask is that you email us your feedback about your study guide. To get your **FREE Test Taking Tips DVD**, email freedvd@studyguideteam.com with "FREE DVD" in the subject line and the following information in the body of the email:

- The title of your study guide.
- Your product rating on a scale of 1-5, with 5 being the highest rating.
- Your feedback about the study guide. What did you think of it?
- Your full name and shipping address to send your free DVD.

Introduction to the PCAT Exam

Function of the Test

The Pharmacy College Admission Test (PCAT) is an admissions test for candidates seeking to attend pharmacy programs at U.S. colleges. It is designed to gauge the academic proficiency of prospective pharmacy curriculum candidates. The PCAT is a prerequisite for most, but not all, pharmacy schools in the United States. From time to time, the test content is modified to make sure that it correctly depicts the current science, mathematics, and language arts requirements specific to pharmacy programs.

Most pharmacy schools do not accept students until they have finished at least two years of undergraduate college courses, but there are some programs that accept students directly from high school. Because of this wide range, PCAT test takers can vary in age from high school students to those attending undergraduate college programs. Most sources agree that it is best to have college-level knowledge of biology, chemistry, and pre-calculus prior to taking the PCAT, and the best time to take the entrance exam is the summer or fall before applying to a pharmacy school.

Test Administration

The PCAT is administered via computer at Pearson VUE test sites in the United States and some international locations several times throughout a test cycle. Registration can be done online or through the mail (although additional fees may be charged). It is important to note that there are two registration deadlines. Test candidates registering by the first deadline are most likely to get the date, time, and location of their choosing. Those who do not register until the second deadline will incur a late fee and are not guaranteed to receive their preferred testing date, time, or location.

The PCAT may be taken up to five times, but on the sixth attempt, restrictions may be placed on successive registrations, and supplementary supporting documents from a pharmacy school, teacher, or official may be required. If this is the case, the candidate cannot register for the PCAT until the required documents are received and he or she is approved to take the exam again.

As per the Americans With Disabilities Act (ADA), testing arrangements for candidates with disabilities are provided by Pearson VUE test centers at no additional cost. Test candidates with physical limitations that are considered disabilities under the ADA may inquire about special testing accommodations.

Test Format

Established by PsychCorp, a brand of Pearson Assessment, Inc., the PCAT contains about 192 multiple-choice questions and a writing test. Candidates are given four hours to finish the exam, as well as instructive time and a brief rest period, approximately halfway through the test-taking process. There are five sections on the PCAT, covering the following topics: writing, biology, chemistry, critical reading, and quantitative reasoning.

PCAT Section	Number of Questions	Time Allocated
Writing (Essay)	1 Prompt	30 minutes
Biological Processes	48	40 minutes
Chemical Processes	48	40 minutes
Rest Break		15 minutes
Critical Reading	48	50 minutes
Quantitative Reasoning	48	45 minutes
Total	192 multiple-choice + 1 prompt	3 hours 25 minutes + 15-min rest break

The PCAT writing prompt is chosen from topics that address health, science, cultural, social, or political issues. The biology subtest includes questions on general biology, microbiology, health, and human anatomy and physiology. The chemistry section covers general chemistry, organic chemistry, and basic biochemistry processes. Content objectives for the critical reading subtest include comprehension (specifically word and idea recognition and understanding); analysis (such as inference and interpretation of writers and ideas); and reasoned judgment evaluation (concepts such as bias, argument support and thesis/conclusion). The quantitative reasoning (mathematics) section covers the topics of basic math, algebra, probability, and statistics.

Scoring

The PCAT is graded on a scale from 200-600, with a median score of 400. Candidates with a score of 430 are usually in 90th percentile range. Percentile rankings are based on the scores of test takers in the present norm group (all candidates who took the test for the first time between July 2011 and January 2015). Scaled scores are based on the number of correctly answered questions on each subtest. Each multiple-choice subtest is calculated separately. Therefore, examinees obtain a grade for each multiple-choice subtest, a total score for the four multiple-choice subtests together, and a writing score. Since each pharmacy school has its own admissions requirements, there is no typical "passing score" on the PCAT exam.

Recent/Future Developments

As of July 2016, the PCAT underwent some structural changes. The biology and chemistry subtests were renamed biological processes and chemical processes. Both also received new reading sections, each with four corresponding questions. In addition, the verbal ability section (which covered analogy and sentence-completion questions) was totally removed from the test. Also, reading comprehension was renamed critical reading, and quantitative ability was renamed quantitative reasoning. The quantitative section now focuses more on word problems and less on pre-calculus and calculus.

Study Prep Plan for the PCAT Exam

1 **Schedule** - Use one of our study schedules below or come up with one of your own.

2 **Relax** - Test anxiety can hurt even the best students. There are many ways to reduce stress. Find the one that works best for you.

3 **Execute** - Once you have a good plan in place, be sure to stick to it.

Sample Study Plans

One Week Study Schedule

Day 1	Writing
Day 2	Biological Processes
Day 3	Chemical Processes
Day 4	Critical Reading
Day 5	Quantitative Reasoning
Day 6	Practice Questions
Day 7	Take Your Exam!

Two Week Study Schedule

Day 1	Writing the Essay	Day 8	Organic Chemistry
Day 2	Practice Prompt	Day 9	Practice Questions
Day 3	General Biology	Day 10	Critical Reading
Day 4	Cellular and Molecular Biology	Day 11	Practice Questions
Day 5	Medical Microbiology	Day 12	Quantitative Reasoning
Day 6	Practice Questions	Day 13	Practice Questions
Day 7	General Chemistry	Day 14	Take Your Exam!

One Month Study Schedule

Day	Topic	Day	Topic	Day	Topic
Day 1	Writing the Essay	Day 11	Microbial Ecology	Day 21	Analysis
Day 2	Conventions of Standard English	Day 12	Medical Microbiology	Day 22	Evaluation
Day 3	Practice Prompt	Day 13	Immunity	Day 23	Practice Questions
Day 4	General Biology	Day 14	Human Anatomy and Physiology	Day 24	Basic Math
Day 5	Cellular and Molecular Biology	Day 15	Practice Questions	Day 25	Algebra
Day 6	Diversity of Life Forms	Day 16	General Chemistry	Day 26	Probability and Statistics
Day 7	Health	Day 17	Organic Chemistry	Day 27	Precalculus
Day 8	Microbiology	Day 18	Basic Biochemistry Processes	Day 28	Calculus
Day 9	Microorganisms	Day 19	Practice Questions	Day 29	Practice Questions
Day 10	Infectious Diseases & Prevention	Day 20	Comprehension	Day 30	Take Your Exam!

Writing

The writing section of the PCAT allows the test taker thirty minutes to write a problem/solution essay. The test will provide a prompt for the test taker outlining a problem, then will ask the test taker to describe a possible solution. The writing section of the PCAT does not include spellcheck or grammar check, but it does offer basic commands such as "cut," "copy," and "paste."

The writing prompt content is divided into three different possibilities. Below is a bulleted list of the content objectives with specific examples:

- Health Issues
  - Public Health
  - Medicine
  - Nutrition
  - Fitness
  - Prevention
  - Treatments
  - Therapies
  - Medications
  - Drugs
  - Attitudes
- Science Issues
  - Research
  - Theories
  - Findings
  - Applications
  - Controversies
  - Education
  - Attitudes
- Social, Cultural, or Political Issues
  - Beliefs
  - Attitudes
  - Behaviors
  - Trends
  - Laws
  - Policies

The two sections below are called "Writing the Essay" and "Conventions of Standard English." The first section is designed to help you structure your essay and employ prewriting strategies that will help you brainstorm and begin writing the essay. The second section is common mistakes used in the English language. Since there is no spellcheck on the PCAT writing portion of the test, it's important to consider these common mistakes in order to prevent them.

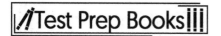

Writing the Essay

Brainstorming

One of the most important steps in writing an essay is prewriting. Before drafting an essay, it's helpful to think about the topic for a moment or two, in order to gain a more solid understanding of what the task is. Then, spending about five minutes jotting down the immediate ideas that could work for the essay is recommended. This is a way to get some words on the page, and it offers a reference for ideas for when drafting. Scratch paper is provided for writers to use for any prewriting techniques such as webbing, free writing, or listing. The goal is to simply get ideas out of the mind and onto the page.

Considering Opposing Viewpoints

In the planning stage, it's important to consider all aspects of the topic, including different viewpoints on the subject. There are more than two ways to look at a topic, and a strong argument considers those opposing viewpoints. Considering opposing viewpoints can help writers present a fair, balanced, and informed essay that shows consideration for all readers. This approach can also strengthen an argument by recognizing and potentially refuting the opposing viewpoint(s).

Drawing from personal experience may help to support ideas. For example, if the goal for writing is a personal narrative, then the story should be from the writer's own life. Many writers find it helpful to draw from personal experience, even in an essay that is not strictly narrative. Personal anecdotes or short stories can help to illustrate a point in other types of essays as well.

Moving from Brainstorming to Planning

Once the ideas are on the page, it's time to turn them into a solid plan for the essay. The best ideas from the brainstorming stage can then be developed into a more formal outline. An outline typically has one main point (the thesis) and at least three sub-points that support the main point. Here's an example:

Main Idea

- Point #1
- Point #2
- Point #3

Of course, there will be details under each point, but this approach is often the best when dealing with timed writing.

Staying on Track

Basing the essay on the outline aids in both organization and coherence. The goal is to ensure that there is enough time to develop each sub-point in the essay, roughly spending an equal amount of time on each idea. Keeping an eye on the time will help. If there are fifteen minutes left to draft the essay, then it makes sense to spend about 5 minutes on each of the ideas. Staying on task is critical to success, and timing out the parts of the essay can help writers avoid feeling overwhelmed.

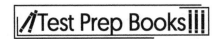

Parts of the Essay

The *introduction* should do a few important things:

- Establish the *topic* of the essay in original wording (i.e., not just repeating the prompt)
- Clarify the significance/importance of the topic or purpose for writing (a brief overview without too many details)
- Offer a *thesis statement* that identifies the writer's own viewpoint on the topic (typically one-two brief sentences as a clear, concise explanation of the main point on the topic)

Body paragraphs reflect the ideas developed in the outline. Three or four points is probably sufficient for a short essay, and they should include the following:

- A *topic sentence* that identifies the sub-point (e.g., a reason why, a way how, a cause or effect)
- A detailed *explanation* of the point, explaining why the writer thinks this point is valid
- Illustrative *examples*, such as personal examples or real-world examples, that support and validate the point (i.e., "prove" the point)
- A *concluding sentence* that connects the examples, reasoning, and analysis to the point being made

The *conclusion*, or final paragraph, should be brief and should reiterate the focus, clarifying why the discussion is significant or important. It is important to avoid adding specific details or new ideas to this paragraph. The purpose of the conclusion is to sum up what has been said to bring the discussion to a close.

Don't Panic!

Writing an essay can be overwhelming, and performance panic is a natural response. The outline serves as a basis for the writing and it helps writers stay focused. Getting stuck can also happen, and it's helpful to remember that brainstorming can be done at any time during the writing process. Following the steps of the writing process is the best defense against writer's block.

Timed essays can be particularly stressful, but assessors are trained to recognize the necessary planning and thinking for these timed efforts. Using the plan above and sticking to it helps with time management. Timing each part of the process helps writers stay on track. Sometimes writers try to cover too much in their essays. If time seems to be running out, this is an opportunity to determine whether all of the ideas in the outline are necessary. Three body paragraphs are sufficient, and more than that is probably too much to cover in a short essay.

More isn't always *better* in writing. A strong essay will be clear and concise. It will avoid unnecessary or repetitive details. It is better to have a concise, five-paragraph essay that makes a clear point, than a ten-paragraph essay that doesn't. The goal is to write one to two pages of quality writing. Paragraphs should also reflect balance; if the introduction goes to the bottom of the first page, the writing may be going off-track or be repetitive. It's best to fall into the one to two page range, but a complete, well-developed essay is the ultimate goal.

The Final Steps

Leaving a few minutes at the end to revise and proofread offers an opportunity for writers to polish things up. Writers can often identify problems by putting themselves in the reader's shoes—it's a movement from the mindset of writer to the mindset of editor. Reading aloud is often a great strategy to identify grammatical errors and confusing wording. The goal is to have a clean, clear copy of the essay. The following areas should be considered when proofreading:

- Sentence fragments
- Awkward sentence structure
- Run-on sentences
- Incorrect word choice
- Grammatical agreement errors
- Spelling errors
- Punctuation errors
- Capitalization errors

The Short Overview

The essay may seem challenging, but following these steps can help writers focus:

- Take one or two minutes to think about the topic.
- Generate some ideas through brainstorming (three to four minutes).
- Organize ideas into a brief outline.
- Selecting just three to four main points to cover in the essay (eventually the body paragraphs).
- Develop the essay in parts:
    - Introduction paragraph, with an intro to the topic and main points
    - Viewpoint on the subject at the end of the introduction
    - Body paragraphs have a main point and support of that point
    - Brief conclusion highlighting the main points and closing
- Read over the essay (last five minutes).
- Look for any obvious errors, making sure that the writing makes sense.

Conventions of Standard English

Errors in Standard English Grammar, Usage, Syntax, and Mechanics

Sentence Fragments

A *complete sentence* requires a verb and a subject that expresses a complete thought. Sometimes, the subject is omitted in the case of the implied *you*, which is particularly the case in sentences that are the command or imperative form—e.g., "Look!" or "Give me that." It is understood that the subject of the command is *you*, the listener or reader, so it is possible to have a structure without an explicit subject. Without these elements, though, the sentence is incomplete—it is a *sentence fragment.* While sentence fragments often occur in conversational English or creative writing, they are generally not appropriate in academic writing. Sentence fragments often occur when dependent clauses are not joined to an independent clause:

> *Sentence fragment*: Because the airline overbooked the flight.

The sentence above is a dependent clause that does not express a complete thought. What happened as a result of this cause? With the addition of an independent clause, this now becomes a complete sentence:

> *Complete sentence*: Because the airline overbooked the flight, several passengers were unable to board.

Sentences fragments may also occur through improper use of conjunctions:

> I'm going to the Bahamas for spring break. And to New York City for New Year's Eve.
>
> While the first sentence above is a complete sentence, the second one is not because it is a prepositional phrase that lacks a subject [I] and a verb [am going]. Joining the two together with the coordinating conjunction forms one grammatically-correct sentence:
>
> I'm going to the Bahamas for spring break and to New York City for New Year's Eve.

Run-ons

A *run-on* is a sentence with too many independent clauses that are improperly connected to each other:

> This winter has been very cold some farmers have suffered damage to their crops.

The sentence above has two subject-verb combinations. The first is "this winter has been"; the second is "some farmers have suffered." However, they are simply stuck next to each other without any punctuation or conjunction. Therefore, the sentence is a run-on.

Another type of run-on occurs when writers use inappropriate punctuation:

> This winter has been very cold, some farmers have suffered damage to their crops.

Though a comma has been added, this sentence is still not correct. When a comma alone is used to join two independent clauses, it is known as a *comma splice*. Without an appropriate conjunction, a comma cannot join two independent clauses by itself.

Run-on sentences can be corrected by either dividing the independent clauses into two or more separate sentences or inserting appropriate conjunctions and/or punctuation. The run-on sentence can be amended by separating each subject-verb pair into its own sentence:

> This winter has been very cold. Some farmers have suffered damage to their crops.

The run-on can also be fixed by adding a comma and a conjunction to join the two independent clauses with each other:

> This winter has been very cold, so some farmers have suffered damage to their crops.

Parallelism

Parallel structure occurs when phrases or clauses within a sentence contain the same structure. Parallelism increases readability and comprehensibility because it is easy to tell which sentence elements are paired with each other in meaning.

> Jennifer enjoys cooking, knitting, and to spend time with her cat.

This sentence is not parallel because the items in the list appear in two different forms. Some are *gerunds*, which is the verb + ing: *cooking, knitting*. The other item uses the *infinitive* form, which is to + verb: *to spend*. To create parallelism, all items in the list will reflect the same form:

> Jennifer enjoys cooking, knitting, and spending time with her cat.

All of the items in the list are now in gerund forms, so this sentence exhibits parallel structure. Here's another example:

> The company is looking for employees who are responsible and with a lot of experience.

Again, the items that are listed in this sentence are not parallel. "Responsible" is an adjective, yet "with a lot of experience" is a prepositional phrase. The sentence elements do not utilize parallel parts of speech.

> The company is looking for employees who are responsible and experienced.

"Responsible" and "experienced" are both adjectives, so this sentence now has parallel structure.

Dangling and Misplaced Modifiers

Modifiers enhance meaning by clarifying or giving greater detail about another part of a sentence. However, incorrectly-placed modifiers have the opposite effect and can cause confusion. A *misplaced modifier* is a modifier that is not located appropriately in relation to the word or phrase that it modifies:

> Because he was one of the greatest thinkers of Renaissance Italy, John idolized Leonardo da Vinci.

In this sentence, the modifier is "because he was one of the greatest thinkers of Renaissance Italy," and the noun it is intended to modify is "Leonardo da Vinci." However, due to the placement of the modifier next to the subject, John, it seems as if the sentence is stating that John was a Renaissance genius, not Da Vinci.

> John idolized Leonard da Vinci because he was one of the greatest thinkers of Renaissance Italy.

The modifier is now adjacent to the appropriate noun, clarifying which of the two men in this sentence is the greatest thinker.

Dangling modifiers modify a word or phrase that is not readily apparent in the sentence. That is, they "dangle" because they are not clearly attached to anything:

> After getting accepted to college, Amir's parents were proud.

The modifier here, "after getting accepted to college," should modify who got accepted. The noun immediately following the modifier is "Amir's parents"—but they are probably not the ones who are going to college.

> After getting accepted to college, Amir made his parents proud.

The subject of the sentence has been changed to Amir himself, and now the subject and its modifier are appropriately matched.

Inconsistent Verb Tense

Verb tense reflects when an action occurred or a state existed. For example, the tense known as *simple present* expresses something that is happening right now or that happens regularly:

> She *works* in a hospital.

Present continuous tense expresses something in progress. It is formed by to be + verb + -ing.

> Sorry, I can't go out right now. I *am doing* my homework.

Past tense is used to describe events that previously occurred. However, in conversational English, speakers often use present tense or a mix of past and present tense when relating past events because it gives the narrative a sense of immediacy. In formal written English, though, consistency in verb tense is necessary to avoid reader confusion.

> I traveled to Europe last summer. As soon as I stepped off the plane, I feel like I'm in a movie! I'm surrounded by quaint cafes and impressive architecture.

The passage above abruptly switches from past tense—*traveled, stepped*—to present tense—*feel, am surrounded.*

> I *traveled* to Europe last summer. As soon as I *stepped* off the plane, I *felt* like I was in a movie! I *was surrounded* by quaint cafes and impressive architecture.

All verbs are in past tense, so this passage now has a consistent verb tense.

Split Infinitives

The *infinitive form* of a verb consists of "to + base verb"—e.g., to walk, to sleep, to approve. A *split infinitive* occurs when another word, usually an adverb, is placed between *to* and the verb:

> I decided *to simply walk* to work to get more exercise every day.

The infinitive *to walk* is split by the adverb *simply.*

> It was a mistake *to hastily approve* the project before conducting further preliminary research.

The infinitive *to approve* is split by *hastily.*

Although some grammarians still advise against split infinitives, this syntactic structure is common in both spoken and written English and is widely accepted in standard usage.

Subject-Verb Agreement

In English, verbs must agree with the subject. The form of a verb may change depending on whether the subject is singular or plural, or whether it is first, second, or third person. For example, the verb *to be* has various forms:

> I am a student.
>
> You are a student.
>
> She is a student.
>
> We are students.
>
> They are students.

Errors occur when a verb does not agree with its subject. Sometimes, the error is readily apparent:

> We is hungry.

Is is not the appropriate form of *to be* when used with the third person plural *we*.

> We are hungry.

This sentence now has correct subject-verb agreement.

However, some cases are trickier, particularly when the subject consists of a lengthy noun phrase with many modifiers:

> Students who are hoping to accompany the anthropology department on its annual summer trip to Ecuador needs to sign up by March 31st.

The verb in this sentence is *needs*. However, its subject is not the noun adjacent to it—Ecuador. The subject is the noun at the beginning of the sentence—students. Because *students* is plural, *needs* is the incorrect verb form.

> *Students* who are hoping to accompany the anthropology department on its annual summer trip to Ecuador *need* to sign up by March 31st.

This sentence now uses the correct agreement between *students* and *need.*

Another case to be aware of is a *collective noun*. A collective noun refers to a group of many things or people but can be singular in itself—e.g., family, committee, army, pair team, council, jury. Whether or not a collective noun uses a singular or plural verb depends on how the noun is being used. If the noun refers to the group performing a collective action as one unit, it should use a singular verb conjugation:

> The family is moving to a new neighborhood.

The whole family is moving together in unison, so the singular verb form *is* is appropriate here.

> The committee has made its decision.

The verb *has* and the possessive pronoun *its* both reflect the word *committee* as a singular noun in the sentence above; however, when a collective noun refers to the group as individuals, it can take a plural verb:

> The newlywed pair spend every moment together.

This sentence emphasizes the love between two people in a pair, so it can use the plural verb *spend*.

> The council are all newly elected members.

The sentence refers to the council in terms of its individual members and uses the plural verb *are*.

Overall though, American English is more likely to pair a collective noun with a singular verb, while British English is more likely to pair a collective noun with a plural verb.

Practice Prompt

Prepare an essay of about 300-600 words on the topic below.

Heart disease is considered the number one cause of death for people in the United States. Heart disease occurs when plaque builds up in the arteries, making it difficult for blood to flow, which creates a heart attack or stroke. Write a solution to the problem of heart disease in the United States.

Biological Processes

General Biology

Biology Basics

Biology is the study of living organisms and the processes that are vital for life. Scientists who study biology are interested in the origin, evolution, structure, function, growth, and distribution of these living organisms. They study these organisms on a cellular level, individually or as populations, and look at the effects they have on their surrounding environment.

There are five foundations of modern biology: cell theory, evolution, genetics, homeostasis, and energy.

Cell theory is the idea that the cell is the fundamental unit of life. Living organisms are made up of one or more cells, and the products that are generated by those cells. Cells have processes that both produce and use energy, known as *metabolism*. They also contain deoxyribonucleic acid (DNA), which is hereditary information that gets passed on to subsequent generations.

Evolution is the theory that all living organisms descended from one common ancestor. Charles Darwin generated a viable scientific model of evolution based on the concept of natural selection. *Natural selection* is the idea that certain individuals of a species (or sometimes a species as a whole) with more advantageous phenotypes are more likely to survive than those individuals with less advantageous phenotypes. Over long periods of time, populations of species can develop phenotypes specialized for their environment.

Genetics is the study of genes. *Genes* are the primary unit of inheritance between generations or organisms. They are regions of DNA that encode ribonucleic acid (RNA) and proteins, all of which have specific forms and functions. DNA is present in all living cells and is important for the cell's own functions, as well as for its ability to divide and pass on information to subsequent daughter cells.

Homeostasis is the ability of a system, such as a cell or organism, to regulate itself so that its internal conditions remain stable even when its external environment may be changing. By maintaining homeostasis, systems are able to function normally even in adverse conditions.

The constant flow of energy is important for the survival of living organisms. All organisms have vital functions that require the input of energy and other functions that release energy. These processes work together to drive all chemical reactions required for life.

Cellular and Molecular Biology

Structure and Function of Cells

The cell is the main functional and structural component of all living organisms. Robert Hooke, an English scientist, coined the term "cell" in 1665. Hooke's discovery laid the groundwork for the cell theory, which is composed of three principals:

1. All organisms are composed of cells.
2. All existing cells are created from other living cells.
3. The cell is the most fundamental unit of life.

Organisms can be unicellular (composed of one cell) or multicellular (composed of many cells). All cells must be bounded by a cell membrane, filled with cytoplasm of some sort, and coded by a genetic sequence.

The cell membrane separates a cell's internal and external environments. It is a selectively permeable membrane, which usually only allows the passage of certain molecules by diffusion. Phospholipids and proteins are crucial components of all cell membranes. The cytoplasm is the cell's internal environment and is aqueous, or water-based. The genome represents the genetic material inside the cell that is passed on from generation to generation.

Prokaryotes and Eukaryotes

Prokaryotic cells are much smaller than eukaryotic cells. The majority of prokaryotes are unicellular, while the majority of eukaryotes are multicellular. Prokaryotic cells have no nucleus, and their genome is found in an area known as the nucleoid. They also do not have membrane-bound organelles, which are "little organs" that perform specific functions within a cell.

Eukaryotic cells have a proper nucleus containing the genome. They also have numerous membrane-bound organelles such as lysosomes, endoplasmic reticula (rough and smooth), Golgi complexes, and mitochondria. The majority of prokaryotic cells have cell walls, while most eukaryotic cells do not have cell walls. The DNA of prokaryotic cells is contained in a single circular chromosome, while the DNA of eukaryotic cells is contained in multiple linear chromosomes. Prokaryotic cells divide using binary fission, while eukaryotic cells divide using mitosis. Examples of prokaryotes are bacteria and archaea while examples of eukaryotes are animals and plants.

Nuclear Parts of a Cell

Nucleus (plural nuclei): Houses a cell's genetic material, deoxyribonucleic acid (DNA), which is used to form chromosomes. A single nucleus is the defining characteristic of eukaryotic cells. The nucleus of a cell controls gene expression. It ensures genetic material is transmitted from one generation to the next.

Chromosomes: Complex thread-like arrangements composed of DNA that is found in a cell's nucleus. Humans have 23 pairs of chromosomes for a total of 46.

Chromatin: An aggregate of genetic material consisting of DNA and proteins that forms chromosomes during cell division.

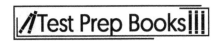

Nucleolus (plural nucleoli): The largest component of the nucleus of a eukaryotic cell. With no membrane, the primary function of the nucleolus is the production of ribosomes, which are crucial to the synthesis of proteins.

Cell Membranes

Cell membranes encircle the cell's cytoplasm, separating the intracellular environment from the extracellular environment. They are selectively permeable, which enables them to control molecular traffic entering and exiting cells. Cell membranes are made of a double layer of phospholipids studded with proteins. Cholesterol is also dispersed in the phospholipid bilayer of cell membranes to provide stability. The proteins in the phospholipid bilayer aid the transport of molecules across cell membranes.

Scientists use the term "fluid mosaic model" to refer to the arrangement of phospholipids and proteins in cell membranes. In that model, phospholipids have a head region and a tail region. The head region of the phospholipids is hydrophilic, which means it is attracted to water, while the tail region hydrophobic, or repelled by water. Because they are hydrophilic, the heads of the phospholipids are facing the water, pointing inside and outside of the cell. Because they are hydrophobic, the tails of the phospholipids are oriented inward between both head regions. This orientation constructs the phospholipid bilayer.

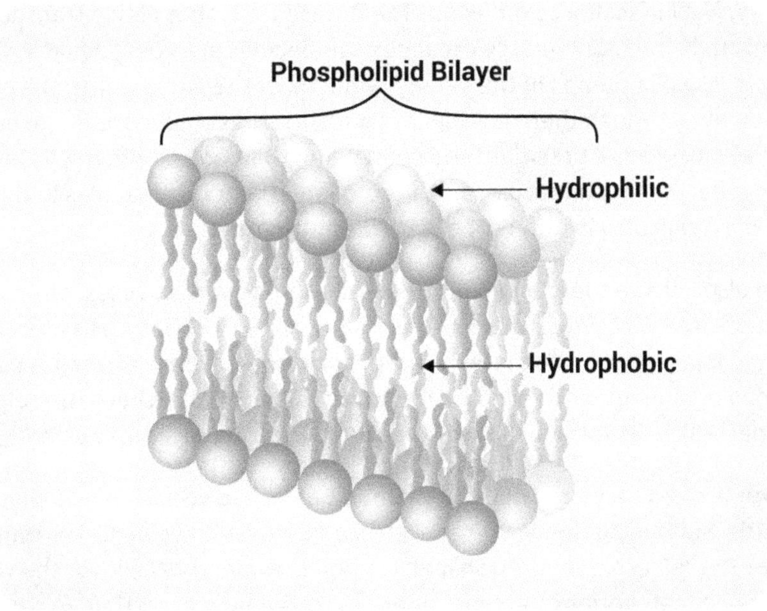

Cell membranes have the distinct trait of selective permeability. The fact that cell membranes are amphiphilic (having hydrophilic and hydrophobic zones) contributes to this trait. As a result, cell membranes are able to regulate the flow of molecules in and out of the cell.

Factors relating to molecules such as size, polarity, and solubility determine their likelihood of passage across cell membranes. Small molecules are able to diffuse easily across cell membranes compared to large molecules. Polarity refers to the charge present in a molecule. Polar molecules have regions, or poles, of positive and negative charge and are water soluble, while nonpolar molecules have no charge and are fat-soluble. *Solubility* refers to the ability of a substance, called a solute, to dissolve in a solvent. A soluble substance can be dissolved in a solvent, while an insoluble substance cannot be dissolved in a solvent. Nonpolar, fat-soluble substances have a much easier time passing through cell membranes compared to polar, water-soluble substances.

Passive Transport Mechanisms

Passive transport refers to the migration of molecules across a cell membrane that does not require energy. The three types of passive transport include simple diffusion, facilitated diffusion, and osmosis.

Simple diffusion relies on a concentration gradient, or differing quantities of molecules inside or outside of a cell. During simple diffusion, molecules move from an area of high concentration to an area of low concentration. *Facilitated diffusion* utilizes carrier proteins to transport molecules across a cell membrane. *Osmosis* refers to the transport of water across a selectively permeable membrane. During osmosis, water moves from a region of low solute concentration to a region of high solute concentration.

Active Transport Mechanisms

Active transport refers to the migration of molecules across a cell membrane that requires energy. It's a useful way to move molecules from an area of low concentration to an area of high concentration. Adenosine triphosphate (ATP), the currency of cellular energy, is needed to work against the concentration gradient.

Active transport can involve carrier proteins that cross the cell membrane to pump molecules and ions across the membrane, like in facilitated diffusion. The difference is that active transport uses the energy from ATP to drive this transport, as typically the ions or molecules are going against their concentration gradient. For example, glucose pumps in the kidney pump all of the glucose into the cells from the lumen of the nephron even though there is a higher concentration of glucose in the cell than in the lumen. This is because glucose is a precious food source and the body wants to conserve as much as possible. Pumps can either send a molecule in one direction, multiple molecules in the same direction (symports), or multiple molecules in different directions (antiports).

Active transport can also involve the movement of membrane-bound particles, either into a cell (endocytosis) or out of a cell (exocytosis). The three major forms of endocytosis are: pinocytosis, where the cell is *drinking* and intakes only small molecules; phagocytosis, where the cell is *eating* and intakes large particles or small organisms; and receptor-mediated endocytosis, where the cell's membrane splits off to form an internal vesicle as a response to molecules activating receptors on its surface.

Exocytosis is the inverse of endocytosis, and the membranes of the vesicle join to that of the cell's surface while the molecules inside the vesicle are released outside. Exocytosis is common in nervous and muscle tissue for the release of neurotransmitters and in endocrine cells for the release of hormones. The two major categories of exocytosis are excretion and secretion. *Excretion* is defined as the removal of waste from a cell. *Secretion* is defined as the transport of molecules, such as hormones or enzymes, from a cell.

Structure and Function of Cellular Organelles

Organelles are specialized structures that perform specific tasks in a cell. The term literally means "little organ." Most organelles are membrane-bound and serve as sites for the production or degradation of chemicals. The following are organelles found in eukaryotic cells:

Nucleus: As mentioned, a cell's nucleus contains genetic information in the form of DNA. The nucleus is surrounded by the nuclear envelope. A single nucleus is the defining characteristic of eukaryotic cells. The nucleus is also the most important organelle of the cell. It contains the nucleolus, which manufactures ribosomes (another organelle), which are crucial in protein synthesis (also called gene expression).

Mitochondria: Mitochondria are oval-shaped and have a double membrane. The inner membrane has multiple folds called *cristae*. Mitochondria are responsible for the production of a cell's energy in the form of adenosine triphosphate (ATP). ATP is the principal energy transfer molecule in eukaryotic cells. Mitochondria also participate in cellular respiration.

Rough Endoplasmic Reticulum: The rough endoplasmic reticulum (RER) is composed of linked membranous sacs called cisternae with ribosomes attached to their external surfaces. The RER is responsible for the production of proteins that will eventually get shipped out of the cell.

Smooth Endoplasmic Reticulum: The smooth endoplasmic reticulum (SER) is composed of linked membranous sacs called cisternae without ribosomes, which distinguishes it from the RER. The SER's main function is the production of carbohydrates and lipids, which can be created expressly for the cell or to modify the proteins from the RER that will eventually get shipped out of the cell.

Golgi Apparatus: The Golgi apparatus is located next to the SER. Its main function is the final modification, storage, and shipment of products (proteins, carbohydrates, and lipids) from the endoplasmic reticulum.

Lysosomes: Lysosomes are specialized vesicles that contain enzymes capable of digesting food, surplus organelles, and foreign invaders such as bacteria and viruses. They often destroy dead cells in order to recycle cellular components. Lysosomes are only found in animal cells.

Secretory Vesicles: Secretory vesicles transport and deliver molecules into or out of the cell via the cell membrane. Endocytosis refers to the movement of molecules into a cell via secretory vesicles. Exocytosis refers to the movement of molecules out of a cell via secretory vesicles.

Ribosomes: Ribosomes are not membrane-bound. They are responsible for the production of proteins as specified from DNA instructions. Ribosomes can be free or bound.

Cilia and Flagella: Cilia are specialized hair-like projections on some eukaryotic cells that aid in movement, while flagella are long, whip-like projections that are used in the same capacity.

Here an illustration of the cell:

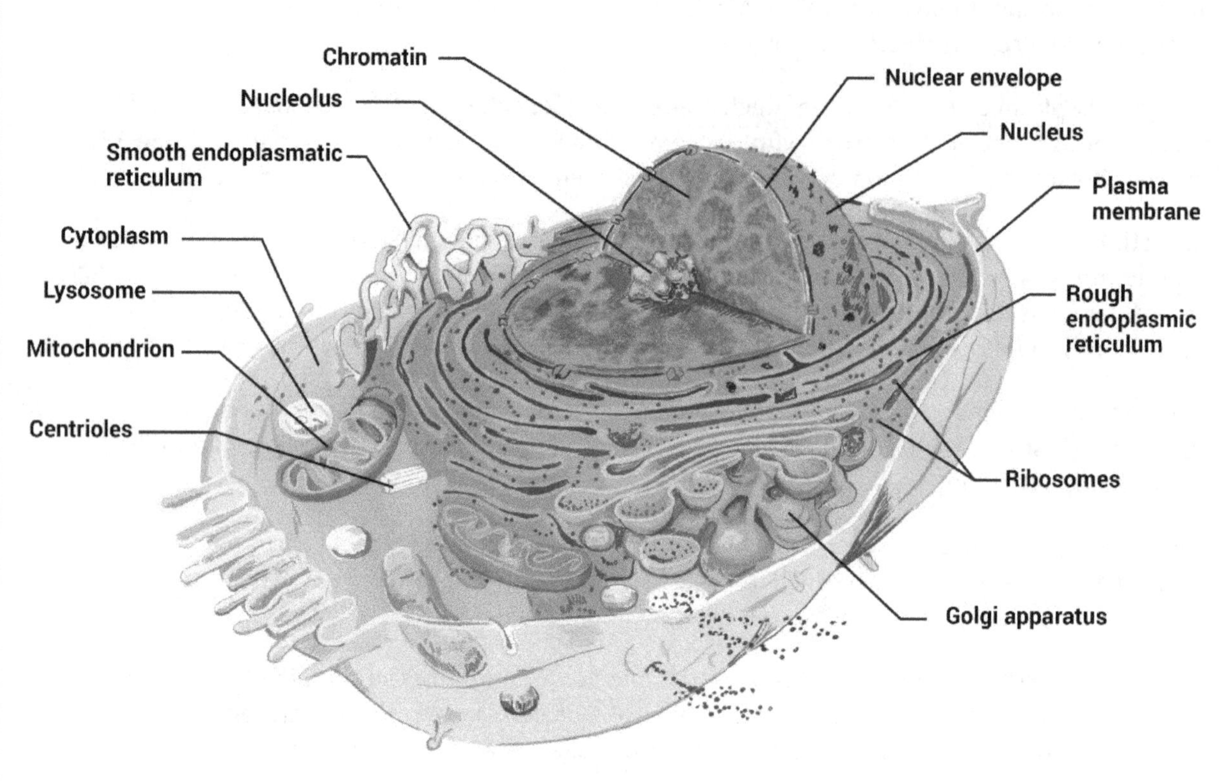

The following organelles are not found in animal cells:

Cell Walls: Cell walls can be found in plants, bacteria, and fungi, and are made of cellulose, peptidoglycan, and lignin, and other substances, depending on the organism it surrounds. Each of these substances is a type of sugar recognized as a structural carbohydrate. The carbohydrates are rigid structures located outside of the cell membrane. Cell walls function to protect the cell, maintain the cell's shape, and provide structural support. The prevent over-expansion of the cell by excess water.

Vacuoles: Plant cells have central vacuoles, which are essentially a membrane surrounding a body of water. They may store nutrients or waste products. Since vacuoles are large, they also help to support the structure of plant cells.

Chloroplasts: Chloroplasts are membrane-bound organelles that perform photosynthesis. They contain structural units called *thylakoids*. Chlorophyll, a green pigment that circulates within the thylakoids, harnesses light energy (sunlight) and helps convert it into chemical energy (glucose).

Gene Expression

Genes are the basis of heredity. The German scientist Gregor Mendel first suggested the existence of genes in 1866. A gene can be pinpointed to a locus, or a particular position, on DNA. It is estimated that humans have approximately 20,000 to 25,000 genes. For any particular gene, a human inherits one copy from each parent for a total of two.

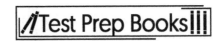

Genotypes and Phenotypes

Genotype refers to the genetic makeup of an individual within a species. Phenotype refers to the visible characteristics and observable behavior of an individual within a species.

Genotypes are written with pairs of letters that represent alleles. *Alleles* are different versions of the same gene, and, in simple systems, each gene has one dominant allele and one recessive allele. The letter of the dominant trait is capitalized, while the letter of the recessive trait is not capitalized. An individual can be homozygous dominant, homozygous recessive, or heterozygous for a particular gene. *Homozygous* means that the individual inherits two alleles of the same type, while *heterozygous* means that one dominant allele and one recessive allele have been inherited.

If an individual has homozygous dominant alleles or heterozygous alleles, the dominant allele is expressed. If an individual has homozygous recessive alleles, the recessive allele is expressed. For example, a species of bird develops either white or black feathers. The white feathers are the dominant allele, or trait (*A*), while the black feathers are the recessive allele (*a*). Homozygous dominant (*AA*) and heterozygous (*Aa*) birds will develop white feathers. Homozygous recessive (aa) birds will develop black feathers.

Genotype (genetic makeup)	Phenotype (observable traits)
AA	white feathers
Aa	white feathers
aa	black feathers

Influence of Phenotype on Genotype

An individual's genotype is determined by the genetic material (DNA) inherited from the individual's parents. Natural selection leads to adaptations within a species, which affects the phenotype. Over time, individuals within a species with the most advantageous phenotypes will survive and reproduce. As result of reproduction, the subsequent generation of phenotypes receives the fittest genotype. Eventually, the individuals within a species with genetic fitness flourish and those without it die out without passing on their traits. As explained above, this is also referred to as the concept of "survival of the fittest." When this process is duplicated over numerous generations, the outcome is offspring with a level of genetic fitness that meets or exceeds that of their parents.

Cell Division and Growth

Cell replication in eukaryotes involves duplicating the genetic material (DNA) and then dividing to yield two daughter cells, which are clones of the parent cell. The cell cycle is a series of stages leading to the growth and division of a cell. The cell cycle helps to replenish damaged or depleted cells. On average, eukaryotic cells go through a complete cell cycle every 24 hours. Some cells such as epithelial, or skin, cells are constantly dividing, while other cells such as mature nerve cells do not divide. Prior to mitosis, cells exist in a non-divisional stage of the cell cycle called interphase. During interphase, the cell begins to prepare for division by duplicating DNA and its cytoplasmic contents. Interphase is divided into three phases: gap 1 (G_1), synthesis (S), and gap 2 (G_2).

DNA Replication

Replication refers to the process during which DNA makes copies of itself. Enzymes govern the major steps of DNA replication.

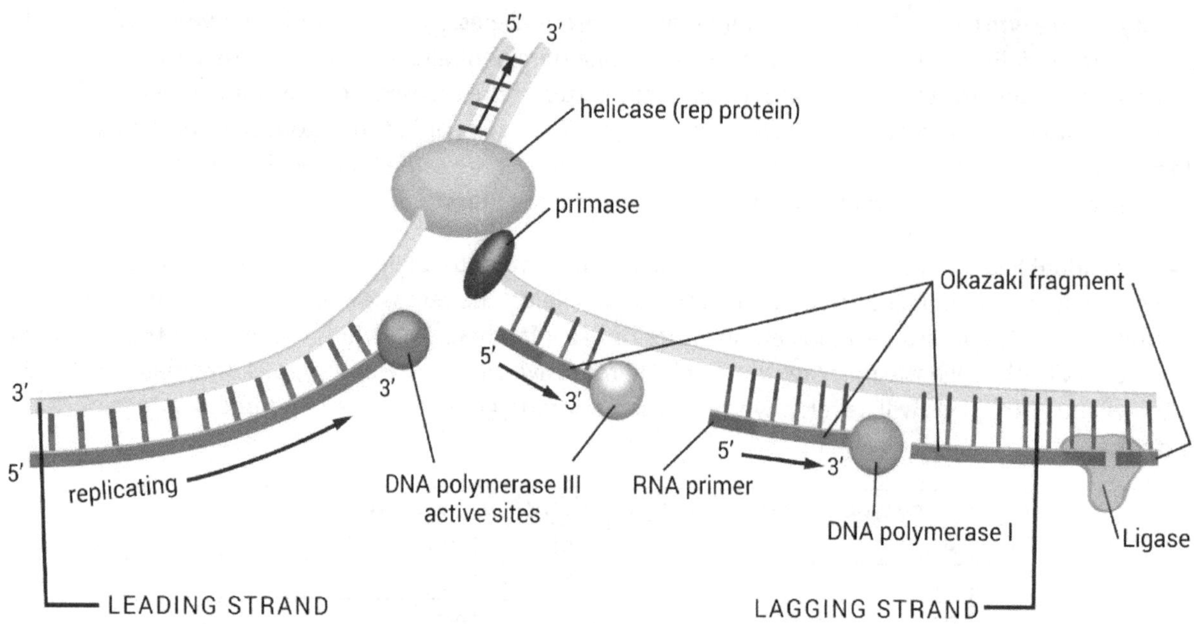

The process begins with the uncoiling of the double helix of DNA. *Helicase*, an enzyme, accomplishes this task by breaking the weak hydrogen bonds uniting base pairs. The uncoiling of DNA gives rise to the replication fork, which has a Y-shape. Each separated strand of DNA will act as a template for the production of a new molecule of DNA. The strand of DNA oriented toward the replication fork is called the *leading strand* and the strand oriented away from the replication fork is named the *lagging strand.*

Replication of the leading strand is continuous. *DNA polymerase*, an enzyme, binds to the leading strand and adds complementary bases. Replication of the lagging strand of DNA, on the other hand, is discontinuous. DNA polymerase produces discontinuous segments, called *Okazaki fragments*, which are later joined together by another enzyme, *DNA ligase*. To start the DNA synthesis on the lagging strand, the enzyme *primase* lays down a strip of RNA, called an *RNA primer*, to which the DNA polymerase can bind. As a result, two clones of the original DNA emerge from this process. DNA replication is considered *semiconservative* due to the fact that half of the new molecule is old, and the other half is new.

Cell Differentiation

Cell differentiation refers to the process of a cell transforming into another type of cell. It most commonly involves a less specialized cell transforming into a more specialized cell.

The human body contains a vast array of cells, which undergo division and differentiation to compose each unique human being. The trillions of cells composing the human body are derived from one cell, a fertilized egg called a zygote. The zygote not only divides, but also differentiates into cells that perform specific tasks.

Genes control the process of cell differentiation during human development. The zygote divides through mitosis into a blastula and then into a gastrula. At this stage, the three embryonic germ layers (endoderm, mesoderm, and ectoderm) are formed. Most of the human body systems develop from one or more of the embryonic germ layers. For example, the digestive system develops from the endoderm, or innermost germ layer; the cardiovascular system develops from the mesoderm, or middle germ layer; and the nervous system develops from the ectoderm, or outer germ layer.

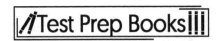

Mitosis

Mitosis, or asexual reproduction, produces two new cells that are genetically identical to the parent cell. It can happen in virtually every healthy adult cell, although some cells like red blood cells and neurons do not divide in general. When a cell is not undergoing cell division, it is in a stage called *interphase* which is characterized by growth, typical maintenance, and DNA synthesis in the nucleus. Each healthy human cell nucleus typically has 46 chromosomes and is said to be *diploid* (2n), as this count comes from 23 pairs of *homologous chromosomes*. Homologous chromosomes are pairs of chromatids with similar sections that correspond to similar genes, as in pairs of chromosome 1 or pairs of chromosome 21.

Mitosis is divided into the following events:

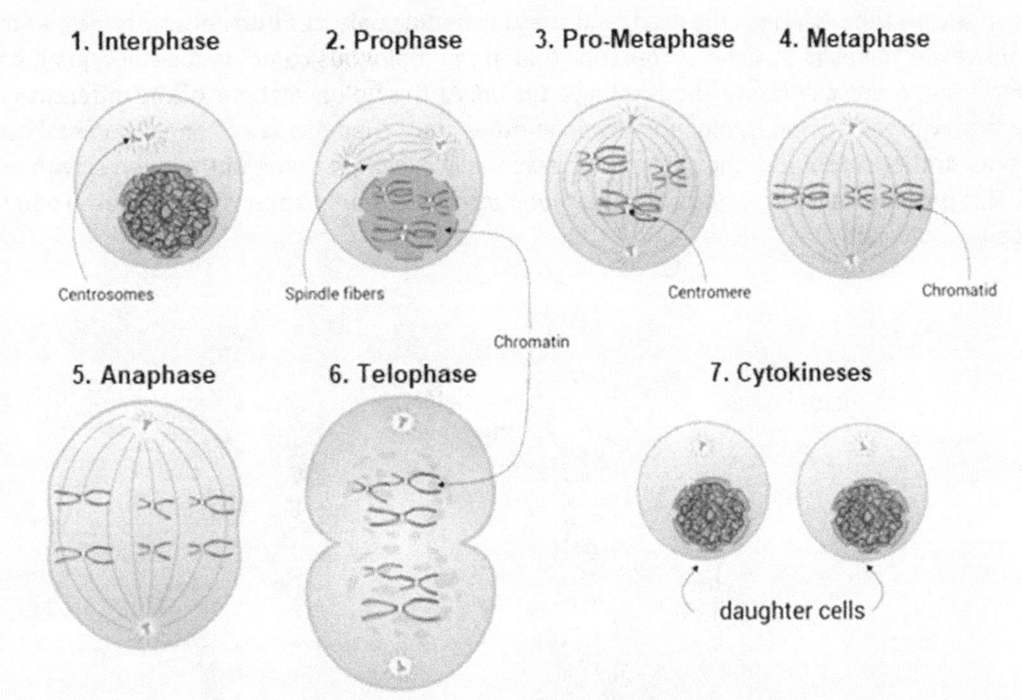

Prophase: Before entering prophase, chromatin duplicates. Prophase begins when the chromatin condenses to form chromosomes. Each new chromosome is made up of two identical sister chromatids joined by a structure called a *centromere*. Then, spindle fibers form and attach to structures called *centrioles*. Afterwards, the centrioles proceed to opposite poles of the cell. Finally, the nuclear envelope begins to degrade.

Pro-metaphase: The centrioles build spindle fibers and attach them to the chromosomes.

Metaphase: Using tension from spindle fibers, the chromosomes align in the middle of the cell.

Anaphase: The spindle fibers contract and separate the chromosomes at their centromere. The single chromatids, pulled by the spindle fibers, begin migrating to opposite poles of the cell.

Telophase: The chromatids arrive at opposite poles of the cell. The spindle fibers disappear, the nuclear envelope reforms, and the chromosomes uncoil back into chromatin.

Cytokinesis: This process refers to the cleaving of the cytoplasm to form two daughter cells genetically identical to the parent cell. In animal cells, this happens via a *cleavage furrow*; a cleavage furrow is a pinching of the cell membrane near the center that deepens until it reaches the point that the cell membrane can recombine and split the entity into two separate cells.

Meiosis

Meiosis, or sexual division, happens only in specialized sex cells, and it produces four cells called gametes. In humans, sex cells are found in the ovaries and in the testes, and are in contrast to somatic cells, which constitute the rest of the body of the organism. Each gamete contains half the number of chromosomes of a normal cell, and each is said to be *haploid* (n), rather than *diploid* (2n). In humans, a gamete has 23 chromosomes instead of the 46 that are typically found in somatic cells. The female gamete is called an *egg* and the male gamete is called a *sperm*.

Preceding meiosis, the DNA is synthesized, and the chromatin coalesces into chromosomes, as in mitosis. However, the pairs of sister chromatids that are homologous combine together, joining their centromeres into a single *chiasma* and forming a *tetrad*. At this point, sections of the different chromatids may break off and rejoin, possibly in another place. Half of a leg of one chromatid may swap with that of another chromatid; the chromatids essentially exchange some of their genes with one another. This process, called *crossing over* or *genetic recombination*, happens in prophase I and leads to greater genetic diversity.

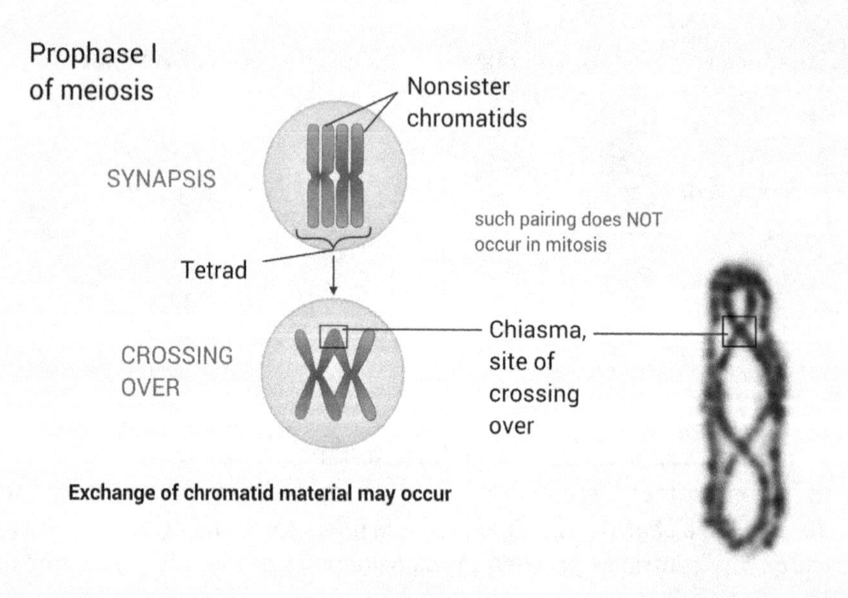

Like mitosis, meiosis is divided into the stages of prophase, metaphase, anaphase, telophase, and cytokinesis. However, as the end products have half the genetic material as the end products of mitosis, another round of division is needed. Therefore, meiosis is first partitioned into meiosis I and meiosis II, each round similar in scope to mitosis. During meiosis I, homologous chromosome pairs are separated into two daughter cells. Each daughter cell is haploid (n) because, although each cell at the end of meiosis I has 46 chromatids, half of them are duplicates of the other and not considered unique genetic material.

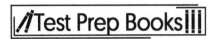

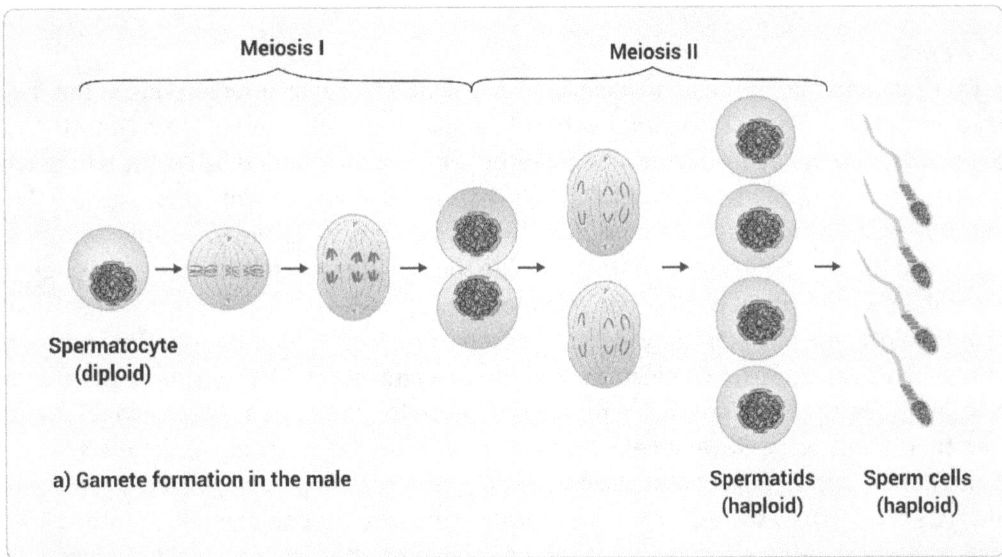

After cytokinesis I, the daughter cells immediately enter prophase II, rather than duplicating DNA or entering interphase. The nucleus disintegrates, the centrioles migrate to the ends of the cell, and the next round of divisions begins. This results in four haploid (n) daughter cells, the gametes of egg and sperm referenced earlier.

A common problem that arises in both meiosis and mitosis, but is especially noticeable in meiosis, is that of *nondisjunction*. Nondisjunction is the failure of homologous chromosomes or sister chromatids to separate during anaphase. This causes the daughter cells to have one more or one fewer chromosomes than usual, which can ultimately result in genetic conditions like Down's syndrome, when a meiotic egg with nondisjunction is fertilized.

Energy Transformations

There is a fundamental law of thermodynamics (the study of heat and movement) called *Conservation of Energy*. This law states that energy cannot be created nor destroyed, but rather, energy is transferred to different forms.

One biological example of energy transformation can be seen in photosynthesis. Photosynthesis is the process of converting light energy into chemical energy that is then stored in sugar and other organic molecules. It can be divided into two stages: the light-dependent reactions and the Calvin cycle. In plants, the photosynthetic process takes place in the chloroplast. Inside the chloroplast are membranous sacs, called thylakoids. Chlorophyll is a green pigment that lives in the thylakoid membranes and absorbs the light energy, starting the process of photosynthesis. The Calvin cycle takes place in the stroma, or inner space, of the chloroplasts. The complex series of reactions that take place in photosynthesis can be simplified into the following equation:

$$6CO_2 + 12H_2O + \text{Light Energy} \rightarrow C_6H_{12}O_6 + 6O_2 + 6H_2O.$$

Basically, carbon dioxide and water combine with light energy inside the chloroplast to produce organic molecules, oxygen, and water. Note that water is on both sides of the equation. Twelve water molecules are consumed during this process and six water molecules are newly formed as byproducts.

The Light Reactions

During the light reactions, chlorophyll molecules absorb light energy, or solar energy. In the thylakoid membrane, chlorophyll molecules, together with other small molecules and proteins, form *photosystems*, which are made up of a reaction-center complex surrounded by a light-harvesting complex. In the first step of photosynthesis, the light-harvesting complex from photosystem II (PSII) absorbs a photon from light, passes the photon from one pigment molecule to another within itself, and then transfers it to the reaction-center complex. Inside the reaction-center complex, the energy from the photon enables a special pair of chlorophyll *a* molecules to release two electrons. These two electrons are then accepted by a primary electron acceptor molecule. Simultaneously, a water molecule is split into two hydrogen atoms, two electrons, and one oxygen atom. The two electrons are transferred one by one to the chlorophyll *a* molecules, replacing their released electrons. The released electrons are then transported down an electron transport chain by attaching to the electron carrier plastoquinone (Pq), a cytochrome complex, and then a protein called plastocyanin (Pc) before they reach photosystem I (PS I). As the electrons pass through the cytochrome complex, protons are pumped into the thylakoid space, providing the concentration gradient that will eventually travel through ATP synthase to make ATP (like in aerobic respiration).

PS I absorbs photons from light, similar to PS II. However, the electrons that are released from the chlorophyll *a* molecules in PS I are replaced by the electrons coming down the electron transport chain (from PS II). A primary electron acceptor molecule accepts the released electrons in PS I and passes the electrons onto another electron transport chain, involving the protein ferredoxin (Fd). In the final steps of the light reactions, electrons are transferred from Fd to Nicotinamide adenine dinucleotide phosphate (NADP+) with the help of the enzyme NADP+ reductase and NADPH is produced. The ATP and nicotinamide adenine dinucleotide phosphate-oxidase (NADPH) produced from the light reactions are used as energy to form organic molecules in the Calvin cycle.

The Calvin Cycle

There are three phases in the Calvin cycle: carbon fixation, reduction, and regeneration of the CO_2 acceptor. Carbon fixation is when the first carbon molecule is introduced into the cycle, when CO_2 from the air is absorbed by the chloroplast. Each CO_2 molecule enters the cycle and attaches to ribulose bisphosphate (RuBP), a five-carbon sugar. The enzyme RuBP carboxylase-oxygenase, also known as rubisco, catalyzes this reaction. Next, two three-carbon 3-phosphoglycerate sugar molecules are formed immediately from the splitting of the six-carbon sugar.

Next, during the reduction phase, an ATP molecule is reduced to ADP and the phosphate group attaches to 3-phosphoglycerate, forming 1,3-bisphosphoglycerate. An NADPH molecule then donates two high-energy electrons to the newly formed 1,3-bisphosphate, causing it to lose the phosphate group and become glyceraldehyde 3-phosphate (G3P), which is a high-energy sugar molecule. At this point in the cycle, one G3P molecule exits the cycle and is used by the plant. However, to regenerate RuBP molecules, which are the CO_2 acceptors in the cycle, five G3P molecules continue in the cycle. It takes three turns of the cycle and three CO_2 molecules entering the cycle to form one G3P molecule.

In the final phase of the Calvin cycle, three RuBP molecules are formed from the rearrangement of the carbon skeletons of five G3P molecules. It is a complex process that involves the reduction of three ATP molecules. At the end of the process, RuBP molecules are again ready to enter the first phase and accept CO_2 molecules.

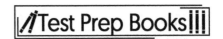

Although the Calvin cycle is not dependent on light energy, both steps of photosynthesis usually occur during daylight, as the Calvin cycle is dependent upon the ATP and NADPH produced by the light reactions, because that energy can be invested into bonds to create high-energy sugars. The Calvin cycle invests nine ATP molecules and six NADPH molecules into every one molecule of G3P that it produces. The G3P that is produced can be used as the starting material to build larger organic compounds, such as glucose.

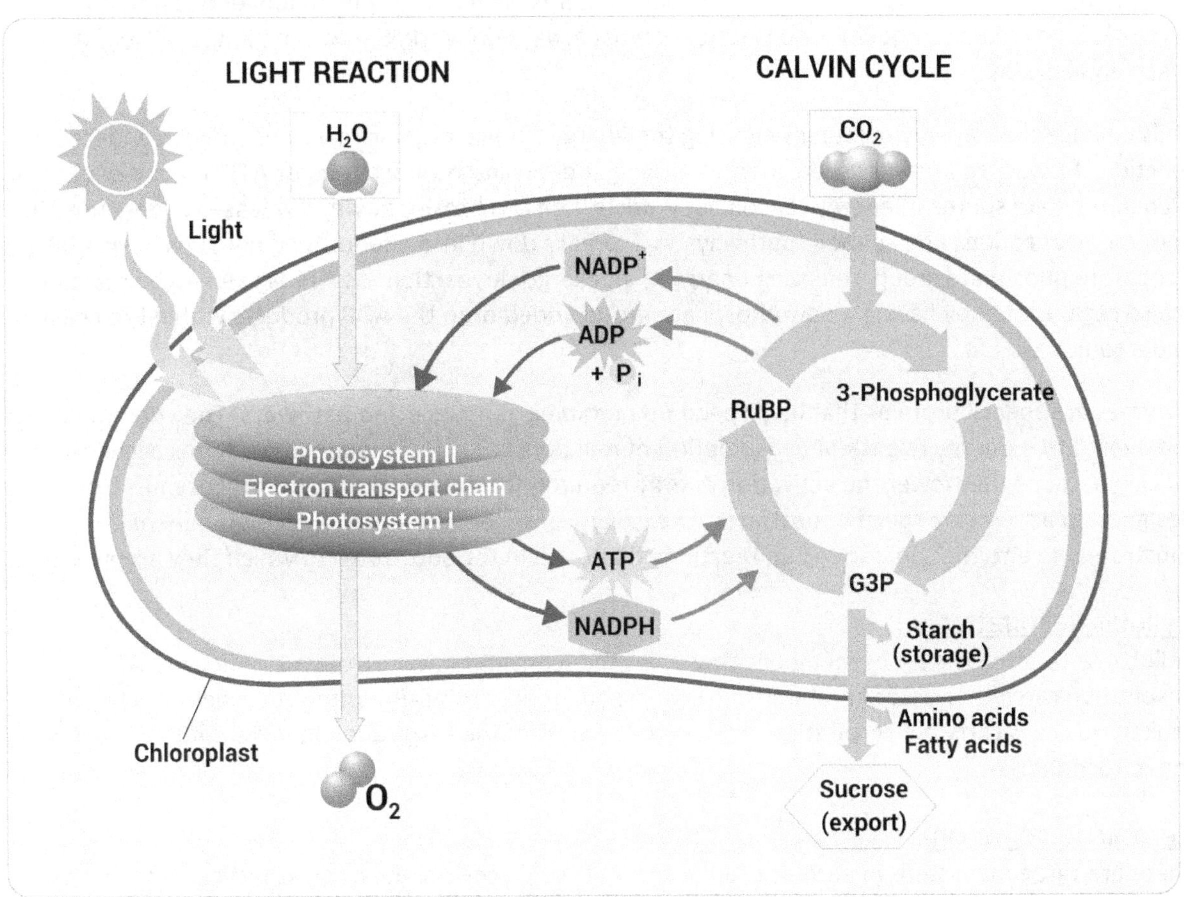

Metabolism

Metabolism is the set of chemical processes that occur within a cell for the maintenance of life. It includes both the synthesizing and breaking down of substances. A metabolic pathway begins with a molecule and ends with a specific product after going through a series of reactions, often involving an enzyme at each step. An enzyme is a protein that aids in the reaction. Catabolic pathways are metabolic pathways in which energy is released by complex molecules being broken down into simpler molecules. Opposite to catabolic pathways are anabolic pathways, which use energy to build complex molecules out of simple molecules. With cell metabolism, remember the first law of thermodynamics: Energy can be transformed, but it cannot be created or destroyed. Therefore, the energy released in a cell by a catabolic pathway is used up in anabolic pathways.

The reactions that occur within metabolic pathways are classified as either exergonic reactions or endergonic reactions. Exergonic reactions end in a release of free energy, while endergonic reactions absorb free energy from its surroundings. Free energy is the portion of energy in a system, such as a living cell, that can be used to perform work, such as a chemical reaction. It is denoted as the capital letter G, and the change in free energy from a reaction or set of reactions is denoted as delta G (ΔG). When reactions do not require an input of energy, they are said to occur spontaneously. Exergonic reactions are considered spontaneous because they result in a negative delta G ($-\Delta G$), where the products of the reaction have less free energy within them than the reactants. Endergonic reactions require an input of energy and result in a positive delta G ($+\Delta G$), with the products of the reaction containing more free energy than the individual reactants. When a system no longer has free energy to do work, it has reached equilibrium. Since cells must always do work, they are no longer alive if they reach equilibrium.

Cells balance their energy resources by using the energy from exergonic reactions to drive endergonic reactions forward, a process called energy coupling. Adenosine triphosphate, or ATP, is a molecule that is an immediate source of energy for cellular work. When it is broken down, it releases energy used in endergonic reactions and anabolic pathways. ATP breaks down into adenosine diphosphate, or ADP, and a separate phosphate group, releasing energy in an exergonic reaction. As ATP is used up by reactions, it is also regenerated by having a new phosphate group added onto the ADP products within the cell in an endergonic reaction.

Enzymes are special proteins that help speed up metabolic reactions and pathways. They do not change the overall free energy release or consumption of reactions; they just make the reactions occur more quickly because they lower the activation energy required for the reaction to occur. Enzymes are designed to act only on specific substrates. Their physical shape fits snugly onto their matched substrates, so enzymes only speed up reactions that contain the substrates to which they are matched.

Cellular Respiration

Cellular respiration is a set of metabolic processes that converts energy from nutrients into ATP. Respiration can either occur aerobically, using oxygen, or anaerobically, without oxygen. While prokaryotic cells carry out respiration in the cytosol, most of the respiration in eukaryotic cells occurs in the mitochondria.

Aerobic Respiration

There are three main steps in aerobic cellular respiration: glycolysis, the citric acid cycle (also known as the Krebs cycle), and oxidative phosphorylation. Glycolysis is an essential metabolic pathway that converts glucose to pyruvate and allows for cellular respiration to occur. It does not require oxygen to be present. Glucose is a common molecule used for energy production in cells. During glycolysis, two three-carbon sugars are generated from the splitting of a glucose molecule. These smaller sugars are then converted into pyruvate molecules via oxidation and atom rearrangement. Glycolysis requires two ATP molecules to drive the process forward, but the end product of the process has four ATP molecules, for a net production of two ATP molecules. Also, two reduced nicotinamide adenine dinucleotide (NADH) molecules are created from when the electron carrier oxidized nicotinamide adenine dinucleotide (NAD^+) peels off two electrons and a hydrogen atom.

In aerobically-respiring eukaryotic cells, the pyruvate molecules then enter the mitochondrion. Pyruvate is oxidized and converted into a compound called acetyl-CoA. This molecule enters the citric acid cycle to begin the process of aerobic respiration.

The citric acid cycle has eight steps. Remember that glycolysis produces two pyruvate molecules from each glucose molecule. Each pyruvate molecule oxidizes into a single acetyl-CoA molecule, which then enters the citric acid cycle. Therefore, two citric acid cycles can be completed and twice the number of ATP molecules are generated per glucose molecule.

Step 1: Acetyl-CoA adds a two-carbon acetyl group to an oxaloacetate molecule and produces one citrate molecule.

Step 2: Citrate is converted to its isomer, isocitrate, by removing one water molecule and adding a new water molecule in a different configuration.

Step 3: Isocitrate is oxidized and converted to α-ketoglutarate. A carbon dioxide (CO_2) molecule is released and one NAD+ molecule is converted to NADH.

Step 4: α-Ketoglutarate is converted to succinyl-CoA. Another carbon dioxide molecule is released and another NAD+ molecule is converted to NADH.

Step 5: Succinyl-CoA becomes succinate by the addition of a phosphate group to the cycle. The oxygen molecule of the phosphate group attaches to the succinyl-CoA molecule and the CoA group is released. The rest of the phosphate group transfers to a guanosine diphosphate (GDP) molecule, converting it to guanosine triphosphate (GTP). GTP acts similarly to ATP and can actually be used to generate an ATP molecule at this step.

Step 6: Succinate is converted to fumarate by losing two hydrogen atoms. The hydrogen atoms join a flavin adenine dinucleotide (FAD) molecule, converting it to $FADH_2$, which is a hydroquinone form.

Step 7: A water molecule is added to the cycle and converts fumarate to malate.

Step 8: Malate is oxidized and converted to oxaloacetate. One lost hydrogen atom is added to an NAD molecule to create NADH. The oxaloacetate generated here then enters back into step one of the cycle.

At the end of glycolysis and the citric acid cycles, four ATP molecules have been generated. The NADH and $FADH_2$ molecules are used as energy to drive the next step of oxidative phosphorylation.

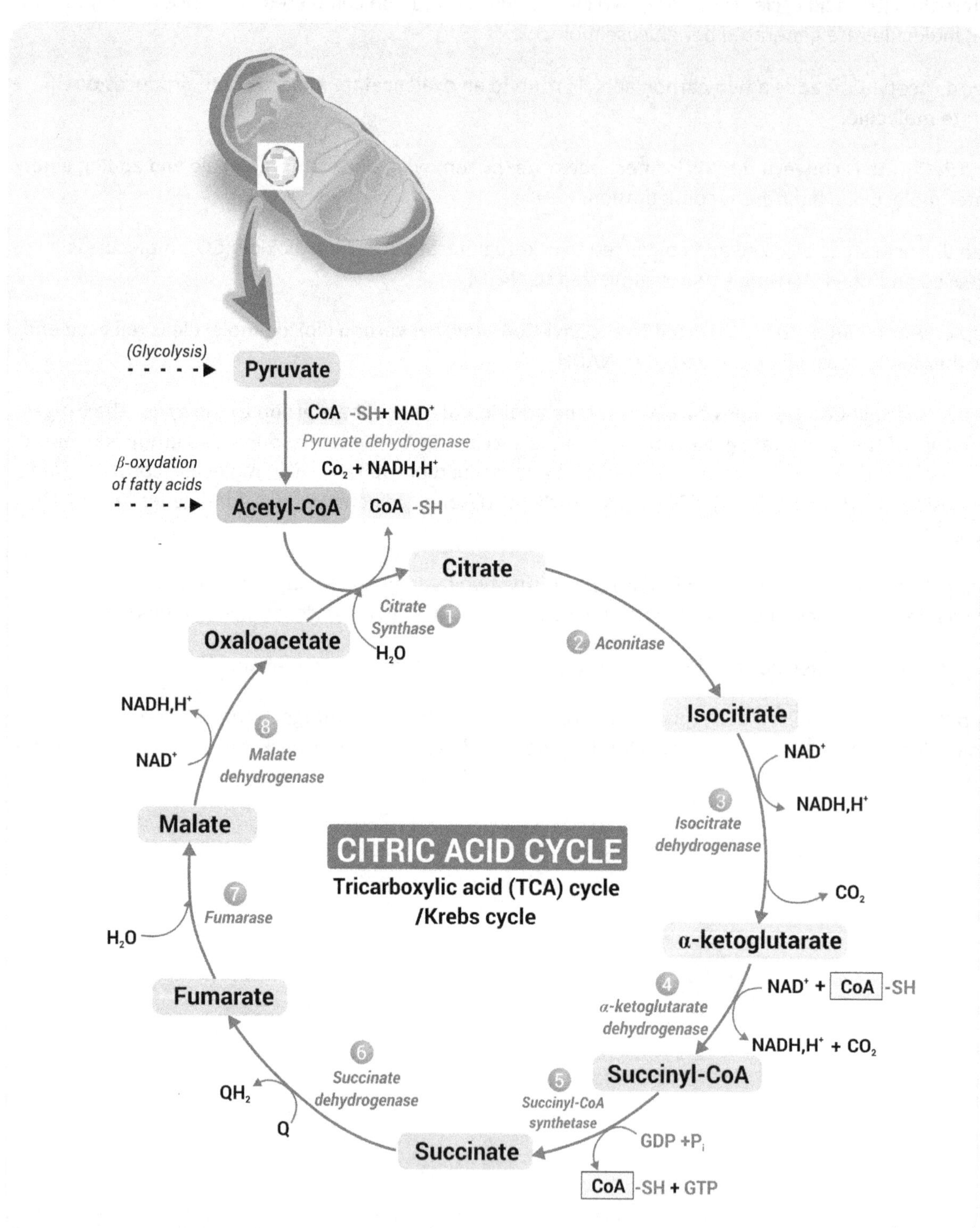

Oxidative Phosphorylation

Oxidative phosphorylation includes two steps: the electron transport chain and chemiosmosis. The inner mitochondrial membrane has four protein complexes, sequenced I to IV, used to transport protons and electrons through the inner mitochondrial matrix. Two electrons and a proton (H+) are passed from each NADH and $FADH_2$ to these channel proteins, pumping the hydrogen ions to the inner-membrane space using energy from the high-energy electrons to create a concentration gradient. NADH and $FADH_2$ also drop their high-energy electrons to the electron transport chain. NAD+ and FAD molecules in the mitochondrial matrix return to the Krebs cycle to pick up materials for the next delivery. From here, two processes happen simultaneously:

1. Electron Transport Chain: In addition to complexes I to IV, there are two mobile electron carriers present in the inner mitochondrial membrane, called ubiquinone and cytochrome C. At the end of this transport chain, electrons are accepted by an O_2 molecule in the matrix, and water is formed with the addition of two hydrogen atoms from chemiosmosis.

2. Chemiosmosis: This occurs in an ATP synthase complex that sits next to the four electron transporting complexes. ATP synthase uses facilitated diffusion (passive transport) to deliver protons across the concentration gradient from the inner mitochondrial membrane to the matrix. As the protons travel, the ATP synthase protein physically spins, and the kinetic energy generated is invested into phosphorylation of ADP molecules to generate ATP. Oxidative phosphorylation produces twenty-six to twenty-eight ATP molecules, bringing the total number of ATP generated through glycolysis and cellular respiration to thirty to thirty-two molecules.

Anaerobic Respiration

Some organisms do not live in oxygen-rich environments and must find alternate methods of respiration. Anaerobic respiration occurs in certain prokaryotic organisms. They utilize an electron transport chain similar to the aerobic respiration pathway; however, the terminal acceptor molecule is an electronegative substance that is not O_2. Some bacteria, for example, use the sulfate ion (SO_4^{2-}) as the final electron accepting molecule and the resulting byproduct is hydrogen sulfide (H_2S), instead of water.

Muscle cells that reach anaerobic threshold go through lactic acid respiration, while yeasts go through alcohol fermentation. Both processes only make two ATP.

Diversity of Life Forms

Genetics

Genetics is the study of heredity, which is the transmission of traits from one generation to the next, and hereditary variation. The chromosomes passed from parent to child contain hereditary information in the form of genes. Each gene has specific sequences of DNA that encode proteins, start pathways, and result in inherited traits. In the human life cycle, one haploid sperm cell joins one haploid egg cell to form a diploid cell. The diploid cell is the zygote, the first cell of the new organism, and from then on, mitosis takes over and nine months later, there is a fully developed human that has billions of identical cells.

The monk Gregor Mendel is referred to as the father of genetics. In the 1860s, Mendel came up with one of the first models of inheritance, using peapods with different traits in the garden at his abbey to test his theory and develop his model. His model included three laws to determine which traits are inherited; his theories still apply today, even after genetics has been studied more in depth.

1. The Law of Segregation: When two parent cells form daughter cells, the alleles segregate and each daughter cell only inherits one of the alleles from each parent.

2. The Law of Independent Assortment: Different traits are inherited independent of one another because in metaphase, the set of chromosomes line up in random fashion – mom's set of chromosomes do not line up all on the left or right, there is a random mix.

3. The Law of Dominance: Each characteristic has two versions that can be inherited. The gene that encodes for the characteristic has two variations, or alleles, and one is dominant over the other.

Dominant and Recessive Traits

Each gene has two alleles, one inherited from each parent. As mentioned, dominant alleles are noted in capital letters (A) and recessive alleles are noted in lower case letters (a). There are three possible combinations of alleles among dominant and recessive alleles: AA, Aa (known as a heterozygote), and aa. Dominant alleles, when mixed with recessive alleles, will mask the recessive trait. The recessive trait would only appear as the phenotype when the allele combination is aa because a dominant allele is not present to mask it.

Although most genes follow the standard dominant/recessive rules, there are some genes that defy them. Examples include cases of co-dominance, multiple alleles, incomplete dominance, sex-linked traits, and polygenic inheritance.

In cases of co-dominance, both alleles are expressed equally. For example, blood type has three alleles: I^A, I^B, and i. I^A and I^B are both dominant to i, but co-dominant with each other. An I^AI^B has AB blood. With incomplete dominance, the allele combination Aa actually makes a third phenotype. An example: certain flowers can be red (AA), white (aa), or pink (Aa).

Mendel's Laws of Genetics and Punnett Squares

Mendel's first law of genetics is the principle of *segregation* and states that alleles will segregate into different cells during the formation of gametes in meiosis. Mendel's second law of genetics is the principle of *independent assortment* and states that genes for different traits will be assigned to different gametes independent of the others. Together, these two laws state the assumptions on which genetic probabilities are based.

Punnett squares are simple graphic representations of all the possible genotypes of offspring, given the genotypes of the parent organisms. For instance, in the above example with the species of bird with black or white feathers, *A* represents a dominant allele and determines white colored feathers on a bird. The recessive allele *a* determines black colored feathers on a bird. If both parents are heterozygous (*Aa*, the x- and y-axis of the square), the offspring will have the possible genotypes *AA*, *Aa*, *Aa*, and *aa*.

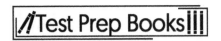

Phenotypically, three offspring would have white feathers and one would have black feathers, as shown in the Punnett square below:

	A	a
A	White	White
a	White	Black

Monohybrid and Dihybrid Genetic Crosses

Genetic crosses represent all possible permutations of gene combinations, or alleles. A monohybrid cross investigates the inheritance pattern of a single gene such as in the above example of the birds with black or white feathers. Both parents must have heterozygous gene pairs in a monohybrid cross.

The phenotypic ratio for a monohybrid cross is 3:1 (*AA*, *Aa*, *Aa*, *aa*) in favor of the dominant gene. A dihybrid cross investigates the inheritance patterns of two genes that are related, for example *A* and *B*. A dihybrid cross has a phenotypic ratio of 9:3:3:1 with nine offspring inheriting both dominant genes, six offspring inheriting a single dominant and a single recessive gene, and one offspring inheriting both recessive genes.

Mutations

Mutations are permanent alterations to an organism's genetic DNA sequence. Mutations can result from DNA failing to replicate accurately. They can also result from environmental influences such as radiation or chemicals. Mutations occur randomly and spontaneously at low rates.

Mutations can occur in reproductive and non-reproductive cells. Those occurring in non-reproductive cells are termed somatic mutations. Those occurring in reproductive cells (eggs or sperm) are termed germ line mutations. Although somatic mutations cannot be transmitted to offspring, germ line mutations are transmitted to offspring and can be advantageous, neutral, or disadvantageous.

In general, single-nucleotide alterations to DNA, or point mutations, can be either silent or same-sense (so that an identical amino acid sequence is encoded), missense (so that a different amino acid sequence is encoded), or nonsense (so that a new stop codon is encoded, and the resultant protein is truncated). They can also either be transitions (a purine base to another purine base or vice versa) or transversions (a purine base to a pyrimidine base or vice versa).

The four common multi-nucleotide mutations are:

1. Insertions: One or more nitrogen bases are added or inserted into the typical DNA sequence.

2. Deletions: One or more nitrogen bases are removed or deleted from the typical DNA sequence.

3. Inversions: A length of DNA is removed and reattached in reverse order from the typical DNA sequence.

4. Translocations: A length of DNA is removed and reattached in an alternate place or chromosome than where found in the typical DNA sequence.

Health

Nutritional Factors Affecting Health

Meal Planning Applications

There are a number of health-related applications that can be used for meal planning, including the United States Department of Agriculture (USDA) Food Patterns, the DASH (Dietary Approaches to Stop Hypertension) Eating Plan, MyPlate, food exchanges, and the glycemic index.

USDA Food Patterns

There are three USDA Food Patterns included in the 2015-2020 Dietary Guidelines: Healthy U.S. Style Eating, Healthy Mediterranean Style Eating, and Healthy Vegetarian Style Eating. One eating pattern is not necessarily superior to another, but rather more of a preference; however, a vegetarian lifestyle has been associated with a decreased risk for some chronic diseases such as heart disease and certain cancers. The USDA Food Patterns are all based on systematic review from scientific research, food pattern modeling, and analysis of intake of the U.S. population. Each USDA Food Pattern is based on the five food groups—vegetables, fruits, grains, dairy, and protein—and can be customized to meet an individual's needs based on age, sex, height, weight, and level of physical activity.

The Healthy U.S. Style Eating Pattern is based on typical foods consumed in Americans' diets with a focus on nutrient-dense foods in portions that are appropriate for the desired caloric intake. The Healthy Mediterranean Style Eating Pattern is based on the Healthy U.S. Style Eating Pattern but adjusted to align with the eating patterns of the Mediterranean diet, which have been associated with positive health outcomes. Specifically, the Healthy Mediterranean Style Eating Pattern has more fruit and seafood, but less dairy, than the U.S. Style Eating Pattern. The Healthy Vegetarian Style Eating Pattern is also based on the Healthy U.S. Style Eating Pattern, but is adjusted to reflect the eating habits of self-reported vegetarians, as identified in the National Health and Nutrition Examination Survey (NHANES).

DASH Eating Plan

The DASH Eating Plan is based on clinical research trials, which found that the plan helped individuals lower their blood pressure and low-density lipoprotein (LDL) cholesterol and improve heart health, while meeting nutrient requirements. The DASH Eating Plan emphasizes whole grains, poultry, fish, and nuts, along with food sources of potassium, calcium, and magnesium. Individuals are encouraged to consume as much as seven to eight servings of grains and four to five servings of fruits and vegetables per day on a 2000-calorie diet. Individuals using the DASH Eating Plan may need to gradually increase the intake of whole grains, fruits, and vegetables, since the increased fiber of these foods can lead to bloating and diarrhea.

MyPlate

MyPlate is a tool developed by the USDA based on the five food groups and healthy eating, focused on variety, appropriate portion sizes, nutrient-dense foods, and low saturated fat, sodium, and added sugar intake. The MyPlate Daily Checklist and the SuperTracker are two specific online tools that allow individuals to customize nutrition planning for their specific needs.

Food Exchanges

Food exchanges are used for meal planning purposes, especially for those with diabetes and/or seeking weight loss. Food exchanges divide food into six categories based on the amount of carbohydrate, fat, and protein they contain: starches/breads, fruits, milk, vegetables, meat, and fat.

- Starches and breads contain 15 grams of carbohydrate and 3 grams of protein per exchange with 80 calories.
- Fruits contain 15 grams of carbohydrate per exchange with 60 calories.
- Milk exchanges contain 12 grams of carbohydrate; 8 grams of protein; 3-8 grams of fat depending on whether the milk exchange is a low-, medium-, or high-fat choice; and 90-150 calories, depending on the fat content.
- Vegetable exchanges contain 5 grams of carbohydrate per serving with 25 calories.
- Meat exchanges contain 7 grams of protein per ounce and 0-8 grams of fat, depending on whether the source of the meat exchange is very lean, lean, medium fat, or high fat, with a range of 35-100 calories.
- Fat exchanges provide 5 grams of fat and 45 calories.

Glycemic Index

Finally, the glycemic index and glycemic load offer insight as to how foods affect blood glucose and insulin levels. Glycemic index and load can be useful tools in meal planning to help individuals better understand the impact specific foods may have on their blood sugar. Carbohydrate counting may also be a useful tool in helping individuals monitor and understand the impact various carbohydrates have on their blood sugar.

Nutritional Needs

Carbohydrates

Carbohydrates provide 4 kilocalories per gram and are a major source of fuel for the body, particularly during moderate- and high-intensity exercise, up to 2 hours in duration. Beyond approximately this duration, stores deplete, and the body relies on fatty acid metabolism for sustained energy. Carbohydrates are used for energy immediately, if needed, but excess carbohydrates are converted to glycogen and stored in skeletal muscles and the liver or converted to fat if the body's glycogen stores are full. The amount of glycogen the body can store is influenced by a variety of factors including physical training status, basal metabolic rate, body size, and eating habits, but in general, the body can store about 15 grams per kilogram of body weight. In general, athletes should consume about 6-10 grams of carbohydrate per kilogram of body weight daily, depending on the intensity, duration, and frequency of their training, as well as their current health and physical goals. This is somewhat higher than recommendations for minimally-active individuals. The standard recommendation for the general population is to consume 45-65% of daily caloric intake from carbohydrates.

Protein

Like carbohydrates, protein provides 4 kilocalories per gram. Protein, which consists of amino acids, is used to support the body in the development of tissues, enzymes, and hormones, and to rebuild and repair muscles after exercise. In general, protein recommendations for athletes fall in the range of 1.5-2.0 grams per kilogram of body weight daily, depending on the type, duration, and frequency of exercise. For the general public, the recommendation is much lower, at 0.8 grams per kilogram of body weight daily. Excessive consumption of protein does not lead to increased muscle mass because protein in excess of physiologic needs is converted and stored as fat.

Protein is essential in the diet and is needed to support the building of connective tissue, cell membranes, and the development of muscle. Protein consists of amino acids, and there are 22 amino acids used in the body. EAAs are required through the diet, since they cannot be synthesized in the body, and the eight of them include isoleucine, leucine, lysine, methionine, phenylalanine, threonine, tryptophan, and valine. There are also seven conditional amino acids that cannot be sufficiently produced in the body, so they should come from the diet: arginine, cysteine, glutamine, histidine, proline, taurine, and tyrosine. There are seven non-EAAs: alanine, asparagine, aspartic acid, citrulline, glutamic acid, glycine, and serine. These amino acids can be produced by the body so are not required in the diet.

Protein can be categorized as complete or incomplete. Complete proteins contain all of the EAAs, while incomplete proteins do not. Protein that comes from animal sources is usually complete and contains all of the EAAs, while incomplete proteins typically come from plant sources and do not contain all the EAAs. Proteins that have a higher amount of the EAAs are considered to have a higher amino acid profile. Good sources of animal protein include meat (beef, chicken, turkey, pork, and lamb), eggs, fish/seafood (tuna, crab, shrimp, lobster), and dairy (milk, yogurt, and cheese). Sources of plant-based protein include grains (brown rice, spelt, quinoa, amaranth, oatmeal), legumes (beans, peas, and lentils—pinto, black kidney, garbanzo, edamame, and tofu), and nuts and seeds (peanut butter, almond butter, peanuts, almonds, pistachios, walnuts, pecans, pumpkin seeds, and sunflower seeds).

Fat

Fat provides 9 kilocalories per gram and contributes significantly to resting energy requirements, as well as requirements during low-intensity and long-duration exercise. Fats can be divided into two basic categories: saturated and unsaturated. Saturated fats, which are primarily found in animal sources, include butyric, lauric, myristic, palmitic, and stearic acid, while unsaturated fats typically come from plant sources, such as soybeans, nuts, seeds, olives, and avocados. Fats should comprise at least 15% of the total caloric intake; as much as 30%-40% can be acceptable, depending on the health, age, and needs of the individual. An intake of 30% fat (10% saturated, 10% polyunsaturated, and 10% monounsaturated) aligns with dietary guidelines and should ensure an adequate—but not excessive—dietary intake.

Vitamins and Minerals

Vitamin and mineral needs vary throughout the lifespan and between sexes, but typically can be met if a balanced, varied diet is consumed with foods such as lean meats/protein, fruits, vegetables, whole grains, and dairy. B vitamins such as thiamin, riboflavin, and niacin are required to support metabolic processes; vitamin D is required for calcium absorption, and vitamins C and E are required to mitigate stress oxidation in the body. Fat-soluble vitamins (A, D, E, and K) are stored in the body, so they should not be consumed in excessive quantities. If an individual is not meeting their vitamins and minerals requirements through diet, a multivitamin-mineral supplement or specific supplementation is needed. Supplementation is also necessary at certain times. For example, a folic acid supplement is recommended to women hoping to conceive as deficiencies in folic acid have been linked to spinal malformations.

Sweating can lower electrolytes and minerals such as sodium, potassium, chloride, iron, calcium, phosphorus, and magnesium. Sodium and potassium help to regulate the body's water balance and also play a significant role in muscle contraction. Chloride also helps with fluid balance and nerve conductions. Iron plays an important role in the body's ability to transport and use oxygen, and calcium is critical for bone formation, nerve conduction, and muscle contraction. Phosphorus is involved in intramuscular oxidation processes, and magnesium helps support energy metabolism. Electrolytes (sodium, potassium, and chloride) and water need to be replaced during extended exercise, particularly in hot and humid environments, because they are excreted in sweat.

Health Risk Factors Associated with Dietary Choices

Dietary choices affect health risks associated with some chronic health conditions.

Saturated fats

Saturated fat is associated with an increased risk for cardiovascular disease, so the Dietary Guidelines for Americans recommends consuming no more than 10% of caloric intake from saturated fats. An emphasis should be made on replacing saturated fats with unsaturated fats, especially polyunsaturated, as this substitution is associated with improved total and LDL cholesterol.

Triglycerides

Circulating triglycerides are also affected by diet. Limiting refined, sugary foods; replacing saturated fats with unsaturated fats; and increasing fiber intake can help to keep triglycerides in the normal range of less than 150 milligrams per deciliter. High triglycerides can lead to increased risk of heart disease and diabetes.

Trans fats

Trans fats are produced through a process called *hydrogenation,* which makes packaged foods (such as coffee creamer, snack foods, store-bought baked goods, vegetable shortening, stick margarines, fast foods, and refrigerated dough products) more shelf stable. In recent years, manufacturers have begun limiting or removing trans fats, per the Food and Drug Administration regulatory requirements, because these fats have been shown to pose a significant risk for heart disease and should be eliminated from the diet.

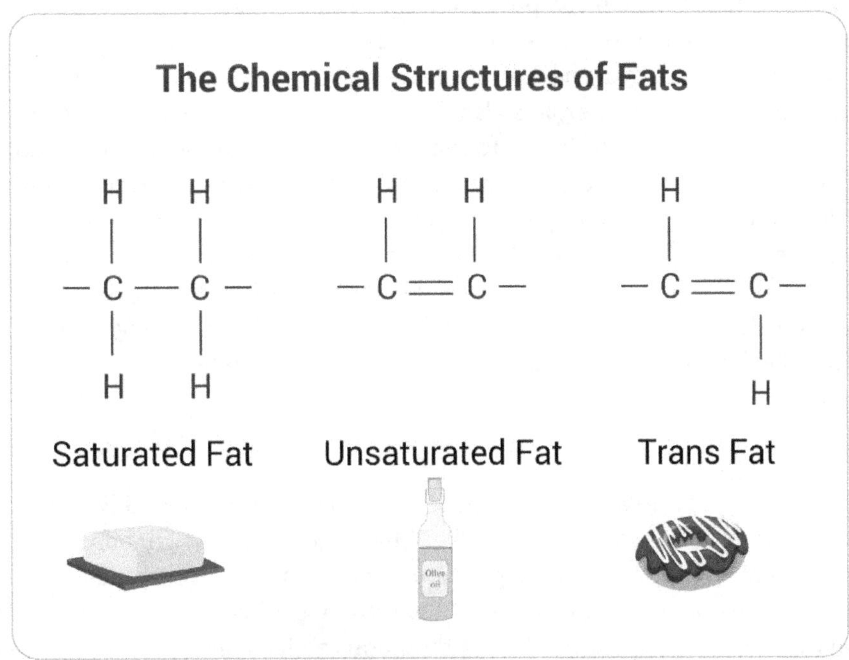

Cholesterol

Cholesterol is required for various physiological and structural functions, such as the production of cells and hormones. However, these requirements are met by the cholesterol produced in the body; little to no additional dietary cholesterol is needed. The upper limit for healthy levels of cholesterol is 200 milligrams per deciliter; high cholesterol is a risk factor for heart disease. Because recent research has failed to find a significant correlation between dietary intake and circulating cholesterol, the 2015-2020 Dietary Guidelines no longer contain recommendations that limit cholesterol intake to 300 milligrams per day. The Institute of Medicine (IOM) still recommends limiting the intake of cholesterol-laden foods such as high-fat meats and dairy, which also contain high amounts of saturated fat.

Calcium

Calcium plays important physiologic roles including vascular contraction, vasodilation, muscle contraction, and nerve impulse transmission. The majority of calcium in the body is stored in bones and teeth. To support bone mineral deposition and avoid bone resorption, it is important to have adequate calcium intake. This is especially true at certain stages of the life cycle, when bones are forming or have the tendency to demineralize, as well as for athletes, who may lose additional calcium through perspiration. Postmenopausal women, especially, need to obtain adequate amounts of calcium in the diet to decrease the risk for osteoporosis. Signs and symptoms of calcium deficiency may be absent or may include muscle weakness, cramping, and increased susceptibility to fractures. Recommended intake varies by gender and throughout the lifespan, with increases for females, adolescents, lactating mothers, and postmenopausal women.

Iron

Iron in the body is primarily combined with hemoglobin, in an iron-protein compound that increases the blood's oxygen-carrying capacity 65 times, as well as in muscle myoglobin. Intensive workout programs put individuals at risk for developing iron-deficiency anemia, which decreases aerobic capacity, since less oxygen can circulate to working tissues, leading to fatigue and reduced athletic performance. Other symptoms of iron-deficiency anemia include brittle nails, sluggishness, headaches, pale skin, and dizziness. Iron recommendations are 1.3-1.7 times higher for athletes than nonathletes and another 1.8 times higher for vegetarian athletes in comparison to those who consume animal protein, due to the lower bioavailability of nonheme iron sources in the vegetarian diet. The Recommended Dietary Allowance (RDA) for iron for men over the age of 18 is 8 milligrams per day; for women ages 19-50, 18 milligrams; for women ages 51 and older, it is also 8 milligrams per day. Females of childbearing age are at a higher risk for iron-deficiency anemia due to red blood cell loss during menstruation. Females often tend to consume less dietary iron as well. Endurance athletes may require additional iron due to foot-strike hemolysis, loss of hemoglobin in urine from strenuous training, and the small amount of iron lost in sweat. Heme sources of iron are more easily absorbed and include beef, pork, and beef liver. Nonheme sources include oatmeal, lentils, dark green leafy vegetables, and fortified cereals. Vitamin C intake can increase the absorption of iron in the small intestine; a glass of orange juice increases nonheme iron bioavailability by three times. It should be noted that excessive iron intake, especially in males, can be toxic.

Hydration and Electrolytes

The adult male body is about 60% water, while the female body is about 50%-55% water. As a result, less than optimal hydration status can affect health. Dehydration can cause headaches, sluggishness, mood changes and loss of cognitive functioning, and muscle cramping. Decreased athletic performance can occur with just a 3% loss in body weight from dehydration. During exercise, perspiration helps mitigate the increase in body temperature. During strenuous activity, individuals can lose as much as

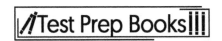

6%-10% of their body weight via sweating, depending on the type and duration of the activity. It is important to maintain adequate hydration before, during, and after exercise; the recommendation is 8-12 cups of water per day plus replacement of fluid loss during exercise. Individual needs may vary, but during exercise, about 6-8 ounces of fluid are usually needed every 15-20 minutes of activity. Within the context of adequate hydration, electrolyte balance must also be preserved. The five major electrolytes that are important to health are sodium, potassium, chloride, calcium, and magnesium. Sodium, which is needed to help maintain fluid balance, nerve function, muscle contractions, and acid-base balance, is the primary electrolyte lost in sweat and must be replaced. It is important to include sodium in fluids or food as part of the rehydration process after exercise so that overhydration, or hyponatremia, does not occur as a result of drinking water alone. Adding sodium to fluids also helps to improve the absorption of water and carbohydrates. Most commercial sports drinks are formulated to provide the optimal levels of sodium and carbohydrates in solution.

Nutrient-dense versus caloric-dense foods

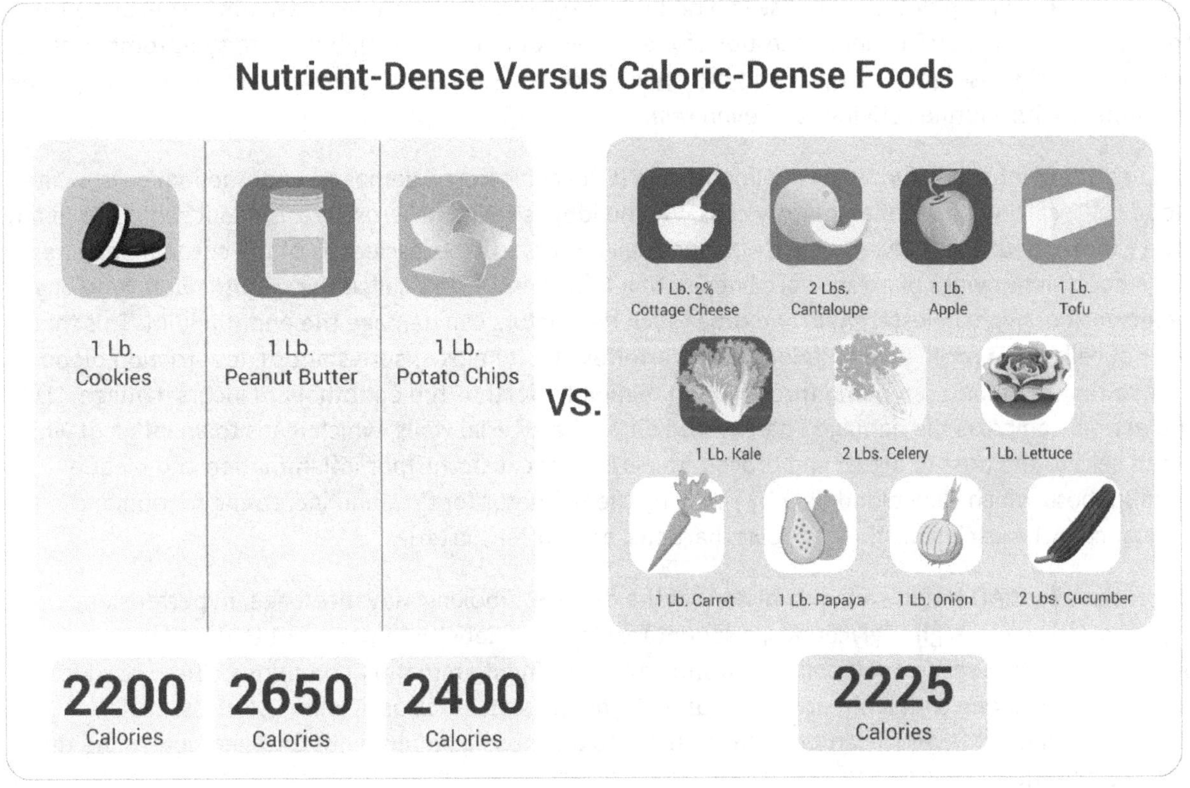

Nutrient-dense foods are rich in essential nutrients, vitamins, and minerals but low in calories, especially in comparison to calorically-dense or energy-dense foods. Calorically-dense foods provide few essential nutrients relative to the number of calories they provide. When focusing on weight loss or optimal health, it is important to focus on nutrient-dense foods. Sources of nutrient-dense foods include fresh vegetables and fruits, specifically dark green leafy vegetables like kale, spinach, and collard greens and fruits like berries, melon, mangoes, and citrus. Other nutrient-dense foods include lean sources of protein, dairy, legumes, and whole grains that have been enriched with vitamins and minerals. Calorically-dense foods include cookies, cakes, pastries, soda, chips, high-fat meats, and fast foods and other highly processed, highly caloric foods.

Diseases

Coronary Artery Disease (CAD)

According to the World Health Organization (WHO), coronary artery disease, or CAD, is the deadliest disease in the world, accounting for 15.5% of all deaths worldwide in 2015. CAD, also known as ischemic heart disease, is a narrowing of the blood vessels that supply blood, oxygen, and nutrients to the heart muscle. This narrowing is usually caused by the buildup of cholesterol-containing plaques along the arterial walls, which then reduces blood flow. Decreased coronary blood flow can cause angina (chest pain) and dyspnea (shortness of breath). Left untreated, overtime, arrhythmias, heart failure, and heart attacks can result, particularly if the blockage completely occludes blood flow.

CAD develops gradually over time, and is often considered insidious in nature because patients can be asymptomatic for years while the plaques are slowly building up in the coronary arterial walls. In these cases, patients may be entirely unaware of their condition until it becomes severe enough to trigger symptoms, at which point, the disease can be fairly progressed. Oftentimes, patients first experience angina and dyspnea during heavy exertion (for example, during exercise), but these symptoms subside with rest. As the disease progresses and the buildup more significantly narrows the arteries, symptoms can appear with routine activities and even rest.

Plaques are composed of low-density lipoprotein (LDL) cholesterol, damaged endothelium cells, white blood cells, calcium, and inflammatory cells. The buildup is called *atherosclerosis* and it can occur in any artery throughout the body, though CAD specifically refers to atherosclerosis of the coronary arteries. The smooth inner walls of arteries are lined with a thin layer of cells called the *endothelium.* Smoking, hypertension, hypocholesteremia, and other such risk factors can damage the endothelium. This thin layer of cells has a protective function for the arteries and it helps ensure smooth, low-friction blood flow so that the blood can pump through with minimal effort. As the endothelium incurs damage, LDL cholesterol can cross the damaged barrier and enter the arterial walls, which leads to an influx of white blood cells to the area to digest and process the LDL. This causes further inflammation and plaque buildup, both which slow blood flow by reducing the diameter for flow and increasing friction and resistance. Atherosclerosis thus narrows, hardens, and stiffens arteries.

Risk factors for CAD include a family history of the disease, smoking, advanced age, hypertension, hypocholesteremia, high triglycerides, a sedentary lifestyle, diabetes, a poor diet that is high in processed foods, obesity, metabolic syndrome, and certain inflammatory conditions. These risk factors are considered along with a physical exam and diagnostic tests, such as an exercise stress test, echocardiogram, EKG, and a cardiac catherization, to diagnose a patient with CAD and determine the best treatment.

Treatment often focuses on lifestyle modifications, including obtaining regular aerobic exercise, smoking cessation, blood sugar control, and adopting a healthy diet with minimal processed foods. Medications, such as statins and aspirin, may be prescribed. Depending on the severity and extent of the blockages and symptoms, surgeries may be indicated. Common procedures for CAD include the insertion of stents, balloon angioplasties, and coronary artery bypass surgeries.

Stroke

The WHO reports that strokes are the second leading cause deaths worldwide, accounting for 11.1% of the total in 2015. Moreover, they are the leading cause of long-term disability. A *stroke* is defined as the death of brain tissue due to ischemic or hemorrhagic injury. Ischemic strokes are more common than hemorrhagic strokes; however, the differential diagnosis of these conditions requires careful attention to the patient's history and physical examination. In general, an acute onset of neurological symptoms and seizures is more common with hemorrhagic stroke, while ischemic stroke is more frequently associated with a history of some form of trauma. The National Institutes of Health (NIH) Stroke Scale represents an international effort to standardize the assessment and treatment protocols for stroke. The scale includes detailed criteria and the protocol for assessment of the neurological system. The stroke scale items are to be administered in the official order listed and there are directions that denote how to score each item.

Ischemic Stroke

Ischemic strokes result from occlusion of the cerebral vasculature as a result of a thrombotic or embolic event. At the cellular level, the ischemia leads to hypoxia that rapidly depletes the ATP stores. As a result, the cellular membrane pressure gradient is lost, and there is an influx of sodium, calcium, and water into the cell, which leads to cytotoxic edema. This process creates scattered regions of ischemia in the affected area, containing cells that are dead within minutes of the precipitating event. This core of ischemic tissue is surrounded by an area with minimally-adequate perfusion that may remain viable for several hours after the event. These necrotic areas are eventually liquefied and acted upon by macrophages, resulting in the loss of brain parenchyma. These affected sites, if sufficiently large, may be prone to hemorrhage, due to the formation of collateral vascular supply with or without the use of medications such as recombinant tissue plasminogen activator (rtPA). The ischemic process also compromises the blood-brain barrier, which leads to the movement of water and protein into the extracellular space within 4 to 6 hours after the onset of the stroke, resulting in vasogenic edema.

Nonmodifiable risk factors for ischemic stroke include age, gender, ethnicity, history of migraine headaches with aura, and a family history of stroke or transient ischemic attacks (TIAs). Modifiable risk factors include hypertension, diabetes, hypercholesterolemia, cardiac disease including atrial fibrillation, valvular disease and heart failure, elevated homocysteine levels, obesity, illicit drug use, alcohol abuse, smoking, and sedentary lifestyle. The research related to the occurrence of stroke in women indicates the need to treat hypertension aggressively prior to and during pregnancy and prior to the use of contraceptives to prevent irreversible damage to the microvasculature. In addition, it is recommended that to reduce their risk of stroke, women with a history of migraine headaches preceded by an aura should ameliorate all modifiable risk factors, and all women over seventy-five years old should be routinely assessed for the onset of atrial fibrillation.

Heredity is associated with identified gene mutations and the process of atherosclerosis and cholesterol metabolism. Hypercholesterolemia and the progression of atherosclerosis in genetically-susceptible individuals are now regarded as active inflammatory processes that contribute to endothelial damage of the cerebral vasculature, thereby increasing the risk for strokes. There are also early indications that infection also contributes to the development and advancement of atherosclerosis.

The presenting manifestations of ischemic stroke must be differentiated from other common diseases, including brain tumor formation, hyponatremia, hypoglycemia, seizure disorders, and systemic infection. The sudden onset of hemisensory losses, visual alterations, hemiparesis, ataxia, nystagmus, and aphasia are commonly, although not exclusively, associated with ischemic strokes. The availability of reperfusion therapies dictates the emergent use of diagnostic imaging studies, including CT and MRI scans, carotid duplex scans, and digital subtraction angiography to confirm the data obtained from the patient's history and physical examination. Laboratory studies include CBC, coagulation studies, chemistry panels, cardiac biomarkers, toxicology assays, and pregnancy testing as appropriate.

The emergency care of the patient who presents with an ischemic stroke is focused on the stabilization of the patient's ABCs, completion of the physical examination and appropriate diagnostic studies, and initiation of reperfusion therapy as appropriate, within 60 minutes of arrival in the emergency department. Reperfusion therapies include the use of alteplase (the only fibrinolytic agent that is approved for the treatment of ischemic stroke), antiplatelet agents, and mechanical thrombectomy. Emergency providers must also be alert for hyperthermia, hypoxia, hypertension or hypotension, and signs of cardiac ischemia or cardiac arrhythmias.

Hemorrhagic Stroke

Hemorrhagic strokes are less common than ischemic strokes; however, a hemorrhagic stroke is more likely to be fatal than an ischemic stroke. A hemorrhagic stroke is the result of bleeding into the parenchymal tissue of the brain due to leakage of blood from damaged intracerebral arteries. These hemorrhagic events occur more often in specific areas of the brain, including the thalamus, cerebellum, and brain stem. The tissue surrounding the hemorrhagic area is also subject to injury due to the mass effect of the accumulated blood volume. In the event of subarachnoid hemorrhage, ICP becomes elevated with resulting dysfunction of the autoregulation response, which leads to abnormal vasoconstriction, platelet aggregation, and decreased perfusion and blood flow, resulting in cerebral ischemia.

Risk factors for hemorrhagic stroke include older age; a history of hypertension, which is present in 60 percent of patients; personal history of stroke; alcohol abuse; and illicit drug use. Common conditions associated with hemorrhagic stroke include hypertension, cerebral amyloidosis, coagulopathies, vascular alterations including arteriovenous malformation, vasculitis, intracranial neoplasm, and a history of anticoagulant or antithrombotic therapy.

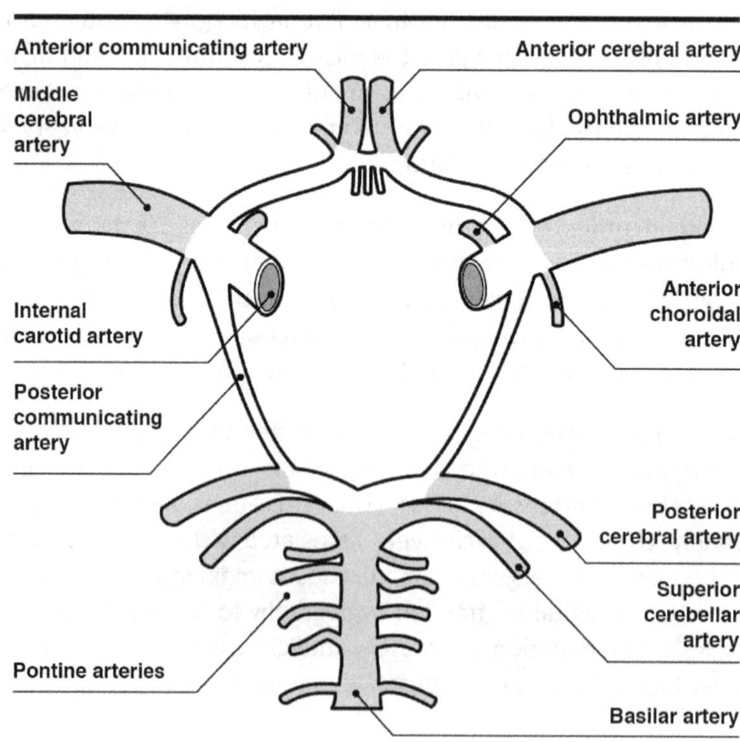

Although the presenting manifestations for hemorrhagic shock differ in some respect from the those associated with ischemic stroke, none of these such manifestations is an absolute predictor of one or the other. In general, patients with hemorrhagic stroke present with a headache that may be severe, significant alterations in the level of consciousness and neurological function, hypertension, seizures, and nausea and vomiting. The specific neurological defects depend on the anatomical site of the hemorrhage and may include hemisensory loss, hemiparesis, aphasia, and visual alterations.

A common site for an aneurysm, or bulging or ballooning in a blood vessel within the brain is where the internal carotid artery (ICA) enters the cranium; it branches into a system of arteries that provide blood flow to the brain, known as the *circle of Willis*. Most small brain aneurysms do not rupture and are found during various tests. An aneurysm may press on brain tissue and present with ocular pain or symptoms. However, a rupture is a medical emergency that can lead to stroke or hemorrhage. The most common symptom described by patients is "the *worst* headache of my life." A sudden, severe headache, stiff neck, blurred or double vision, photophobia, seizure, loss of consciousness, and confusion may also be reported.

Diagnostic studies include CBC, chemistry panel, coagulation studies, and blood glucose. Non-contrast CT scan or MRI are the preferred imaging studies. CT or magnetic resonance angiography may also be used to obtain images of the cerebral vasculature. Close observation of the patient's vital signs, neurological vital signs, and ICP is necessary.

The emergency management of the patient with hemorrhagic shock is focused on the ABC protocol, in addition to the control of bleeding, seizure activity, and increased ICP. There is no single medication used to treat hemorrhagic stroke; however, recent data suggests that aggressive emergency management of hypertension initiated early and aimed at reducing the systolic BP to less than 140 millimeters of mercury may be effective in reducing the growth of the hematoma at the site, which decreases the mass effect. Beta-blockers and ACE inhibitors are recommended to facilitate this reduction. Endotracheal intubation for ventilatory support may be necessary.

Patients who present with manifestations of hemorrhagic stroke with a history of anticoagulation therapy present a special therapeutic challenge due to the extension of the hematoma formation. More than 50 percent of patients taking warfarin who suffer a hemorrhagic stroke will die within thirty days. This statistic is consistent in patients with international normalized ratio (INR) levels within the therapeutic range, with increased mortality noted in patients with INRs that exceed the therapeutic level. Emergency treatment includes fresh frozen plasma, IV vitamin K, prothrombin complex concentrates, and recombinant factor VIIa (rFVIIa). There are administration concerns with each of these therapies that must be addressed to prevent any delays in the reversal of the effects of the warfarin.

Transient Ischemic Attack

A *transient ischemic attack* (TIA) is defined as a short-term episode of altered neurological function that lasts for less than one hour; it may be imperceptible to the patient. The deficit may be related to speech, movement, behavior, or memory and may be caused by an ischemic event in the brain, spinal cord, or retina. The patient's history and neurological assessment according to the NIH Stroke Scale establish the diagnosis. Additional diagnostic studies include CBC, glucose, sedimentation rate, electrolytes, lipid profile, toxicology screen, 12-lead ECG, and CSF analysis. Imaging studies include non-contrast MRI or CT, carotid Doppler exam, and angiography.

The $ABCD^2$ stroke risk score calculates the patient's risk for experiencing a true stroke within two days after the TIA based on five factors (see the table below). Interventions aimed at stroke prevention in relation to the risk stratification as calculated by the ABCD^2 score are specific to underlying comorbidities; however, treatment with ASA and clopidogrel is commonly prescribed.

ABCD^2 Stroke Risk Score		
	1 Point	2 Points
***A*ge**	≥ 60 years	
***B*lood Pressure**	SBP ≥ 140 mmHg DBP ≥ 90 mmHg	
***C*linical Features**	Speech impairment but no focal weakness	Focal weakness
***D*uration of Symptoms**	≤ 59 minutes	≥ 60 minutes
***D*iabetes**	Diagnosed	
Total Score (denotes risk for stroke (CVA) within 2 days after TIA)	0-3 points = 1% risk 4-5 points = 4.1% risk 6-7 points = 8.1% risk	

Cancer

Cancer is a general term that refers to a disease characterized by abnormal cells that can development in any number of body tissues, organs, or systems that divide uncontrollably and that can infiltrate, crowd out, and kill healthy body cells. Cancer of the lung, pancreas, testicles, cervix, brain, and blood are just a few of the many tissues that may incur cancerous growth. Regardless as to the initial site of the development of cancer cells, cancer, unlike benign tumors, can usually spread throughout one's body. There are over 100 distinct types of recognized cancers and when all types are aggregated, cancer is the second-leading cause of death in the United States. Signs and symptoms vary widely, depending on the specific cancer; however, common symptoms include unexplained weight loss, the presence of a palpable lump or mass, notable changes in bowel habits or appetite, abnormal bleeding, and persistent cough or fever.

Tobacco use, including smoking, is the single greatest risk factor for the development of most cancers. Family history, obesity, exposure to ionizing radiation and certain chemicals and environmental pollutants, poor diet, sedentary lifestyle, drug or alcohol abuse, and infections such as hepatitis and HPV can also increase one's risk of developing cancer. Any of these factors or others may initiate genetic changes that precede and place the individual at risk for the development of abnormal cell growth. Cancer may be suspected from laboratory results, patient symptoms, and a physical exam and then detected through imaging studies, such as CT scans and MRIs. These scans may also be used to assess the spread of the malignancy. Biopsies are often used to confirm the diagnosis.

Treatment typically involves surgery to remove malignant tissue, chemotherapy, radiation therapy, targeted cell therapy, and supportive palliative care for pain reduction, disease- and treatment-symptom management, restoration of overall health, and emotional care. Survival rates depend on several factors, mainly the specific type of cancer, the extent to which it is confined or spread, and the patient's age and general health status. Early detection is critical for the most favorable treatment outcomes.

Diabetes Mellitus

This is a condition that affects how the body responds to the presence of glucose. Glucose is needed for cell functioning, and all consumable calories eventually are converted to glucose in the body. A hormone produced by the pancreas, called *insulin,* is needed to break down food and drink into glucose molecules. In patients with type 1 diabetes, the pancreas fails to produce insulin, leading to high levels of glucose in the bloodstream. This can lead to organ damage, organ failure, or nerve damage. Patients with type 1 diabetes receive daily insulin injections or have a pump that continuously monitors their blood insulin levels and releases insulin as needed. These patients need to be careful to not administer excess insulin, as this will cause their blood sugar to become too low. Low blood sugar can lead to fainting and exhaustion and may require hospitalization. In patients with type 2 diabetes, the pancreas produces insulin, but the body is unable to use it effectively. Patients with type 2 diabetes typically need to manage their condition through lifestyle changes, such as losing weight and eating fewer carbohydrate-rich and sugary foods. There are also some medications that help the body use the insulin that is present in the bloodstream. Gestational diabetes is a form of diabetes that some women develop during the second to third trimester of pregnancy, when their systems temporarily become resistant to insulin. High blood sugar in a pregnant woman can affect fetal growth and influence the baby's risk of becoming obese. Pregnant women with gestational diabetes are encouraged to exercise daily, avoid excessive weight gain, and carefully monitor their diet. Gestational diabetes is similar to type 2 diabetes in the way symptoms present and in treatment options.

Diabetic Ketoacidosis

This is an acute complication that primarily occurs in patients with type 1 diabetes who lack adequate insulin. When the body does not have enough insulin in the blood to break down macronutrients into glucose, it defaults to breaking down fatty acids into ketones for energy. This typically does not cause major issues in a person who does not have diabetes, as eventual insulin production and uptake will balance the level of ketones in the blood. In a patient with diabetes who cannot produce enough insulin, the body will continue to release fatty acids into the bloodstream. Eventually, this will result in too many ketones in the blood and will shift the body's pH level to an excessively acidic one. This is a crisis situation, and the patient may eventually go into a coma if left untreated. Symptoms include dehydration, nausea, sweet-smelling breath, confusion, and fatigue. Treatment includes oral or IV electrolyte and insulin administration. Diabetic ketoacidosis can occur with type 2 diabetes but occurs more frequently with type 1 diabetes. Often, a ketoacidosis event is the first indicator that a person may have diabetes.

Metabolic Syndrome/Syndrome X

Metabolic syndrome, or *Syndrome X,* refers to the presence of comorbid cardiovascular and insulin-related conditions. Patients diagnosed with metabolic syndrome must have three or more of the following conditions: hypertension, elevated fasting blood glucose levels, low HDL cholesterol, high triglycerides, and excess belly fat. This syndrome is believed to result from insulin resistance, causing high blood glucose, insulin, and lipid levels. Patients with metabolic syndrome tend to be overweight or obese and at an increased risk of organ failure, heart attacks, and strokes. They often suffer from another underlying condition, such as diabetes or polycystic ovary syndrome, that leads to metabolic syndrome. Metabolic syndrome is often treated with prescription medications that lower cholesterol and blood pressure, but diet and exercise changes are strongly recommended. Weight loss is a key component in managing metabolic syndrome.

Chronic Obstructive Pulmonary Disease (COPD)

Chronic Obstructive Pulmonary Disease (COPD) is characterized by an airflow obstruction that's not fully reversible. It's usually progressive and is associated with an abnormal inflammatory response in the lungs. The primary cause of COPD is exposure to tobacco smoke, and is one of the leading causes of death in the United States. COPD includes chronic bronchitis, emphysema, or a combination of both. Though asthma is part of the classic triad of obstructive lung diseases, it is not part of COPD. However, someone with COPD can have an asthma component to their disease. Chronic bronchitis is described as a chronic productive cough for three or more months during each of two consecutive years. Emphysema is the abnormal enlargement of alveoli (air sacs) with accompanying destruction of their walls. Signs and symptoms of COPD can include:

- Dyspnea
- Wheezing
- Cough (usually worse in the morning and that produces sputum/phlegm)
- Cyanosis
- Chest tightness
- Fever
- Tachypnea
- Orthopnea
- Use of accessory respiratory muscles
- Elevated jugular venous pressure (JVP)
- Barrel chest
- Pursed lip breathing
- Altered mental status

A diagnosis of COPD can be made through pulmonary function tests (PFTs), a chest x-ray, blood chemistries, ABG analysis, or a CT scan. A formal diagnosis of COPD can be made through a PFT known as spirometry, which measures lung function. PFTs measure the ratio of forced expiratory volume in one second over forced vital capacity (FEV_1/FVC) and should normally be between 60% and 90%. Values below 60% usually indicate a problem. The other diagnostic tests mentioned are useful in determining the acuity and severity of exacerbations of the disease. In acute exacerbations of COPD, ABG analysis can reveal respiratory acidosis, hypoxemia, and hypercapnia. Generally, a pH less than 7.3 indicates acute respiratory compromise. Compensatory metabolic alkalosis may develop in response to chronic respiratory acidosis. A chest x-ray can show flattening of the diaphragm and increased retrosternal air space (both indicative of hyperinflation), cardiomegaly, and increased bronchovascular markings. Blood chemistries can suggest sodium retention or hypokalemia. A CT scan is more sensitive and specific than a standard chest x-ray for diagnosing emphysema. Treatment for acute exacerbations of COPD can include oxygen supplementation, short-acting Beta-2 agonists, anticholinergics, corticosteroids, and antibiotics.

Acute Respiratory Tract Infections

Acute Bronchitis

Acute bronchitis is inflammation of the bronchial tubes (bronchi), which extend from the trachea to the lungs. It is one of the top five reasons for visits to healthcare providers and can take from ten days to three weeks to resolve. Common causes of acute bronchitis include respiratory viruses (such as influenza A and B), RSV, parainfluenza, adenovirus, rhinovirus, and coronavirus. Bacterial causes include Mycoplasma species, Streptococcus pneumoniae, Chlamydia pneumoniae, Haemophilus influenzae, and Moraxella catarrhalis. Other causes of acute bronchitis are irritants such as chemicals, pollution, and tobacco smoke.

Signs and symptoms of acute bronchitis can include:

- Cough (most common symptom) with or without sputum
- Fever
- Sore throat
- Headache
- Nasal congestion
- Rhinorrhea
- Dyspnea
- Fatigue
- Myalgia
- Chest pain
- Wheezing

Acute bronchitis is typically diagnosed by exclusion, which means tests are used to exclude more serious conditions such as pneumonia, epiglottitis, or COPD. Useful diagnostic tests include a CBC with differential, a chest x-ray, respiratory and blood cultures, PFTs, bronchoscopy, laryngoscopy, and a procalcitonin (PCT) test to determine if the infection is bacterial.

Treatment of acute bronchitis is primarily supportive and can include:

- Bedrest
- Cough suppressants, such as codeine or dextromethorphan
- Beta-2 agonists, such as albuterol, for wheezing
- Nonsteroidal anti-inflammatory drugs (NSAIDs) for pain
- Expectorants, such as guaifenesin

Although acute bronchitis should not be routinely treated with antibiotics, there are exceptions to this rule. It's reasonable to use an antibiotic when an existing medical condition poses a risk of serious complications. Antibiotic use is also reasonable for treating acute bronchitis in elderly patients who have been hospitalized in the past year, have been diagnosed with congestive heart failure (CHF) or diabetes, or are currently being treated with a steroid.

Pneumonia

Pneumonia is an infection that affects the functional tissue of the lung. Microscopically, it is characterized by consolidating lung tissue with exudate, fibrin, and inflammatory cells filling the alveoli (air sacs). Pneumonia can represent a primary disease or a secondary disease (e.g., post-obstructive pneumonia due to lung cancer), and the most common causes of pneumonia are bacteria and viruses. Other causes of pneumonia include fungi and parasites.

Pneumonia can be categorized according to its anatomic distribution on a chest x-ray or the setting in which it is acquired. Pneumonia categorized according to its anatomic distribution on chest x-ray can be:

- Lobar: Limited to one lobe of the lungs. It can affect more than one lobe on the same side (multilobar pneumonia) or bilateral lobes ("double" pneumonia).

- Bronchopneumonia: Scattered diffusely throughout the lungs

- Interstitial: Involving areas between the alveoli

Pneumonia categorized according to the setting in which it is acquired can be:

- Community-Acquired Pneumonia (CAP): Pneumonia in an individual who hasn't been recently hospitalized, or its occurrence in less than 48 hours after admission to a hospital.
- Hospital-Acquired (Nosocomial) Pneumonia: Pneumonia acquired during or after hospitalization for another ailment with onset at least 48 hours or more after admission.
- Aspiration Pneumonia: Pneumonia resulting from the inhalation of gastric or oropharyngeal secretions.

Community-Acquired Pneumonia (CAP)

Common causes of community-acquired pneumonia (CAP) include:

- Streptococcus pneumoniae
- Haemophilus influenzae
- Moraxella catarrhalis
- Atypical organisms (such as Legionella species, Mycoplasma pneumoniae, and Chlamydia pneumonia)
- Staphylococcus aureus
- Respiratory viruses

Streptococcus Pneumoniae

Streptococcus pneumonia (also known as S. pneumonia or pneumococcus) is a gram-positive bacterium and the most common cause of CAP. Due to the introduction of a pneumococcal vaccine in 2000, cases of pneumococcal pneumonia have decreased. However, medical providers should be aware there is now evidence of emerging, antibiotic-resistant strains of the organism. Signs and symptoms of pneumococcal pneumonia can include:

- Cough productive of rust-colored sputum (mucus)
- Fever with or without chills
- Dyspnea
- Wheezing
- Chest pain
- Tachypnea
- Altered mental status
- Tachycardia
- Rales over involved lung
- Increase in tactile fremitus
- E to A change
- Hypotension
- Lung consolidation

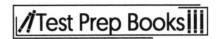

Diagnosis of pneumococcal pneumonia can include:

- CBC with differential
- Chest x-ray
- CT scan (if underlying lung cancer is suspected)
- Sputum gram stain and/or culture
- Blood cultures
- Procalcitonin and C-reactive protein blood level tests
- Sputum, serum, and/or urinary antigen tests
- Immunoglobulin studies
- Bronchoscopy with bronchoalveolar lavage (BAL)

Treatment of pneumococcal pneumonia can include:

- Antibiotics, such as ceftriaxone plus doxycycline, or azithromycin
- Respiratory quinolones, such as levofloxacin (Levaquin®), moxifloxacin (Avelox®), or gemifloxacin (Factive®)
- Supplemental oxygen
- Beta-2 agonists, such as albuterol via nebulizer or metered-dose inhaler (MDI), as needed for wheezing
- Analgesics and antipyretics
- Chest physiotherapy
- Active suctioning of respiratory secretions
- Intubation and mechanical ventilation

Mycoplasma Pneumoniae

Mycoplasma pneumonia, also known as M. pneumoniae, is a bacterium that causes atypical CAP. It is one of the most common causes of CAP in healthy individuals under the age of forty. The most common symptom of mycoplasmal pneumonia is a dry, nonproductive cough. Other signs and symptoms can include diarrhea, earache, fever (usually $\leq 102^0$F), sore throat, myalgias, nasal congestion, skin rash, and general malaise. Chest x-rays of individuals with mycoplasmal pneumonia reveal a pattern of bronchopneumonia. Cold agglutinin titers in the blood can be significantly elevated (> 1:64). Polymerase chain reaction (PCR) is becoming the standard confirmatory test for mycoplasmal pneumonia, though currently it is not used in most clinical settings.

Treatments for mycoplasmal pneumonia are no different than for CAP, except for the specific antibiotics used in treatment are usually different.

Methicillin-Resistant Staphylococcus Aureus

Community-Acquired Methicillin-Resistant Staphylococcus Aureus (CA-MRSA) has emerged as a significant cause of CAP over the past twenty years. It also remains a significant cause of hospital-acquired pneumonia. The majority (up to 75%) of those diagnosed with CA-MRSA pneumonia are young, previously healthy individuals with influenza as a preceding illness. Symptoms are usually identical to those seen with other causes of CAP. Chest x-ray typically reveals multilobar involvement with or without cavitation/necrosis. Gram staining of sputum and/or blood can reveal gram-positive bacteria in clusters.

Treatment of CA-MRSA should be prompt as it has a high mortality rate. Supportive measures are needed as in other cases of CAP. CA-MRSA is notoriously resistant to most antibiotics with the exception of vancomycin and linezolid, but even aggressive courses of these drugs can be unsuccessful.

Viral Pneumonia

Viral pneumonia is more common at the extremes of age (young children and the elderly). It accounts for the majority of cases of childhood pneumonia. Cases of viral pneumonia have been increasing over the past decade, mostly as a result of immunosuppression (weakened immune system). Common causes of viral pneumonia in children, the elderly, and the immunocompromised are the influenza viruses (most common), RSV, parainfluenza virus, and adenovirus.

Signs and symptoms of viral pneumonia largely overlap those of bacterial pneumonia and can include:

- Cough (nonproductive)
- Fever/chills
- Myalgias
- Fatigue
- Headache
- Dyspnea
- Tachypnea
- Tachycardia
- Wheezing
- Cyanosis
- Hypoxia
- Decreased breath sounds
- Respiratory distress

Viral pneumonia is diagnosed via a chest x-ray and viral cultures. The chest x-ray usually reveals bilateral lung infiltrates, instead of the lobar involvement commonly seen in bacterial causes. Viral cultures can take up to two weeks to confirm the diagnosis. Rapid antigen testing and gene amplification via polymerase chain reaction (PCR) have been recently incorporated into the diagnostic mix to shorten the diagnosis lag.

Treatment of viral pneumonia is usually supportive and can include:

- Supplemental oxygen
- Rest
- Antipyretics
- Analgesics
- Intravenous fluids
- Parenteral nutrition
- Intubation and mechanical ventilation

Specific causes of viral pneumonia can benefit from treatment with antiviral medications. Influenza pneumonia can be treated with oseltamivir (Tamiflu®) or zanamivir (Relenza®). Ribavirin® is the only effective antiviral agent for the treatment of RSV pneumonia.

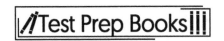

Meningitis

Meningitis is defined as the infection and resulting inflammation of the three layers of the meninges, the membranous covering of the brain and spinal cord. The causative agent may be bacterial, viral, parasitic, or fungal. The most common bacterial agent is *S. pneumoniae*. Meningococcal meningitis is common in crowded living spaces. However, the development and use of the meningococcal vaccine (MCV 4) has reduced the incidence in college students and military personnel. The Haemophilus influenza vaccine (Hib) has decreased the incidence and morbidity of the HI meningitis in infants, and the pneumococcal polysaccharide vaccine (PPSV) is being used to prevent meningitis in at-risk populations, such as immunocompromised adults, smokers, residents in long-term care facilities, and adults with chronic disease.

General risk factors for bacterial infection of the meninges include loss of, or decreased function of, the spleen; hypoglobinemia; chronic glucocorticoid use; deficiency of the complement system; diabetes; renal insufficiency; alcoholism; chronic liver disease; otitis media; and trauma associated with leakage of the CSF. Bacterial meningitis is infectious, and early diagnosis and treatment are essential for survival and recovery. Emergency providers understand that even with adequate treatment, 50 percent of patients with bacterial meningitis will develop complications within two to three weeks of the acute infection, and long-term deficits are common in 30 percent of the surviving patients. The complications are specific to the causative organism, but may include hearing loss, blindness, paralysis, seizure disorder, muscular deficiencies, ataxia, hydrocephalus, and subdural effusions. In contrast, the incidence of viral meningitis is often associated with other viral conditions such as mumps, measles, herpes, and infections due to arboviruses such as the West Nile virus. The treatment is supportive, and the majority of patients recover without long-term complications; however, the outcome is less certain for patients who are immunocompromised, or less than two years old or more than sixty years old.

The classic manifestations of bacterial meningitis include fever, nuchal rigidity, and headache. Additional findings may include nausea and vomiting, photophobia, confusion, and a decreased level of consciousness. Patients with viral meningitis may report the incidence of fatigue, muscle aches, and decreased appetite prior to the illness. Infants may exhibit a high-pitched cry, muscle flaccidity, irritability, and bulging fontanels.

The diagnosis of meningitis is determined by lumbar puncture; CSF analysis; cultures of the blood, nose, and respiratory secretions and any skin lesions that are present; complete blood count (CBC); electrolytes; coagulation studies; serum glucose to compare with CSF glucose; and procalcitonin to differentiate bacterial meningitis from aseptic meningitis in children. There is a small risk of herniation of the brain when the CSF is removed during the lumbar puncture, but effective antibiotic treatment must be initiated as quickly as possible to prevent the morbidity associated with bacterial meningitis. The results of the Gram stain of the CSF and blood will dictate the initial antibiotic therapy, which will be modified when the specific agent is identified. Additional interventions include seizure precautions, cardiac monitoring, and ongoing assessment of respiratory and neurological function. Patients with bacterial meningitis may require long-term rehabilitation.

Seizure Disorders

A *seizure* is defined as a chaotic period of uncoordinated electrical activity in the brain, which results in one of several characteristic behaviors. Although the exact cause is unknown, several possible triggers have been proposed as noted below. The recently revised classification system categorizes seizure activity according to the area of the brain where the seizure initiates, the patient's level of awareness during the seizure, and other descriptive features such as the presence of an aura. The unclassified category includes seizure patterns that do not conform to the primary categories. Seizures that originate in a single area of the brain are designated as *focal* seizures, while seizures that originate in two or more different networks are designated as *generalized* seizures. The remaining seizures in the onset category include seizures without an identified point of onset and seizures that progress from focal seizures to generalized seizures.

Risk factors associated with seizures include genetic predisposition, illnesses with severe temperature elevation, head trauma, cerebral edema, inappropriate use or discontinuance of antiepileptic drugs (AEDs), intracerebral infection, an excess or deficiency of sodium and glucose, toxin exposure, hypoxia, and acute drug or alcohol withdrawal. Patients are encouraged to identify any conditions that may be triggers for their seizure activity. Although the triggers vary greatly from one patient to another, commonly identified events include increased physical activity, excessive stress, hyperventilation, fatigue, acute ETOH (ethyl alcohol) ingestion, exposure to flashing lights, and inhaled chemicals, including cocaine.

The tonic phase presents as stiffening of the limbs for a brief period, while the clonic phase is evidenced by jerking motions of the limbs. These manifestations may be accompanied by a decreased level of consciousness, respiratory alterations and cyanosis, incontinence, and biting of the tongue. Absence seizures are manifested by a decreased level of awareness without abnormal muscular activity. The manifestations of the postictal phase include alterations in consciousness and awareness and increased oral secretions. Seizure disorders are diagnosed by serum lab studies to assess AED levels and to identify excess alcohol and recreational drugs, metabolic alterations, and kidney and liver function. Electroencephalography (EEG) and the enhanced magnetoencephalography are used to identify the origin of the altered electrical activity in the brain, and MRI, skull films, and CSF analysis are used to rule out possible sources of the seizure disorder such as tumor formation.

Dementia

Dementia is a general term used to describe a state of general cognitive decline. Although Alzheimer's disease accounts for up to 80 percent of all cases of dementia in the United States, the remaining two million cases may result from any one of several additional causes. The destruction of cortical tissue resulting from a stroke, or more commonly from multiple small strokes, often results in altered cognitive and physical function, while repetitive head injuries over an extended period also potentially result in permanent damage, limiting normal brain activity. Less common causes of dementia include infection of the brain by prions (abnormal protein fragments) as in Creutzfeldt-Jakob disease or the human immunodeficiency virus (HIV) as in AIDS, deposition of Lewy bodies in the cerebral cortex as in Parkinson's disease, and reversible conditions such as vitamin B-12 deficiency and altered function of the thyroid gland. The onset and progression of the disease relate to the underlying cause and associated patient comorbidities.

Alzheimer's Disease

Alzheimer's disease is a chronic progressive form of dementia with an insidious onset that is caused by the abnormal accumulation of amyloid-β plaque in the brain. The accumulation of this plaque eventually interferes with neural functioning, and the progressive manifestations of the disease. Although the exact etiology is unknown, environmental toxins, vascular alterations due to hemorrhagic or embolic events, infections, and genetic factors have all been proposed as the triggering mechanism for the plaque formation. The progression of the disease and the associated manifestations are specific to the individual; however, in all individuals, over time, there is measurable decline in cognitive functioning, including short-term and long-term memory, behavior and mood, and the ability to perform activities of daily living (ADLs).

The diagnosis is based on the patient's presenting history and manifestations, imaging studies of the brain, protein analysis of the cerebrospinal fluid (CSF), and cognitive assessment with measures such as the Mini-Mental State Exam. Current treatments are only supportive, although cholinesterase inhibitors and N Methyl D aspartate receptor antagonists may slow the progression of the manifestations for a limited period if administered early in the course of the disease. All patients will suffer an eventual decline in all aspects of cognitive functioning, with the average survival rate dependent on the presence of comorbidities and the level of care and support available to the patient.

Multiple Sclerosis

Multiple sclerosis (MS) is a chronic disease manifested by progressive destruction of the myelin sheath and resulting plaque formation in the central nervous system (CNS). The precipitating event of this autoimmune disease is the migration of activated T cells to the CNS, which disrupts the blood-brain barrier. Exposure to environmental toxins is considered to be the likely trigger for this immune response. These alterations facilitate the antigen-antibody reactions that result in the demyelination of the axons. The onset of this disease is insidious, with symptoms occurring intermittently over a period of months or years. Sensory manifestations may include numbness and tingling of the extremities, blurred vision, vertigo, tinnitus, impaired hearing, and chronic neuropathic pain. Motor manifestations may include weakness or paralysis of limbs, trunk, and head; diplopia; scanning speech; and muscle spasticity. Cerebellar manifestations include nystagmus, ataxia, dysarthria, dysphagia, and fatigue.

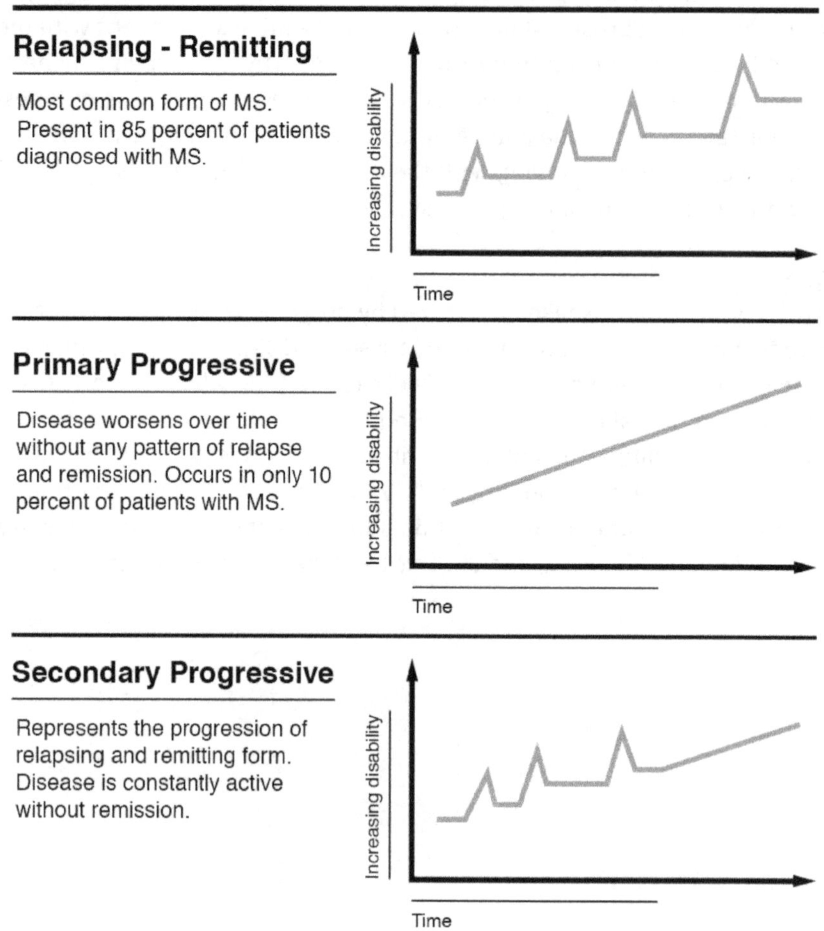

Forms of Multiple Sclerosis
Relapsing - Remitting
Most common form of MS. Present in 85 percent of patients diagnosed with MS.
Increasing disability
Time
Primary Progressive
Disease worsens over time without any pattern of relapse and remission. Occurs in only 10 percent of patients with MS.
Increasing disability
Time
Secondary Progressive
Represents the progression of relapsing and remitting form. Disease is constantly active without remission.
Increasing disability
Time

The progress of the disease and presenting clinical manifestations vary greatly from one individual to another; however, there are common forms of the disease that relate to the expression of the clinical manifestations or disability and the disease activity over time. An initial episode of neurological manifestations due to demyelination that lasts for at least 24 hours is identified as a clinically-isolated episode of MS. The potential for progression of the disease to the relapsing-remitting form of MS is predicted by magnetic resonance imaging (MRI) studies indicating the presence or absence of plaque formation. The remaining forms of MS are all associated with increasing disability related to the disease over time.

The relapsing-remitting form is common to 85 percent of all patients diagnosed with MS and presents a variable pattern of active and inactive disease. The manifestations may resolve, decrease in severity, or become permanent after a relapse. In the primary-progressive form of MS that affects 10 percent of patients diagnosed with MS, the disease is constantly active without periods of remission. The secondary- progressive form of MS is identified as the progression of the relapsing-remitting form to a state of permanently active disease without remission.

Myasthenia Gravis

Myasthenia gravis is also an autoimmune disease of the CNS that is manifested by severe muscle weakness resulting from altered transmission of acetylcholine at the neuromuscular junction due to antibody formation. Relapses and remissions are common, and these relapses may be triggered by infection, stress, pregnancy, and increases in body temperature (such as those induced by immersion in hot water). Subjective manifestations include weakness, diplopia, dysphagia, fatigue on exertion, and bowel and bladder dysfunction. Objective manifestations include unilateral or bilateral ptosis of the eye, impaired respiratory function, impaired swallowing, and decreased muscle strength. Tensilon testing and electromyography, which measure muscle activity over time, are used to diagnose this disorder, while anticholinesterase agents and immunosuppressant agents are the mainstays of treatment. Additional treatments include plasmapheresis to decrease circulating antibodies and removal of the thymus gland to slow T-cell production.

Guillain-Barré Syndrome

The most common form of *Guillain-Barré syndrome (GBS)* is acute immune-mediated demyelinating polyneuropathy. This rare syndrome may develop two to four weeks after a bacterial or viral infection of the respiratory or GI systems or following surgery. The most common causative organisms are *C. jejuni* and cytomegalovirus that may produce a subclinical infection that occurs unnoticed by the patient prior to the development of the acute onset of GBS. Other causative agents that are associated with GBS include the Epstein-Barr virus, *Mycoplasma pneumoniae*, and varicella-zoster virus. There is also an association between GBS and HIV. Current research is focused on investigating any association between the Zika virus and GBS; however, to date, there is little evidence of that relationship because there are few laboratories in the United States with the technology needed to identify the virus. The incidence of GBS has also been associated with vaccine administration; however, accumulated data does not support these claims.

The manifestations present as an acute onset of progressive, bilateral muscle weakness of the limbs that begins distally and continues proximally. The syndrome is the result of segmental demyelination of the nerves with edema, resulting from the inflammatory process. Additional presenting manifestations include pain, paresthesia, and abnormal sensations in the fingers. The progressive muscle weakness peaks at four weeks and potentially involves the arms, the muscles of the core, the cranial nerves, and the respiratory muscles. Involvement of the cranial nerves may result in facial drooping, diplopia, dysphagia, weakness or paralysis of the eye muscles, and pupillary alterations. Alterations in the autonomic nervous system also may result in orthostatic hypotension, paroxysmal hypertension, heart block, bradycardia, tachycardia, and asystole. Respiratory manifestations include dyspnea, shortness of breath, and dysphagia. In addition, as many as 30 percent of patients will progress to respiratory failure requiring ventilatory support due to the demyelination of the nerves that innervate the respiratory muscles.

The syndrome is diagnosed by the patient's history and laboratory studies to include electrolytes, liver function analysis, erythrocyte sedimentation rate (ESR), pulmonary function studies, and the assessment of CSF for the presence of excess protein content. In addition, electromyography and nerve conduction studies are used to identify the signs of demyelination, which confirms the diagnosis.

Gastritis

Gastritis may be acute or chronic, and acute gastritis is further differentiated as erosive or nonerosive. Involvement of the entire stomach lining is termed *pangastritis*, while regional involvement is termed *antral gastritis*. Acute gastritis may be asymptomatic or may present with nonspecific abdominal pain, nausea, vomiting, anorexia, belching, and bloating. The most common causes of acute gastritis include use of NSAIDs and corticosteroids and infection by the *H. pylori* bacteria. Acute gastritis may also be associated with alcohol abuse. Double-contrast barium studies, endoscopy, and histological examination of biopsy samples most often confirm the diagnosis and the causative agent. Treatment includes normalization of fluid and electrolyte balance, discontinuance of causative agents such as NSAIDs, and corticosteroids, H^2 blockers, PPIs, and appropriate antibiotic therapy in the event of *H. pylori* infection.

Chronic gastritis is an inflammatory state that has not responded to therapy for acute gastritis. Chronic *H. pylori* infection is associated with the development of peptic ulcers, gastric adenocarcinoma, and mucosal-related lymphoid tissue (MALT) lymphoma. In addition to endoscopy and barium studies, gastric biopsy for assessment of antibiotic sensitivity is done because the initial antibiotic therapy was unsuccessful in eradicating the organism. Autoimmune gastritis is related to vitamin B-12 deficiency due to intrinsic factor deficiency and is associated with megaloblastic anemia and thrombocytopenia. Chemical or reactive gastritis is due to chronic NSAID and steroid use and is manifested by mucosal epithelial erosion, ulcer formation, and mucosal edema and possible hemorrhage. Chronic gastritis is diagnosed by endoscopy, biopsy, and histological studies. Treatment is specific to the causative agent, and in the instance of *H. pylori* infection, a course of three antibiotics will be administered. *H. pylori* infection also requires long-term surveillance for reoccurrence of infection.

Hepatitis

Hepatitis is an inflammatory condition of the liver, which is further categorized as infectious or noninfectious. Causative infectious agents for hepatitis may be viral, fungal, or bacterial, while noninfectious causes include autoimmune disease, prescription and recreational drugs, alcohol abuse, and metabolic disorders. More than 50 percent of the cases of acute hepatitis in the United States are caused by a virus. Transmission routes include fecal-oral, parenteral, sexual contact, and perinatal transmission.

There are four phases of the course of viral hepatitis. During phase 1, which is asymptomatic, the host is infected, and the virus replicates; the onset of mild symptoms occurs in phase 2; progressive symptoms of liver dysfunction appear in phase 3; and recovery from the infection occurs in phase 4. These phases are specific to the causative agent and the individual.

The most common viral agents are hepatitis A (HAV), hepatitis B (HBV), and hepatitis C (HCV). Less commonly, hepatitis D (HDV), hepatitis E (HEV), CMV, Epstein-Barr virus, and adenovirus may cause hepatitis. HAV and HBV often present with nausea, jaundice, anorexia, right upper quadrant pain, fatigue, and malaise. HCV may be asymptomatic or, alternatively, may present with similar symptoms. Approximately 20 percent of acute infections with HBV and HCV result in chronic hepatitis, which is a risk factor for the development of cirrhosis and liver failure. The care of the patient with acute hepatitis due to HAV and HCV is focused on symptom relief, while the antiviral treatment for HBV is effective in decreasing the incidence of adenocarcinoma.

Chronic hepatitis is a complication of acute hepatitis and frequently progresses to hepatic failure, which is associated with deteriorating coagulation status and the onset of hepatic encephalopathy, due to alterations in the blood-brain barrier that result in brain cell edema.

Inflammatory Bowel Disease

Inflammatory bowel disease (IBD) is an idiopathic disease that results from a harmful immune response to normal intestinal flora. Two types of IBD include Crohn's disease and ulcerative colitis (UC). Crohn's disease is characterized by inflammatory changes in all layers of the bowel. Although the entire length of the GI tract may be involved, the ileum and colon are affected most often. The inflamed areas are commonly interrupted by segments of normal bowel. Endoscopic views reveal the cobblestone appearance of these affected segments. UC is characterized by inflammatory changes of the mucosa and submucosa of the bowel that affect only the colon. There is a genetic predisposition for Crohn's disease, and there is also an increased incidence of cancer in patients with either form of IBD. Additional risk factors include a family history of IBD or colorectal cancer, NSAID and antibiotic use, smoking, and psychiatric disorders. IBD is diagnosed by a patient's history, including details of any recent foreign travel or hospitalization to rule out tuberculosis or *C. difficile* as the precipitating cause, in addition to endoscopy, CT and magnetic resonance imaging (MRI), serum and stool studies, and histologic studies.

Manifestations are nonspecific and are most often associated with the affected bowel segment. Common manifestations of IBD include diarrhea with blood and mucous and possible incontinence; constipation primarily with UC that is associated with progression to obstipation and bowel obstruction; rectal pain with associated urgency and tenesmus; and abdominal pain and cramping in the right lower quadrant with Crohn's disease, and in the umbilical area or left lower quadrant with UC. In addition, anemia, fatigue, and arthritis may be present.

The treatment of IBD focuses on attaining periods of remission and preventing recurrent attacks by modifying the inflammatory response. The stepwise treatment protocol begins with aminosalicylates and progresses to antibiotics, corticosteroids, and immunomodulators.

Ulcers

Ulcers of the GI tract are categorized as to the anatomical site of injury. Gastric ulcers are located in the body of the stomach, and peptic ulcers are located in the duodenum. The presenting symptom is abdominal pain 2 to 4 hours after eating for duodenal ulcers, in addition to hematemesis and melena. The defect is due to erosion of the mucosal lining by infectious agents, most commonly *H. pylori;* extreme systemic stress such as burns or head trauma; alcohol abuse; chronic kidney and respiratory disease; and psychological stress. Untreated, the mucosal erosion can progress to perforation, hemorrhage, and peritonitis.

Laboratory studies include examination of endoscopic tissue samples for the presence of the *H. pylori* organism, urea breath test, CBC, stool samples, and metabolic panel. Endoscopy, which is used to obtain tissue samples and achieve hemostasis, and double barium imaging studies made be obtained. The treatment depends on the extent of the erosion and will be focused on healing the ulcerated tissue and preventing additional damage. The treatment protocol for *H. pylori* infection includes the use of a PPI, amoxicillin, and clarithromycin for a minimum of seven to fourteen days. Subsequent testing will be necessary to ensure that the organism has been eradicated. Patients infected with *H. pylori* also must discontinue the use of NSAIDs or continue the long-term use of PPIs. Surgery may be indicated for significant areas of hemorrhage that were not successfully treated by ultrasound, and the procedure will be specific to the anatomical area of ulceration.

Tuberculosis (TB)

Tuberculosis (TB) is a highly communicable disease caused by the infectious bacteria *Mycobacterium tuberculosis*. *M. tuberculosis* is an acid-fast rod that secretes niacin; when the bacteria reach a vulnerable site, they multiply quickly. Because it is an aerobic bacterium, meaning it grows in the presence of oxygen, it principally affects the upper lobes of the lungs where the O_2 concentration is the greatest. It can also affect the brain, intestines, peritoneum, kidneys, joints, and liver. It is transmitted via the airborne route by droplet infection, with the primary source of the virus being saliva and lung secretions. TB has a dangerous onset, and many individuals are not aware of infection until it is well advanced. TB infection progresses as follows:

- Infected droplets enter the lungs, and the bacteria form a tubercle lesion.
- The body's defense systems capture the tubercle, leaving a blemish.
- If capture does not occur, the bacteria may enter the lymph system and travel to the lymph nodes, causing an inflammatory response called granulomatous inflammation.
- Initial lesions form and may become dormant, but can be revived and become a secondary infection when re-exposure to the bacterium occurs.
- Once active, TB is known to cause necrosis and cavitation (formation of a hole) in the lesions, which leads to rupture, the spread of necrotic tissue, and destruction to various areas of the body.

Rapid identification of those in close contact with the infected individual is important so that they may be tested and receive necessary treatment, and once identified, they will be assessed with a tuberculin skin test and chest x-rays to determine if they have been infected with TB. The risk of transmission of the infection is significantly decreased once the infected individual has been taking TB medication for two to three weeks.

TB infection generally manifests as fatigue, lethargy, anorexia, weight loss, low-grade fever, chills, night sweats, incessant cough with the production of mucoid and mucopurulent sputum (sometimes blood streaked), chest tightness, and chest pain that is dull and achy. In the advanced stages of the illness, dullness with percussion over affected parenchymal areas, bronchial breath sounds, rhonchi, and crackles will be present. Partial obstruction of a bronchus caused by endobronchial disease or compression by edematous lymph nodes may create localized wheezing and dyspnea.

The main goals of treatment involve preventing transmission, managing symptoms, and inhibiting progression of the disease. Diagnosis consists of many factors, including collection of an all-inclusive patient history, which will detail the following:

- History of TB exposure
- Country of origin and travel to regions in which the incidence of TB is increased
- Recent history of flu, pneumonia, febrile illness, or foul-smelling sputum production
- Previous tests performed to determine the presence of *M. tuberculosis* in the body and the results of those tests
- Recent bacilli Calmette-Guerin vaccine, a vaccine that contains attenuated (dead) tubercle bacilli and is usually administered to those who reside in foreign countries or are traveling to foreign countries to create increased resistance to TB

Diagnostic efforts will also revolve around results of a physical examination of the chest, auscultation of breath sounds, and inquiring about chest tightness or a dull, achy chest pain. A chest x-ray is not considered a definitive diagnostic tool, but the presence of multinodular infiltrates with deposits of calcium phosphate in the upper lung lobes is suggestive of TB. If the disease is active, it will appear on a chest x-ray as lung inflammation, and it will form a TB-specific necrosis, in which diseased tissue devolves into a firm, dry mass (caseation), also apparent on an x-ray. Additionally, the attending physician will most likely order a specific blood analysis test to determine the presence of TB in the body (QuantiFERON-TB Gold). This test is quite sensitive and rapid, and results can be available in as little as 24 hours. Sputum cultures positive for *M. tuberculosis* are considered confirmatory of the diagnosis, and after the administration of medications has begun, sputum samples are obtained again to establish the effectiveness of therapy. A positive TB skin test does not mean that active TB is present, but it is indicative of previous exposure or the presence of inactive disease. Once it is positive, it will remain so throughout an individual's lifetime.

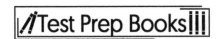

Once diagnosis has confirmed infection, the patient with active TB infection is admitted and placed under airborne isolation precautions in a negative-pressure room (to maintain this, the room door must be tightly closed). The room should have at least six exchanges of fresh air per hour and be ventilated to the outside, if possible. The patient's nurse wears a particulate respirator (special individually fitted mask) and a gown when the probability of clothing contamination exists. Thorough handwashing is required before and after caring for the patient, as well as after leaving his or her room. The patient should be required to wear a surgical mask if he or she needs to leave the room for a test or procedure. Respiratory isolation is discontinued after the patient is no longer considered contagious.

The medications used for active TB infection consist of first-line and second-line drugs. First-line medications include isoniazid, rifampin, ethambutol, pyrazinamide, rifabutin, and rifapentine. These medications provide the most effective anti-TB activity. Second-line agents (amikacin, ciprofloxacin, and kanamycin) are used in conjunction with first-line agents but are more toxic to the body's systems. Active TB is treated with a combination of medications to which it is vulnerable, and this approach is instituted because of resistant strains of the organism.

Education upon discharge consists of the following:

- Providing the patient and caregivers with information about TB and allaying concerns about the contagious aspect of the illness
- Encouraging the patient to follow the medication regimen exactly as prescribed
- Advising the patient that the medication regimen is continued over a six- to twelve-month period, depending on the situation
- Informing the patient of the side effects/adverse effects of the medications and ways to minimize them to maintain compliance
- Instructing the patient to resume activities gradually, as he or she is still in the recovery period
- Instructing the patient to cover his or her mouth and nose when coughing/sneezing and to place used tissues into plastic bags for disposal
- Informing the patient that a sputum culture is necessary every two to four weeks once medication therapy is initiated, and once the results of three consecutive cultures (about three months of treatment) are negative, he or she is no longer considered infectious

- Advising the patient to avoid excessive exposure to silicone or dust because these materials can cause further lung damage
- Informing the patient of the importance of compliance with treatment, follow-up care, and collection of sputum cultures as prescribed

Mononucleosis

Mononucleosis is a common infection caused by the Epstein-Barr virus. It is transferrable via direct intimate contact; its most customary source is oral secretions, but it can also be spread through the secretions from the nasal cavity and oropharynx, and sometimes tears. Incubation may be anywhere from four to six weeks, and the communicable period is unknown. It is most often assessed in teenagers and young adults, particularly those who are sexually active. It is important to remember that those who have been exposed to mononucleosis will always carry the virus, even after infection indicators have resolved. Signs and symptoms usually manifest as a high fever, severe sore throat, swollen lymph nodes/tonsils, nausea, abdominal pain, weakness, and fatigue. Hepatosplenomegaly (enlargement of the liver and spleen) may occur, and the patient may also present with a distinct macular rash that is most prominent over the trunk.

Childhood Diseases

Rubeola (measles), mumps, pertussis (whooping cough), chicken pox (varicella), and diphtheria are all common, contagious viruses that usually strike during childhood.

Measles

Measles (rubeola) is caused by the infectious agent paramyxovirus. It is transmitted via airborne particles and direct contact with infectious droplets, and it also crosses the placental barrier to the fetus. The highest concentration of the measles virus resides in the respiratory tract secretions, blood, or urine of an infected individual. It has an incubation period of ten to twenty days but is considered communicable between four days before the rash appears to five days after. Signs and symptoms of measles virus are fever, malaise, coryza (head cold with a runny nose), cough, conjunctivitis, and a rash that is red, erythematous, and maculopapular. These eruptions normally start on the face and spread downward to the feet and will gradually turn a brownish color. The individual may also display "Koplik's spots," which are small red spots with a bluish-white center and red base, commonly located in the mouth.

Mumps

Mumps is another infection caused by paramyxovirus. It is transmitted the same way as measles, with the highest concentration of the virus existing in an infected individual's saliva or urine. The incubation period is fourteen to twenty-one days, and mumps is communicable immediately before and after the beginning of parotid gland swelling. The patient presenting with mumps will have a fever, headache and malaise, anorexia, jaw or ear pain aggravated by chewing, followed by parotid gland swelling, and orchitis (inflammation of one or both testicles), as well as aseptic meningitis.

Pertussis

Pertussis, otherwise referred to as "whooping cough," is caused by the infectious agent *Bordatella pertussis*. It is spread through direct contact or droplets from an infected person and incidental contact with recently tainted items of clothing and bedclothes; the main source of the virus is discharge from the respiratory tract of the infected individual. Incubation can be anywhere from five to twenty-one days but is generally ten days. The communicable period is greatest during the time when discharge from respiratory secretions ensues. Physical indicators of pertussis include symptoms of respiratory infection followed by increased severity of cough, with a loud "whooping" respiration, possible cyanosis, respiratory distress, restlessness, irritability, and anorexia.

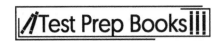

Implementation of care focuses on compliance with strict airborne and droplet precautions during the catarrhal stage (when respiratory secretion discharge is present), especially if the individual is hospitalized. Administration of antimicrobial therapy as prescribed, reduction of cough-causing environmental factors (dust, smoke, sudden alterations in temperature), and encouragement of adequate hydration/nutrition. Monitoring of vital signs, cardiopulmonary status, and pulse oximetry are other interventions involved.

Chicken Pox

Chicken pox (varicella) is a result of the highly contagious varicella-zoster virus. It is transferred via direct contact, droplet (airborne), and contaminated items. The concentration is greatest in the respiratory tract secretions and skin lesions of the infected individual. Incubation is anywhere from thirteen to seventeen days and is transmissible from one to two days before the onset of the rash to six days after the first vesicles appear and when skin lesion crusts have formed. Signs and symptoms of infection include slight fever, malaise, and anorexia, followed by a macular skin outbreak that first develops on the trunk and scalp and then moves to the face and extremities. The rash may also appear in the mouth and genital and rectal areas. Lesions become eruptions, begin to dry out, and create a crust.

The antiviral agent acyclovir (Zovirax®) may be used to treat chicken pox in vulnerable, immunocompromised individuals to lessen the number of lesions, shorten fever time, and decrease itching, lethargy, and anorexia. The use of VCZ immune globulin (VariZIG®) or IV immune globulin (IVIG) is suggested for immunocompromised children who have no previous history of varicella and are most susceptible to contracting the virus and have complications as a result.

Diphtheria

Diphtheria is caused by the contagious *Corynebacterium diphtheriae* and is virulent during direct contact with the infected person, carrier, or contaminated articles. Its source is the discharge from the mucous membrane of the nose and nasopharynx, skin, and other lesions of the infected. The incubation period is between two and five days, with the transferrable period being variable and dependent on the absence of virulent bacilli (three cultures of discharge from the nose, nasopharynx, skin, and other lesions must be negative), usually two to four weeks.

The person presenting with diphtheria infection will experience a low-grade fever; malaise; sore throat; foul-smelling, mucopurulent nasal discharge; lymphadenitis (inflammation of lymph gland); and neck edema.

Care consists of isolation of the hospitalized individual, administration of antibiotics and diphtheria antitoxin as prescribed (after a skin or conjunctival test to rule out sensitivity to horse serum), and tracheostomy care if a tracheotomy is required.

Herpes Zoster

Herpes zoster, also referred to as shingles, normally attacks individuals with a history of chicken pox infection. It usually occurs in adulthood and is a result of the reactivation of the varicella-zoster virus. The possibility of infection is especially likely in persons who are immunocompromised. Flare-ups occur in a segmental distribution pattern on the skin area along the infected nerve (the once-dormant virus is located in the dorsal nerve root ganglia of the sensory cranial and spinal nerves) and will appear after several days of irritation in the area. It is contagious to those who have never had chicken pox and have not been vaccinated against the virus.

The patient with shingles will present with unilaterally clustered skin lesions along peripheral sensory nerves on the trunk, thorax, or face. The person will generally be suffering fever, malaise, burning and pain in the affected area(s), paresthesia (numbness and tingling), and pruritus. Diagnosis is determined by visual evaluation, Tzanck smear, and a viral culture that is specific to the identification of the causative agent.

Fever

Normal body temperature averages around 98.6 degrees Fahrenheit. A fever is an increase in body temperature. It is often the first indicator that the body is fighting an infection or injury, as most bacteria and viruses cannot survive high temperatures. Mild fevers can be treated with over-the-counter pain and fever relievers, such as ibuprofen or acetaminophen. Increased risks for more serious fevers include hospitalization, surgery, travel to high-risk countries, a suppressed immune system, drug abuse, and some medications. These are risk factors due to the increase in exposure to viruses and bacteria that can cause a fever.

Drugs

The following section will discuss different classes of medications. It is important to recognize that drugs with a similar therapeutic effect might have different mechanisms/modes of action. For example, ACE inhibitors (e.g. ramipril), calcium channel blockers (e.g. amlodipine), and antihypertensive agents have similar therapeutic effects, but their mechanisms of action are different. When filling a prescription, it is important for pharmacists understand how a drug works. Not only does knowledge about the pharmacology of a medicine help to identify possible drug interactions, but it also helps to facilitate patients' understanding of why medications are prescribed for them.

Medications Acting on the Nervous System

Antidepressants and Anxiolytics

Antidepressants are used to treat different mood disorders including depression, anxiety, phobias, and obsessive-compulsive disorder (OCD). Treatment for depression includes various medications, in addition to cognitive behavioral therapy (e.g. counseling).

The following are some of the symptoms frequently observed with depression:

- Difficulty concentrating
- Decreased interest or no interest in activities that used to be enjoyable
- Fatigue or lack of energy
- Sense of worthlessness or hopelessness
- Difficulty sleeping
- Changes in appetite
- Suicidal thoughts

Antidepressants exert their therapeutic effects by modulating the release or action of various neurotransmitters in the brain. Neurotransmitters are chemical messengers that transmit signals from one neuron to another. The common side effects of antidepressants are serotonin syndrome (headache, agitation, tremor, hallucination, tachycardia, hyperthermia, shivering and sweating), sexual dysfunction, weight changes, gastric acidity, diarrhea, sleep disturbances, and suicidal ideation.

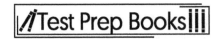

Commonly prescribed antidepressant medications include:

- Sertraline
- Fluoxetine
- Paroxetine
- Citalopram
- Escitalopram
- Venlafaxine
- Desvenlafaxine
- Duloxetine
- Trazodone
- Bupropion
- Amitriptyline
- Nortriptyline

Benzodiazepines are a class of medications used for the short-term treatment of anxiety. They are often combined with antidepressants during initial treatment to increase treatment compliance. Benzodiazepines have the potential for significant physical dependence and withdrawal symptoms. These drugs can be used as sedatives and hypnotics and are also utilized as an add-on therapy with anti-convulsant medications. Benzodiazepines are often used to treat symptoms from alcohol withdrawal. The majority of benzodiazepines are labeled as Class IV controlled substances. The common side effects of these medications include physical dependence, sedation, drowsiness, dizziness, and lack of coordination.

The following are commonly prescribed benzodiazepines:

- Diazepam
- Lorazepam
- Clonazepam
- Alprazolam
- Midazolam
- Temazepam

Antipsychotics

Antipsychotics are used to treat psychosis, including schizophrenia and bipolar disorder. Psychosis is often characterized by a cluster of symptoms including delusions (false beliefs), paranoia (fear or anxiety), hallucinations, and disordered thoughts. The most common side effects of antipsychotics are dyskinesia (movement disorder), loss of libido or sex drive, gynecomastia (breast enlargement) in males, weight gain, heart diseases (QT prolongation), and metabolic disorders, including type 2 diabetes.

The following are examples of commonly prescribed antipsychotics:

- Chlorpromazine
- Fluphenazine
- Haloperidol
- Aripiprazole
- Olanzapine
- Risperidone

- Ziprasidone
- Clozapine

Stimulant Medications

Stimulant medications are also called sympathomimetic agents, as they work by augmenting the sympathetic neurotransmitter activity (e.g. epinephrine and norepinephrine). These drugs are often used during emergencies to treat cardiac arrest and shock. Stimulant medications are more commonly used to treat attention-deficit hyperactivity disorder (ADHD). The common side effects of such medications include irritability, weight loss, insomnia, dizziness, agitation, headache, abdominal pain, tachycardia, growth retardation, hypertension, and cardiovascular disturbances, and death.

The following are examples of sympathomimetic drugs that are used in the treatment of ADHD:

- Methylphenidate
- Dextroamphetamine
- Lisdexamfetamine
- Mixed salts of amphetamine
- Atomoxetine

Anticonvulsant Medications

Anticonvulsants are also called antiepileptic or anti-seizure medications. They are used in the treatment of epileptic seizures. They suppress excessive firing of neurons and therefore, prevent the initiation and spread of seizures. This class of medications is often used to stabilize mood in bipolar disorder or for the treatment of neuropathic pain. The common side effects are dizziness, sedation, weight gain, hepatotoxicity, hair loss, blood disorders, etc. Anticonvulsants are teratogenic and can cause significant harm to a fetus and result in birth defects. Therefore, female patients on anticonvulsant therapy should consult with their physicians before planning pregnancy.

The common medications in this class include the following:

- Carbamazepine
- Oxcarbazepine
- Phenytoin
- Valproic acid
- Divalproex
- Levetiracetam
- Lamotrigine
- Topiramate
- Clobazam

Medications Acting on the Cardiovascular System

Lipid-Lowering Medications

Lipid-lowering medications are used for the treatment of high blood lipids (hyperlipidemia), including high cholesterol (hypercholesterolemia) and high triglycerides (hypertriglyceridemia). Although a patient with hypercholesterolemia typically will not experience symptoms, the condition leads to the accumulation of fatty deposits, called atherosclerotic plaques, in the blood vessels and liver. As time progresses, the deposits slow, impede, or block the flow of blood through the vessels. When blood flow is compromised to the heart muscle, ischemic heart disease can result. If the blood flow to the brain decreases, there is a possibility of ischemic stroke. Compromised blood supply in peripheral tissues and limbs can cause the development of peripheral vascular diseases (PVD). Lifestyle changes, such as a healthy diet and regular exercise, can significantly reduce the risk of hypercholesterolemia, even in the presence of predisposing genetic risk factors. Total cholesterol is determined from two components: high-density lipoproteins (HDL) cholesterol, considered the "good" cholesterol, and low-density lipoproteins (LDL) cholesterol, considered the "bad" cholesterol. Although it is helpful to keep a lower total cholesterol level for health and reduced disease risk, it is more critical to keep the ratio of HDL to LDL elevated.

Examples of lipid-lowering agents include:

- Statins: pravastatin, simvastatin, atorvastatin, rosuvastatin
- Cholesterol absorptions inhibitors: ezetimibe, cholestyramine, colestipol
- Fibrates: gemfibrozil, fenofibrate

Antihypertensive Medications

Antihypertensive medications are used to treat high blood pressure. Although hypertensive individuals generally do not have symptoms, some people experience headaches, blurred vision, and dizziness. When high blood pressure is left untreated, it can lead to different clinical conditions including coronary artery disease, heart failure, kidney failure, or stroke. There are two values that comprise a blood pressure measure. The top number is the systolic pressure (the pressure exerted on the arterial walls when the heart muscle contracts) and the bottom number is the diastolic pressure (the pressure on the arterial walls when the heart muscle relaxes). Normal, healthy blood pressure in adults should be a systolic reading less than 120 mmHg and a diastolic pressure less than 80 mmHg.

There are three stages of high blood pressure, as outlined below:

- Prehypertension is characterized by systolic pressure between 120-139 mmHg and diastolic pressure between 80-89 mmHg

- Stage 1 hypertension is characterized by systolic pressure between 140-159 mmHg and diastolic pressure between 90-99 mmHg

- Stage 2 hypertension is characterized by systolic pressure of 160 mmHg and higher and diastolic pressure of 100 mmHg and higher

ACE Inhibitors (ACEIs): "ACE inhibitors," or angiotensin-converting enzyme inhibitors, are used to treat hypertension and cardiovascular diseases. The most common side effect of ACE inhibitors is a chronic dry cough, which, in many cases, is so annoying for a patient that it results in switching the medication to a different class. Other frequent side effects are low blood pressure (hypotension), dizziness, fatigue, headache, and hyperkalemia (increased blood potassium levels).

Examples of some ACE Inhibitors include:

- Ramipril
- Enalapril
- Lisinopril
- Captopril
- Quinapril
- Perindopril

Angiotensin Receptor Blockers (ARBs): ARBs have similar therapeutic effects as ACE Inhibitors; however, they tend to have better compliance, due to their lower incidence of persistent cough. They block the effect of angiotensin at the receptor site and are widely used for hypertension and cardiovascular disease. The common side effects are hypotension, fatigue, dizziness, headache, and hyperkalemia.

Examples of ARBs include:

- Losartan
- Irbesartan
- Valsartan
- Candesartan
- Telmisartan
- Olmesartan

Calcium Channel Blockers (CCBs): CCBs work by decreasing calcium entry through calcium channels. By regulating the movement of calcium, contraction of vascular smooth muscle is controlled, which causes blood vessels to dilate. This reduces blood pressure and workload on the heart, so this type of medication is used to treat hypertension and angina, and to control heart rate. Common side effects of CCBs include dizziness, flushing of the face, headache, edema (swelling), tachycardia (fast heart rate), bradycardia (slow heart rate), and constipation. In combination with other medications that treat hypertension, calcium channel blocker toxicity is possible. Combinations, like verapamil with beta-blockers, can lead to severe bradycardia.

The following are examples of common calcium channel blockers:

- Amlodipine
- Nifedipine
- Felodipine
- Verapamil
- Diltiazem

Beta Blockers: Beta blockers are an important class of antihypertensive medications, and are widely used to treat hypertension and cardiovascular disease. Some of them are also used to treat migraines, agitation, and anxiety. The side effects of beta blockers include hypotension, dizziness, bradycardia, headache, bronchoconstriction (trouble breathing), and fatigue.

Commonly prescribed beta blockers include:

- Atenolol
- Metoprolol
- Propranolol
- Sotalol
- Nadolol
- Carvedilol
- Labetalol

Vasodilators: Vasodilators cause blood vessels to dilate, lowering resistance to flow and reducing the workload on the heart. Vasodilators are used to treat hypertension, angina, and heart failure. The common side effects associated with their use include lightheadedness, dizziness, low blood pressure, flushing, reflex tachycardia, and headache. Vasodilators should not be combined with medications for erectile dysfunction, as this interaction can cause a fatal drop in blood pressure.

Examples of common vasodilators include:

- Nitroglycerin (available as sublingual tablets, sprays, patches, and extended release capsules)
- Isosorbide mononitrate
- Isosorbide dinitrate
- Hydralazine
- Minoxidil (limited use)

Alpha-1 Receptor Blockers: Alpha-blockers decrease the norepinephrine-induced vascular contraction, causing relaxation of blood vessels and a resultant reduction in blood pressure. This type of medication is used to treat high blood pressure and benign prostatic hyperplasia (BPH). The common side effects of this class of medications include hypotension, dizziness, headache, tachycardia, weakness, and nausea.

Examples of alpha blockers include:

- Prazosin
- Doxazosin
- Terazosin
- Tamsulosin (primarily used to treat BPH)
- Alfuzosin (primarily used to treat BPH)

Diuretics: Diuretics are used alone and in combination with other medications to treat hypertension. They are often used to eliminate excess body fluid to treat swelling/edema. Diuretics inhibit the absorption of sodium in renal tubules, resulting in increased elimination of salt and water. This action increases urine output, decreases blood volume, and lowers blood pressure. Side effects of diuretics include hypotension, dizziness, hypokalemia, dehydration, hyperglycemia, polyuria (frequent or excessive urination), fatigue, syncope (fainting), and tinnitus (ringing in ears).

Examples of commonly prescribed diuretics include:

- Furosemide
- Bumetanide
- Hydrochlorothiazide
- Spironolactone
- Amiloride
- Triamterene

Medications Acting on the Respiratory System

Antiasthmatics

Antiasthmatics are used to prevent and treat the acute symptoms of asthma, which is a disease characterized by wheezing, cough, chest tightness, and shortness of breath. Acute asthma can be life-threatening and needs to be treated promptly. Asthma is caused by inflammation and constriction of the airways, which results in difficulty breathing. Acute asthma may be exacerbated by certain triggering factors including environmental allergens, certain medications (e.g. aspirin), stress or exercise, smoke, and lung infections. It is important to avoid the triggering factors to prevent acute symptoms. The common side effects of antiasthmatics are cough, hoarseness, decreased bone mineral density, growth retardation in children, mouth thrush, agitation, tachycardia, and a transient increase in blood pressure.

There are two categories to asthma medications that can be used alone or in combination:

1. Bronchodilators (dilate the airway to ease breathing)
    - Salbutamol
    - Formoterol (generally used in combination with inhaled corticosteroids)
    - Salmeterol (generally used in combination with inhaled corticosteroids)
2. Anti-inflammatory agents
    - Fluticasone (inhaled corticosteroid)
    - Budesonide (inhaled corticosteroid)
    - Beclometasone (inhaled corticosteroid)
    - Montelukast
    - Zafirlukast

Medication to Treat COPD (Chronic Obstructive Pulmonary Disease)

COPD is an obstructive airway disease that is characterized by coughing, wheezing, shortness of breath, and sputum production. COPD is a progressive disease and it worsens over time. COPD is a combination of two common conditions: chronic bronchitis and emphysema. Chronic bronchitis is inflammation of the smooth lining of bronchial tubes. These tubes are responsible for carrying air to the alveoli, which are the air sacs in the lungs responsible for gaseous exchange between the lungs and blood. Emphysema results from alveolar damage, reducing the ability for healthy gas exchange. These two pathologies cause breathing difficulties in patients with COPD. The contributing factors for the development of COPD include smoking, environmental pollutions, and genetic risk factors. The side effects of COPD medications are similar to that of antiasthmatics.

The medications commonly used to treat COPD include the following:

1. Bronchodilators (dilate the airway to ease breathing)
    - Salbutamol
    - Formoterol (generally used in combination with inhaled corticosteroids)
    - Salmeterol (generally used in combination with inhaled corticosteroids)
2. Anti-inflammatory agents
    - Ipratropium (Atrovent®)
    - Tiotropium (Spiriva®)
    - Fluticasone
    - Budesonide

Medications Acting on the Digestive System

Gastric acid Neutralizers/Suppressants

Gastric acid neutralizers/suppressants either neutralize stomach acid or decrease acid production, and therefore, provide relief of symptoms associated with hyperacidity. They are also used to treat gastroesophageal reflux disease, or GERD. In GERD, the lower esophageal sphincter does not close properly, which causes the contents of the stomach to back up into the esophagus. This leads to irritation, which is why the common symptoms of GERD include heartburn, coughing, nausea, difficulty swallowing, and a strained voice. There are many factors that can cause or exacerbate GERD including obesity, pregnancy, eating a large meal, acidic foods, a hiatal hernia, and smoking. Lifestyle modifications such as avoiding trigger foods, losing weight (if obesity is a component), decreasing meal size, and trying not to lie down immediately after eating, can reduce symptoms.

The medications used to treat hyperacidity in stomach include the following:

- Antacids (e.g. calcium carbonate)
- Ranitidine
- Famotidine
- Omeprazole
- Esomeprazole
- Lansoprazole
- Rabeprazole
- Pantoprazole

Medications Acting on the Endocrine System

Anti-Diabetic Medications

Anti-diabetic medications are used to treat diabetes, which is a chronic metabolic disease in which the body cannot properly regulate blood sugar levels. This dysregulation is caused by either inadequate or absent insulin production from the pancreas (Type 1 diabetes) or inadequate action of insulin in peripheral tissues (i.e. insulin resistance in Type 2 diabetes). Type 1 diabetes usually occurs in early childhood and is typically treated with insulin injections or medications. Type 2 diabetes generally develops later in adolescence or adulthood, and is related to poor diet, lack of physical activity, and obesity. Diabetes often does not to cause daily symptoms, but symptoms do arise when blood sugar is either too high (from inadequate control) or too low (from inappropriate dosing of hypoglycemic (antidiabetic) agents, including insulin). A few of the symptoms of diabetes include increased thirst and hunger, fatigue, blurred vision, a tingling sensation in the feet, and frequent urination.

Examples of some antidiabetic medications include:

- Insulin
- Metformin
- Acarbose
- Gliclazide, glyburide, glimepiride
- Rosiglitazone, pioglitazone
- Sitagliptin, saxagliptin

Drug and Non-Drug Therapy in Type 2 Diabetes: The most effective way of treating Type 2 diabetes is to combine both drug and non-drug therapies. As a part of the treatment, drug therapy can stimulate the pancreas to produce more insulin or help the body better use the insulin produced by the pancreas. As part of the non-drug therapy, counseling is necessary to help patients understand the important diet and lifestyle modifications. Patients with Type 2 diabetes should try to decrease their consumption of processed foods, simple carbohydrates and refined sugars, and overall caloric intake, while increasing physical activity. These interventions help to decrease the requirement of antidiabetic medications and prevent long-term diabetes-related complications.

Glucometer: Patients with diabetes should test their blood sugar regularly to ensure that it is well-controlled. Glucometers are used to measure blood sugar. Patients insert a testing strip into the glucometer, prick a finger with a lancet, and then apply a drop of blood to the test strip. Upon applying the blood, the meter gives a blood sugar reading. Most modern machines need a very small amount of blood to obtain an accurate reading and can generate the result in seconds. Some more advanced meters can store readings for a period of time, so patients can present it to their physicians for review.

Female Hormones

Hormonal medications are generally used as oral contraceptives to prevent pregnancy. Female hormonal medications are also used to treat premenstrual symptoms (PMS), post-menopausal symptoms, acne, and endometriosis. They are also used as emergency contraceptives to prevent unwanted and accidental pregnancy. Oral contraceptives can provide hormones (estrogen and/or progestin), which suppress the egg maturation and ovulation process. Additionally, hormonal contraceptives prevent the endometrium from thickening in preparation to hold the fertilized egg. A mucus barrier is created by progestin, which stops the sperm from migrating to the fallopian tubes and fertilizing the egg.

There are many side effects associated with oral contraceptives, including increasing the risk of fatal blood clots, especially in women older than 35 or in women who smoke. More common and less severe side effects include:

- Nausea and stomach upset
- Headache
- Weight gain
- Spotting between periods
- Mood changes
- Lighter periods
- Aching or swollen breasts

More serious side effects that need immediate emergency care include:

- Chest pain
- Blurred vision
- Stomach pain
- Severe headaches

Examples of some commercially available brands of contraceptive include:

- Yasmin
- Ortho Tri-Cyclen
- TriNessa
- Sprintec
- Ovcon
- Plan B (emergency contraceptive)

Medications Acting on the Immune System

Antivirals

Antivirals are used to fight viruses in the body, by either stopping replication or blocking the function of a viral protein. They are used to treat HIV, herpes, hepatitis B and C, and influenza, among other viruses. Vaccines are also available to prevent some viral infections. Side effects of antivirals include headache, nausea, blood abnormalities including anemia and neutropenia (low neutrophil count), dizziness, cough, runny or stuff nose, etc.

Some examples of disease-specific antivirals include:

- Acyclovir, valaciclovir: Herpes simplex, herpes zoster, and herpes B
- Ritonavir, indinavir, darunavir: Protease inhibitor for HIV
- Tenofovir (Viread®): Hepatitis B and HIV infection
- Interferon: Hepatitis C
- Oseltamivir (Tamiflu®): Influenza

Antibiotics

Antibiotics are antimicrobial agents that are used for treatment and prevention of bacterial infections. The mechanism of action of an antibiotic involves either killing bacteria or inhibiting their growth. Antibiotics are not effective against viruses, and therefore, they should not be used to treat viral infections. Antibiotics are often prescribed based on the result of a bacterial culture to ascertain which class of antibiotic(s) the respective strain will respond to. The common side effects of antibiotics include allergies, hypersensitivity reactions or anaphylaxis, stomach upset, diarrhea, candida (fungal) infections, and bacterial resistance (superinfection, in which a strain of bacteria develops resistance to a broad classes of antibiotics).

Commonly prescribed antibiotics include:

- Penicillin V
- Amoxicillin (with or without clavulinic acid)
- Ampicillin
- Cloxacillin
- Cephalexin
- Cefuroxime
- Cefixime
- Tetracycline
- Doxycycline
- Minocycline
- Gentamicin
- Tobramycin
- Ciprofloxacin
- Levofloxacin
- Erythromycin
- Azithromycin
- Clarithromycin
- Clindamycin

Antimetabolites

Antimetabolites are used to treat diseases including severe psoriasis, rheumatoid arthritis, and several types of cancer (breast, lung, lymphoma, and leukemia). The most commonly used medication of this class is methotrexate, which suppresses the growth of abnormal cells and the action of the immune system. Methotrexate is widely used to treat rheumatoid arthritis. This medication is typically prescribed as once a week dose, and it should not be prescribed for daily dosing because overdosing can be lethal. Pharmacists should be alerted to any prescriptions for daily methotrexate, as the doctor must be contacted to confirm and correct the dosing.

The following are the potential side effects of methotrexate:

- Dizziness
- Drowsiness
- Headache
- Swollen gums
- Increased susceptibility to infections
- Hair loss
- Confusion
- Weakness

Steroids

Steroids are used to treat allergies, asthma, rashes, swelling, and inflammation. These medications are available in different forms, such as oral tablets, nasal sprays, eye drops, topical creams and ointments, inhalants, and injections. The common side effects of steroids include insulin resistance and diabetes, osteoporosis, depression, hypertension, edema, glaucoma, etc.

The following are examples of commonly prescribed corticosteroids:

- Prednisone
- Hydrocortisone
- Fluticason
- Triamcinolone
- Mometasone
- Budesonide
- Fluocinolone
- Betamethasone
- Dexamethasone

Total Parenteral Nutrition: Total parenteral nutrition is used in situations where a patient cannot orally ingest food or digest food through the stomach and intestines. In such cases, total parental nutrition is essential to maintain patient nourishment and to prevent wasting or malnutrition.

The clinical conditions requiring total parenteral nutrition include the following:

- Any cause of malnourishment
- Failure of liver or kidneys
- Short bowel syndrome
- Severe burns

- Enterocutaneous fistulas
- Sepsis
- Chemotherapy and radiation
- Neonates
- Conditions requiring full bowel rest, such as pancreatitis, ulcerative colitis, or Crohn's disease

Microbiology

Physiologic Responses to Toxins

All plants and animals have some sort of innate immunity. Even bacteria have restriction enzymes that have evolved as a primitive defense against viruses. These are enzymes that recognize specific palindromic sequences of DNA along a molecule and cleave them at specific sites, dissecting them into smaller, non-harmful fragments.

Lysozymes, enzymes with natural antibiotic properties, protect against foreign invaders by damaging bacterial cell walls. They are found in many secretions, including tears, saliva, mucus, milk, and even egg whites. Insects have lysozymes in their digestive tracts that protect them from disease. Their exoskeletons, made of chitin, also serve as an effective barrier against foreign invaders. Should a pathogen evade these defenses, hemocytes travel in the hemolymph, the insect circulatory system, and ingest alien particles via phagocytosis. Some hemocytes trigger production of chemicals that kill parasites, bacteria, and fungi.

Mammals have an advanced immune system. Skin epithelial cells, as well as the epithelial lining of the inner mucous membranes, provide protective physical barriers. Mucus traps microbes and washes them away, along with saliva and tears. These physical defenses are enhanced by innate chemical defenses as well. Mucous, tears, and saliva contain lysozymes. The stomach, oil glands, and sweat glands produce acidic fluid that is hostile to many pathogens. Another non-specific chemical defense is stimulated by infected cells themselves. They release chemicals called interferons that provide a localized alarm to surrounding cells. These signals stimulate neighbors to produce substances that inhibit viral replication. Some interferons also recruit and activate white blood cells.

Inflammation

The inflammatory response is also nonspecific and part of the innate defense of mammals. It is characterized by heat, swelling, histamine release, redness, pain, and white blood cell recruitment.

At the site of an injury—a cut, for example—pathogens are released, and cells called mast cells release histamine, which causes the dilation of capillaries, allowing them to become more permeable and to increase blood flow to the area. This results in redness and swelling. Clotting elements then move from the blood to the injury, while a tiny army of white blood cells are recruited to the site due to increased circulation and are attracted to the injury via chemical signals called cytokines released by macrophages. The white blood cells, primarily neutrophils, phagocytose ("eat") the pathogens, allowing the wound to heal. It is very common to feel pain during the inflammatory response, as the pressure caused by swelling stimulates nerves.

Other white blood cells play a role in this non-specific immune response. Dendritic cells are phagocytic cells that reside in tissues. Eosinophils are in mucous membranes and detect multicellular parasites, such as worms, and secrete toxic enzymes to destroy them. Finally, natural killer cells circulate and identify viral-infected and cancer cells and secrete toxins to destroy them.

This highly advanced homeostatic system has another component. If a pathogen is still not destroyed, there is a complicated specific immune response that ensues.

Pain, though deeply uncomfortable, is beneficial. It alerts the organism that there is an issue and helps to prevent further damage. For example, an animal that has a broken leg will not be able to run on it because this would damage an already vulnerable bone. A cat that licks its wounds does so in order to stimulate blood clotting. Without pain receptors, these adaptive responses wouldn't happen.

Fever, an increase in body temperature as a result of the immune system's defense against infection, helps to destroy bacteria and viruses that are sensitive to temperature change, as well as increase the number of lymphocytes capable of killing pathogens. The benefit of a fever may also be to increase enzymatic reactions to stave off infection. As temperature increases, the kinetic energy of substrates and enzymes increase, collisions happen faster, and reaction rates increase. If temperature exceeds a certain point, however, it can be very dangerous because enzymes begin to denature and completely lose functionality.

Immune Responses in Plants

The last section discussed animal innate immunity, but plants have defenses as well. Physical defenses, such as thorns and poison, are defenses against consumers.

Plants also have chemical defenses against microbes. It is not likely that plants will ever develop immune systems as complex as those in animals because it requires a costly energy investment. However, plants that have no immune system are unlikely to survive. Therefore, plants have co-evolved with avirulent strains of pathogens, which are much less harmful than virulent strains. Harmful viruses would decimate plants due to their weak immune systems, and in doing so, they would quickly destroy their host and then be homeless and starving. Less-damaging plant pathogens are, therefore, the norm, since they enable both the plant and the parasitic organism to survive.

Avirulent pathogens have protein effectors (Avr genes) that cause infection in plants that lack the specific resistance (R) protein—a gene responsible for resistance against pathogens. If the R protein is present and the pathogen effector protein binds to it, it initiates a signal transduction cascade that mounts a strong immune response. Part of that response is called the hypersensitive (HR) response, a localized general chemical defense that kills cells surrounding the site of infection. Additionally, modification to the surrounding cells' walls prohibits spreading of the pathogen. There is also a distal immune response; the dying cells secrete methylsalicylic acid that is delivered to non-infected areas and converted to salicylic acid, which signals a systemic, or "whole-plant," immune response.

This description of a plant's general response is akin to innate immunity in animals. Mammals also have an adaptive, or specific, immune response. The cells involved in the adaptive immune response originate in bone marrow and are called B lymphocytes and T lymphocytes. The ones that mature in the bone marrow are B cells and the ones that travel to the thymus to mature are the T cells.

Antigens are anything that activates B and T cells by binding a small region called an epitope to one of their antigen-specific receptors. This may include pathogens, such as bacteria or viruses, toxins or foreign cells introduced by transplantation, or even an organism's own cells in autoimmune responses.

B cells and T cells are different in structure and function, so antigen binding is different between them.

Upon an epitope binding to a B cell's binding site, the B cell proliferates, and its daughter cells secrete its characteristic antigen receptor. This antigen receptor is referred to as an antibody or an immunoglobulin (Ig). T cells behave differently in that they only recognize host cells that present fragments of a pathogen's antigen after ingestion.

There are millions of different B and T cell receptors, and this diversity is due to the many possible combinations of a transcribed immunoglobulin gene. The gene contains light and heavy chains of the B cell receptors, and each one can be arranged in several different structures due to *recombinase*, an important enzyme in antibody development.

These lymphocytes are involved with two different immune responses: cell-mediated and humoral. The cell-mediated response involves T cell destruction of host cells, as outlined below.

1. An antigen-presenting dendritic cell, macrophage, or B-lymphocyte engulfs the pathogen and digests it. The pieces of digested antigens are displayed on MCH (major histocompatibility complex) class II on the surface of antigen-presenting cells. MCH class I complex contains the host cell's peptides, allowing lymphocytes to recognize them. This ensures that the immune system does not attack its own cells when the antigen is not being presented, and is seen on all host cells. The white blood cells with both kinds of MHC molecules are the specific activators of the helper T cells.

2. Helper T cells bind to the antigen and stimulate the humoral and cell-mediated response via the cytokine release.

3. Cytotoxic T cells are activated by helper T cell signals.

4. Cytotoxic T cells recognize MHC class I molecules on host cells and secrete proteins that trigger cell death.

The humoral immune response includes B cell activation and involves antibody neutralization of pathogens in the circulatory and lymphatic vessels. It begins the same way as the cell-mediated immune response with antigen presentation and helper T cell signaling. In this response, B cells proliferate into memory B cells and effector cells, called plasma cells, that secrete antibodies.

Antibodies are tags that mark invaders for destruction. They neutralize surface proteins of a pathogen, preventing them from binding to and affecting its host cell. Antibodies can also cause apoptosis (programmed cell death) in infected body cells. Host cells that present epitopes recruit antibodies, which recruit natural killer cells.

Cell Death

Cells die via two different mechanisms: necrosis and apoptosis. Necrosis is involuntary cell death, in which the cell is damaged via external forces, such as an injury, exposure to toxins, or lack of oxygen, and usually is the cause of the inflammatory response. Apoptosis, however, is when the cell essentially kills *itself* when it is no longer needed, by breaking itself down and then being engulfed by macrophages. Apoptosis is most common in embryonic and fetal development. For example, the webbing in-between the toes and fingers of the fetus in the womb gets broken down via apoptosis before the baby is born. These cells respond to signals in the body that instruct them to commit suicide.

B cell activation not only produces antibody-making cells, but it also produces memory B cells that keep circulating and are not transient. They remain behind and, should the pathogen be encountered again, they immediately recognize the invader and divide quickly to produce many more effector cells. This results in a much faster and stronger secondary immune response because there is no lag time while B cells are proliferating into plasma cells. Vaccines manipulate the immune systems of animals by delivering inactive pathogens that enable these memory cells to develop.

Microorganisms

Microorganisms are tiny single-celled or multicellular organism that can only be seen through a microscope. They include all bacteria and archaea (prokaryotes that live in extreme environmental conditions), and almost all protozoa, fungi, algae, and some rotifers (round microorganisms that reside in freshwater and have three-layered body cavities). Microorganisms have an important role in the environment, as they're found all over and help to recycle nutrients and energy.

Biodiversity

Biodiversity refers to the variety of life and species on Earth. There are many types of microorganisms on our planet. Four main classes of microorganisms are viruses, bacteria, protozoa, and fungi. Although *viruses* are acellular, they use a host species to replicate themselves, allowing for the cycling of nutrients, bacteria, and algae. They can also be pathogens and spread diseases. *Bacteria* are unicellular and obtain energy through photosynthesis, chemosynthesis (the synthesis of organic material from inorganic material for use as energy particularly in the absence of sunlight), and heterotropism (the ability to only produce organic material from carbon derived from animal or plant biosynthesis). *Protozoa* are a diverse group of unicellular organisms that carry out complex metabolic activities. They're also non-photosynthetic, so they cannot use light as an energy source. Amoebae, flagellates, and ciliates are all protozoa. *Fungi* can be unicellular or multicellular and they convert organic matter into nutrients. They are the primary decomposers of an ecological system.

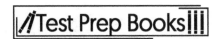

Microbial Systematics

Microbial systematics is the scientific study of the types of microorganisms and the relationships between them. It can be divided into three areas: classification, nomenclature, and identification. This area of discipline allows microbiologists to further study genomic similarities between different species or microorganisms.

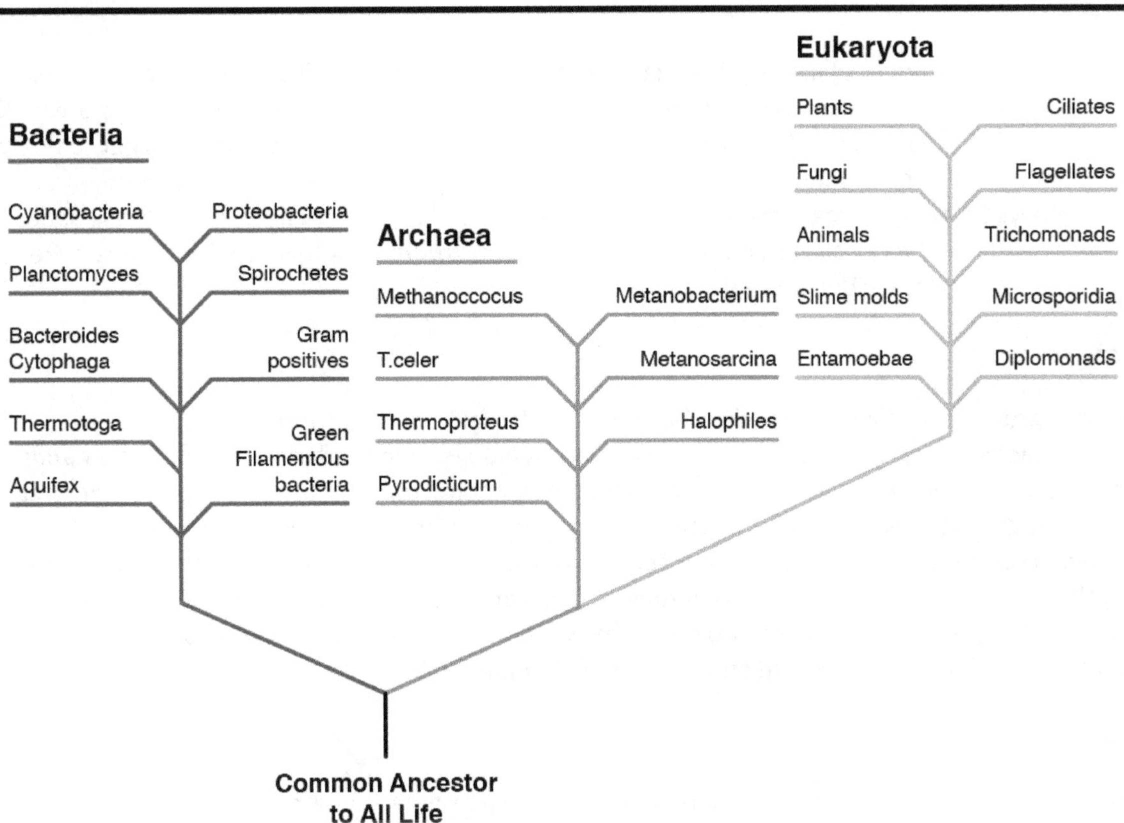

Domain Bacteria

The domain *Bacteria* includes many of the prokaryotic species that people encounter daily. Most are *heterotrophic*, which means they acquire their food from organic matter. Some are *parasitic*, which means they live within a host and cause disease. Some are *autotrophic* and synthesize their own food, such as by photosynthesis or chemosynthesis. They can be aerobic or anaerobic. Bacteria can also be beneficial to the environment by turning nitrogen from the air into organic compounds available to plants. They also help with the decay of landfill materials and other environmental debris. Bacteria swap genetic material through horizontal gene transfer, which can happen by transformation, transduction, or conjugation. *Transformation* involves the naturally-transforming bacteria taking up short fragments of naked DNA. *Transduction* involves the uptake of DNA by bacteriophages. *Conjugation* requires cell-to-cell contact and DNA is transferred by sexual pilus.

Domain Archaea

The domain *Archaea* is comprised of single-cell *prokaryotes*, which means that they don't have a cell nucleus or any membrane-bound organelles within them. Although they are similar in size and shape to bacteria, they contain genes on a single circular chromosome and have several metabolic pathways including transcription and translation. There are three types of archaeal species that use different sources of energy: *Phototrophs* use sunlight for energy, *lithotrophs* use inorganic compounds for energy, and *organotrophs* use organic compounds for energy.

Protists

Protists are a diverse group of unicellular eukaryotic organisms. They are often grouped by convenience and because they are not an animal, plant, or fungus. As eukaryotes, they have a nucleus and organelles. Photosynthetic protists contain plastids, which are organelles responsible for converting light to energy. Protists that use oxygen for energy contain mitochondria. Those that live in hypoxic environments, which lack oxygen, have hydrogenosomes, which appear to be like modified mitochondria. Protists can gain nutrition in many ways, such as photosynthesis or heterotrophism. A few common protists are euglena, amoeba, paramecium, and volvox.

Fungi

Fungi are a group of microorganisms that includes yeasts, molds, and mushrooms. They have the distinct characteristic of having chitin in their cell walls. *Chitin* is a long carbohydrate chain that adds rigidity to the walls of the fungi cells. Fungi are also solely heterotrophic; they break down dead organic material and use the released nutrients. They play an important role in cycling nutrients throughout an ecosystem. Many vascular plants only grow because of the symbiotic fungi that inhabit their roots and supply them with essential nutrition. Some fungi are responsible for the production of antibiotics, such as penicillin. Contrastingly, fungi can also cause many diseases in plants and animals, such as rusts and stem rot in plants and ringworm and athlete's foot in humans.

Helminths

Helminths are large multicellular organisms generally known as parasitic worms. Many worms classified as helminths are the cause of intestinal infections. They live in and feed off their living hosts. They disrupt their host's nutrient absorption, causing them to feel weak and be ridden with disease. Although they share a similar form, many species classified as helminths are not actually evolutionarily related.

Viruses and Virus-Like Agents

Viruses are acellular units comprised of a nucleic acid core surrounded by a layer of protein. As they are acellular and therefore non-living, they cannot reproduce or metabolize on their own—they must use a host organism to do both. Viruses can have a variety of effects on their host. Many viruses disable their hosts and cause cell death. Other viruses are latent and don't show signs of infection within their host.

Microbial Growth, Nutrition, and Metabolism

Most microorganisms reproduce by binary fission, a process where a cell grows to twice its normal size and then divides in half to produce two equally-sized daughter cells. These two cells can eventually divide again and become four cells, and the four cells can grow and divide to become eight total cells, and so on, to make the microorganism population larger. The growth of the microorganisms depends on intake and metabolism of appropriate nutrients. The most important nutrients are carbon, oxygen, nitrogen, and hydrogen. Different microorganisms can metabolize these elements for use as both food and energy. The flagella of protozoa are like those of human sperm and can aid in the study of human reproduction.

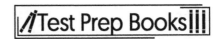

Microbial Genetics

Microbial genetics looks at the genotype and phenotypic expression of microorganisms. Because microorganisms have a rapid growth rate and a short generation time, they have been used for centuries to study different processes and pathways. The distinct traits of microorganisms allow for a variety of things to be studied. Bacteria have been used to study gene transfer systems. Archaea can withstand harsh environments and are used to study extreme environmental conditions *in vitro*. Fungi are used to study cell cycle regulation, chromatin structure, and gene regulation. Although their gene function isn't well understood, it is thought that both archaea and fungi have horizontal gene transfer functions like bacteria. Viruses are important for the study of genetics, as well as the study of viral pathogenic properties. Molecular biologists often use viral vectors to insert genetic material into cells.

Physical and Chemical Methods of Controlling Microorganisms

It is important to be able to control microorganisms to prevent the transmission and spread of diseases, and to stop decomposition of organisms and food spoilage. They can be controlled by both physical and chemical methods. Physical control can occur through changes in temperature, humidity, osmotic pressure, and by filtration. These changes can inhibit microorganism growth and make the environment less ideal for their survival. Filtration includes the physical removal of microorganisms by preventing their passage through a porous material. Chemical control occurs using disinfectants, antibiotics, antiseptics, and antimicrobial chemicals, which all work by selective toxicity. These agents seek out and kill the microorganisms without harming anything else.

Tools for Studying Microorganisms

Microorganisms cannot be seen by the naked eye and can only be visualized using a microscope. Certain types of microscopy, such as bright field, phase-contrast, and dark field, allow the cells to be seen without staining. Cells can also be stained and then viewed under a microscope so that different characteristics of the cell can be illuminated. Electron microscopy uses a beam of electrons to magnify specimens so that their details can be seen more clearly.

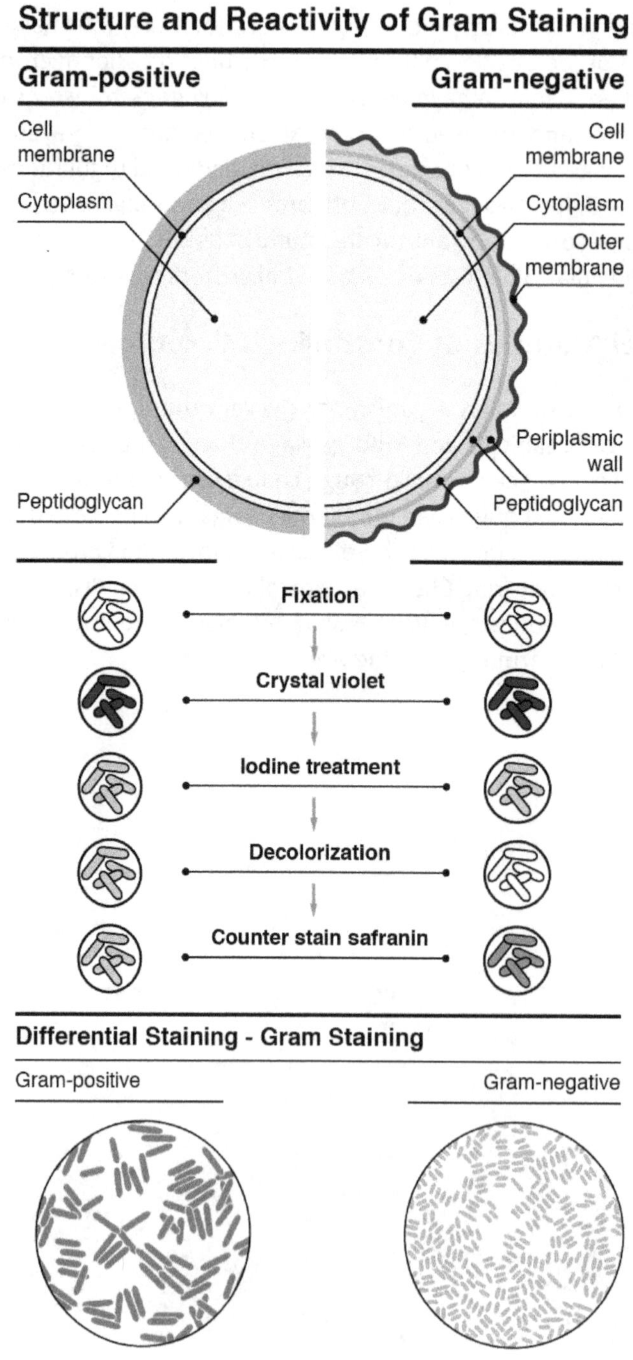

Infectious Diseases & Prevention

Infectious diseases are caused by the spread of microorganisms from one person to another, either directly or indirectly. *Direct contact* involves that exchange of bodily fluids or droplets between an infected person and another person. *Indirect contact* involves airborne spread or touching a contaminated object. Individuals with compromised immune systems are often more susceptible hosts than healthy individuals. The spread of infectious diseases can be prevented by thorough sanitization and disinfection, such as hand washing, vaccination, and the use of disinfectants while cleaning surfaces.

Immunity and Serology

Serology is the study of *blood serum*, the clear fluid that separates when blood clots, and how it relates to the immune system. The body's immune system is the network of cells, tissues, and organs that helps fight off infections. *Immunity* is the ability of an organism to use specific antibodies to fight an infection or toxin. Serology includes identifying these antibodies present in blood serum and investigating problems with the immune system. Three important serology tests include those for immunoglobulins (proteins responsible for antibody activity), rheumatoid factor (involved in certain types of arthritis), and human leukocyte antigen (HLA) typing (which determines organ, tissue, and bone marrow transplant compatibility).

AIDS and Immune Disorders

Immunodeficiency disorders occur when the body's immune system is unable to defend itself against foreign cells that can cause infection. This can cause unusual, prolonged, and/or frequent infections or cancers. There are two types of immunodeficiency disorders: primary and secondary. Primary disorders are generally hereditary and present at birth. Secondary disorders develop later in life and result from the use of certain drugs or from another disorder. Acquired immune deficiency syndrome (AIDS) is a secondary disorder that develops from the human immunodeficiency virus (HIV). AIDS develops from HIV when a specific set of T cells, CD4+, from the immune system are depleted. The absence of these cells prevents the body from effectively fighting infections or killing cancerous cells. Immunodeficiency disorders can also include autoimmune disorders, which occur when the body's immune system attacks itself as if it were a foreign pathogen.

Antimicrobial Medications and Drugs

An antimicrobial medication or drug is used to treat a microbial infection. It can be antibiotic, antifungal, antiprotozoal, or antiviral. These drugs work by penetrating the cell wall of the microorganism and then disrupting the inside of the cell. They work to inhibit microbial growth and reproduction. The *therapeutic index* of a drug is a measure of its relative toxicity to a patient. It is calculated by taking the lowest dose that is toxic to a patient and dividing it by the dose typically used for therapy. Drugs that have antimicrobial selective toxicity are more harmful to microorganisms than patients. Some strains of microorganisms can change and become antimicrobial-resistant. When this happens, the microorganisms are no longer harmed by the medications, so they continue to survive, multiply, and harm the patient.

Systemic Infectious Diseases

Systemic infections are infections that occur in the bloodstream and therefore affect the whole body. As the infection is carried in the blood, it can affect multiple organs and tissues and cause multiple systemic infectious disease syndrome (MSIDS). Patients affected by MSIDS can have a variety of concurrent symptoms, making it hard to identify the source of the infection and thus also making it hard to treat the infection. The flu is an example of a systemic infection, and hypertension is an example of a systemic disease.

Infectious Diseases Affecting the Cardiovascular, Respiratory, Lymphatic and Nervous Systems

Infections of the cardiovascular system affect the blood, blood vessels, and the heart. *Septicemia* is the general term given to a microbial infection of the blood and blood vessels. If this infection reaches the heart valves, it results in endocarditis. Generally, this can be treated with antibiotics, but if there's too much damage to the heart, surgery may be needed. Common infections of the respiratory tract are the common cold and flu. *Bacterial infections* are less common than viral infections in the respiratory system. These affect the sinuses, throat, airways, or lungs. *Pneumonia* is an example of a bacterial infection of the lower respiratory tract. When microorganisms infect the lymphatic system, the lymph, lymph vessels, lymph nodes, and lymphoid organs—such as the spleen, tonsils, and thymus—are affected. Infectious lymphangitis occurs when viruses or bacteria invade the vessels of the lymphatic system through an infected wound. Infections of the central nervous system can be very serious, as they affect the brain and spinal cord. Brain abscesses and bacterial meningitis are caused by bacteria or fungi, while viral meningitis and encephalitis are caused by viruses.

Infectious Diseases Affecting the Digestive, Urinary, and Reproductive Systems

When microorganisms enter the digestive tract, they cause gastrointestinal infections, which are an inflammation of the gastrointestinal (GI) tract that involves the stomach and the small intestine. Dehydration is the largest worry with GI infections, as the patient may not be absorbing enough water while affected by the virus, bacteria, or parasite. Infections of the urinary tract (UTIs) are most often caused by bacteria. They are often the result of bacteria from the large intestine entering the urethra and traveling up to the bladder. If they are not treated in a timely manner, the infection can also continue up to the kidneys and cause a serious infection. Symptoms of a kidney infection can include chills, fever, back pain, and nausea. There are three types of reproductive tract infections: sexually-transmitted diseases, endogenous infections, and iatrogenic infections. Sexually-transmitted diseases (STDs), such as chlamydia, gonorrhea, and HIV, are transmitted from one person to another by bodily fluids that are part of the reproductive system. Endogenous infections are caused by the abnormal growth of organisms that are normally present, such as bacterial vaginosis. Iatrogenic infection of the reproductive system occurs when microorganisms are introduced during an unsterile medical procedure. Serious reproductive infections may result in infertility.

Infectious Diseases Affecting the Skin and Eyes

Although the skin provides a barrier from infection, it sometimes gets infected. Bacterial infections include cellulitis and impetigo. Viral infections include shingles, warts, and herpes simplex virus. These infections can start with a rash, itching, pain, and tenderness. Most can be treated with antibiotics. Fungal infections include yeast infections, athlete's foot, and ringworm. They often occur when there is a cut on the skin's surface and the body's immune system is weakened. Microorganisms can also affect the surface or interior of the eyes. The most common eye infection is *conjunctivitis*, or pink eye, which is caused by the viruses and bacteria that cause the common cold. *Bacterial keratitis* is an infection of the cornea. When microorganisms reach the interior of the eyes, pain is not usually felt, but vision starts to deteriorate.

Microbial Ecology

Microbial ecology is the study of microorganisms and their relationship to each other and the environment. Microorganisms play a significant role in the cycling of environments and biological systems.

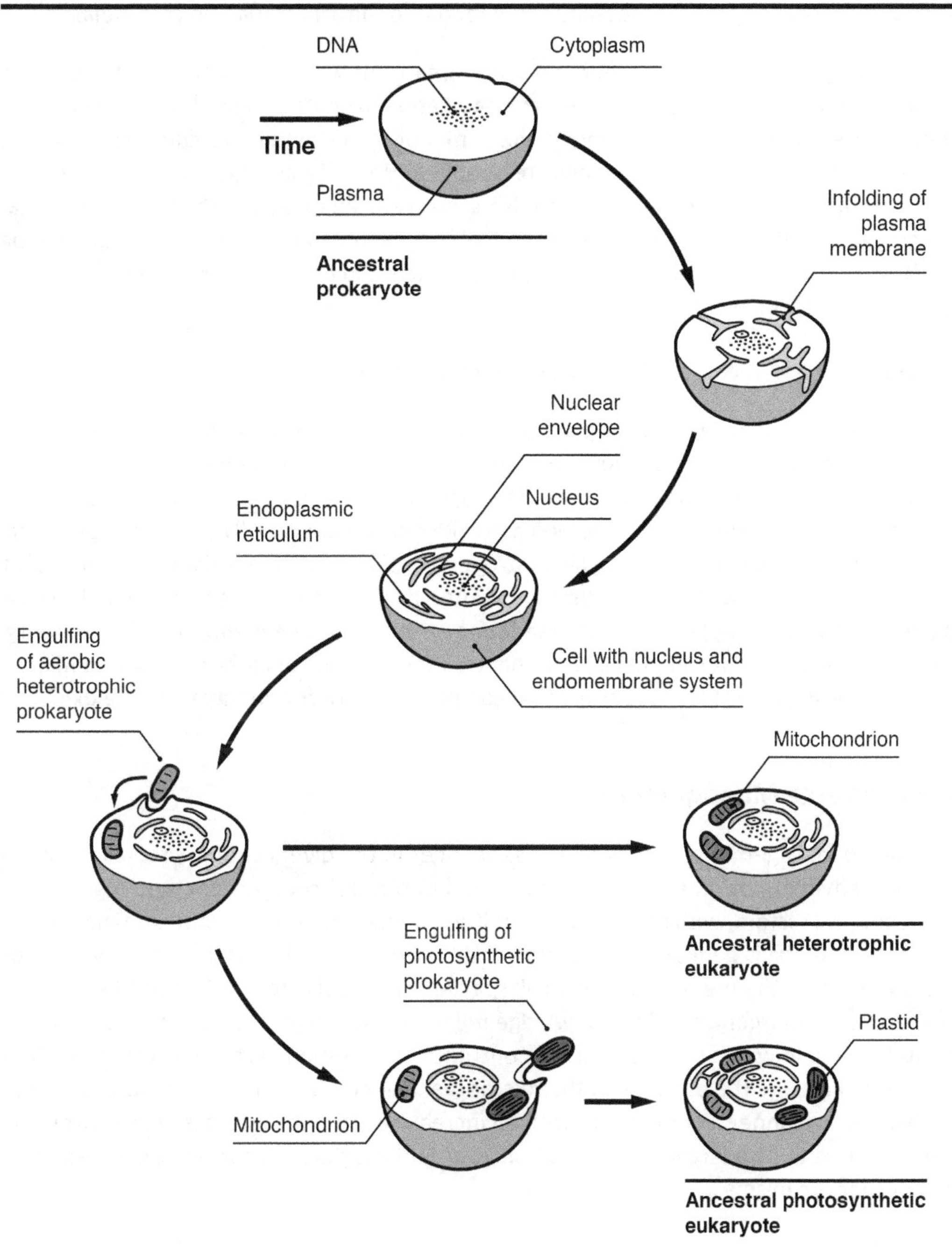

There are three major domains of life: *Eukaryota*, *Archaea*, and *Bacteria*. *Eukaryota* includes all organisms made up of one or more cells that contain a cell nucleus and organelles enclosed by a membrane. *Archaea* comprises single-celled organisms called *prokaryotes*, which means that they do not have a cell nucleus or organelles bound by membranes. Bacteria is also made up of prokaryotic cells but unlike the species of *Archaea*, they do not have genes or metabolic pathways. *Viruses* are microscopic parasites that can only live and reproduce within a host body. They are often even smaller than bacteria. Eukaryotes, archaea, bacteria, and viruses have a symbiotic relationship. The *endosymbiosis* theory of evolution states that eukaryotes developed from larger prokaryotes engulfing smaller prokaryote cells without breaking them up. The small prokaryotes provided the larger prokaryotes with extra energy and eventually developed into mitochondria and chloroplasts.

Microorganisms help to provide each other and other organisms with energy sources to sustain the environment and biosphere. They play specific roles to keep nutrients cycling throughout the environment. In areas that lack light, chemosynthetic microorganisms can provide carbon and energy to organisms, as photosynthetic microorganisms are unable to do so. Microorganisms that are decomposers can use nutrients from other organisms' waste as an energy source. Different organisms get their energy from different forms of the primary elements, mainly carbon, oxygen, and nitrogen. Microorganisms have a large diversity of metabolic pathways and can therefore provide other organisms with whichever form of the elements they need.

The Metabolic Processes and Impact of Microorganisms

Microorganisms perform many metabolic processes that provide energy to other organisms. They can take the elements of an environment and turn them into usable nutrients for other organisms. When microorganisms function as a *carbon sink*, they take carbon dioxide (CO_2) from the atmosphere and store it for the long-term underground. Bacteria can take nitrogenous gas (N_2) from the atmosphere and convert it to ammonia (NH_3) in a process called *nitrogen fixation*. This allows plants and animals to access nitrogen from the atmosphere in a usable manner, as they cannot use nitrogen in the gaseous form. Nitrogen fixation also replenishes nitrogen found in soil. *Methane metabolism* by microorganisms is important for organisms that can only use methane as their source of carbon energy. Similarly, oxidation of sulfur is important for organisms that can produce ATP for energy from the oxidation process.

Microbial Resource Management

Microbial resource management is a way to assess changes in the diversity of microbial communities over time. In the environment, there are thousands of different microorganisms working together to sustain the ecological system, with each playing a different role. Microbial resource management has three main parts. The first is genetic identification of different species in a mixed microbe environment. The second is to identify the metabolic roles of all species. The third is to distinguish the relationships between different microorganisms. This knowledge helps microbiologists to further understand the environmental cycling to which microorganisms contribute. In addition, as the environment changes, microbiologists can change the diversity of the microorganism population to keep the environment cycling in a beneficial manner. For example, with an increase in greenhouse gases in the atmosphere, it is important for there to be a larger presence of microorganisms that can convert the gases to usable resources for other organisms.

Microbes and Human Health

Microorganisms can be a major threat to human health. They can be especially dangerous for people who have compromised immune systems, infants, and elderly individuals. However, they are also harmful for healthy individuals. When humans come in contact with microorganisms, the microbes can enter the body and multiply. They may also release toxins and then damage cells, which leads to disease conditions. *Transmission* is the process by which a person gets infected by a microorganism. *Direct transmission* occurs when a person comes in direct contact with something infected with the microbe, such as soil or another person. *Indirect transmission* occurs when the microbe must travel to the person before they are infected. These microorganisms can be airborne, vector-borne, or vehicle-borne. *Airborne microbes* are suspended in the air between the source of the infection and potential recipients of the infection. *Vector-borne microbes* are carried in living organisms, such as mosquitos, fleas, and ticks. *Vehicle-borne microbes* are carried by inanimate objects, such as food, blood, or surgical instruments. The immune system tries to fight off the infection but isn't always successful.

Food Microbiology

Microorganisms are a large part of the food industry. Some are considered good, such as probiotics and the microorganisms that create cheese, yogurt, and fermented food and drinks. Others contaminate food and cause it to spoil. Food microbiology is an area of study about all of these helpful and harmful bacteria.

Spoilage, Food Preservation, and Fermented Foods

Testing the safety of food products is very important. Microbiological tests are performed at every stage of the food production supply chain to ensure the product is free of contamination and will not spoil unexpectedly. These tests can detect spoilage organisms, determine germ content, and identify yeasts, molds, and salmonella. All of these precautions are imperative preventative measures for food poisoning outbreaks.

There are many techniques used in both home and industrial settings to prevent spoilage and preserve food products. Food preservation prevents or slows the growth of microorganisms that would cause the food to spoil. Some traditional techniques often used in home kitchens are curing, freezing, boiling, sugaring, and canning. Modern techniques used in the food industry are pasteurization, vacuum packing, artificial food additives, and irradiation.

Some foods actually use small amounts of specific microorganisms to prevent spoilage from occurring from other more harmful organisms. This process is called *fermentation.* These microorganisms convert starch and sugars into alcohol to create an environment that's toxic for themselves and other microorganisms to live and multiply in.

Water Pollution

Water pollution occurs when pollutants enter large bodies of water and adequate processes aren't in place to remove the contaminants. Some microorganisms that contaminate water can carry diseases that spread through contact with water. These diseases include salmonella, norovirus, and giardia lamblia. Microorganisms can enter the water from sanitation systems, such as septic tanks, or inadequately-treated sewage discharge. Water pollution occurs more often in less-developed countries, where the infrastructure may be old and resources are limited to fix the problems.

Antimicrobial Agents

Antimicrobial agents include substances that act against microorganisms. They can be natural or synthetic, and can kill or inhibit growth of microbes without affecting the host organism. Antibacterial agents work against bacteria, antiviral agents work against viruses, antifungal agents work against fungi, and antiprotozoal agents work against protozoa. Antibacterial agents are the largest and most studied class of antimicrobial agents. Antibiotics are a specific type of antibacterial agent produced by one type of microorganism to act against another type. They can be used preventatively in populations with weakened immune systems, such as those with HIV, or to treat a current infection, such as an ear infection.

Medical Microbiology

Role of Microorganisms in Disease

Microorganisms can enter the body and make a person ill. These types of microbes are called *pathogens*. They cause infectious diseases such as the common cold and measles. Different pathogens cause different illnesses. A pathogen can enter the body in one of four ways—through the respiratory tract, the gastrointestinal tract, the urogenital tract, or through a break in the skin's surface. To cause an infection, the microorganism must attach to its target site in the body. Then, it must multiply rapidly, obtain its nutrients from its host, and avoid any harm from the host's immune system. Once the pathogen starts causing damage to a person's vital functions and systems, it progresses from an infection to a disease. Diseases have specific signs and symptoms that are a result of the pathogen invading a specific location within the body.

Infectious Disease	Causative Microbe	Microbe Type
Cold	Rhinovirus	Virus
Chickenpox	*Varicella zoster*	Virus
German measles	Rubella	Virus
Whooping cough	*Bordatella pertussis*	Bacterium
Bubonic plague	*Yersinia pestis*	Bacterium
TB (Tuberculosis)	*Mycobacterium tuberculosis*	Bacterium
Malaria	*Plasmodium falciparum*	Protozoan
Ringworm	*Trichophyton rubrum*	Fungus
Athletes' foot	*Trichophyton mentagrophytes*	Fungus

Germ Theory

The germ theory of disease is a belief that microorganisms are the cause of many diseases. Once they invade a living organism, they grow and multiply within their host, causing localized damage to tissues and therefore, disease. Louis Pasteur was one of the first scientists to prove the germ theory of disease in the 1860s. Before his work, it was believed that microorganisms spontaneously generated. He isolated nutrient broth and proved that without outside access, no living organisms appeared in the broth. Following Pasteur, Robert Koch demonstrated that diseases are caused by specific microorganisms. He helped build the framework for isolating and identifying specific pathogens to see how they were related to different infectious diseases.

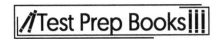

Vaccine Strategies

A vaccine is an agent that helps the body develop an immunity to a disease as a preventative measure. It looks like a disease-causing pathogen, but it is usually a weakened or dead form of it, and stimulates the body's immune system to react against it. The body then gets programmed to remember that microorganism and destroy it during any future encounters. There are several different types of vaccines:

- Live: A living microbe that has been weakened in a lab so that it can cause an immune response but will not cause the disease associated with it; examples include chicken pox, measles, and mumps vaccines.
- Inactivated: Previously-threatening microorganisms treated to become inactive by chemicals, heat, radiation, or antibiotics; examples include influenza, hepatitis A, and rabies vaccines.
- Toxoid: Made from inactivated toxic compounds (not microorganisms) that cause diseases; examples include tetanus and diphtheria vaccines.
- Subunit: A fragment of the whole microorganism, which can still cause an immune response; examples include hepatitis B and HPV vaccines.
- Conjugate: A polysaccharide that resembles the outer coat of certain bacteria and is linked to toxic proteins that cause an immune response; an example includes the Haemophilus influenza type B vaccine
- DNA: A genetically-engineered strand of DNA that causes cells to produce an antigen to a microbe directly; these are still in the experimental stages for human use against diseases such as influenza and herpes.
- Recombinant vector: Microbial DNA is inserted into a harmless virus, which stimulates an immune response; these are still in the experimental stages for diseases such as HIV, rabies, and measles.

Laboratory Diagnostic Methods

There are several laboratory methods that can help to identify a microbial infection. Direct examination with a microscope can identify specific microorganisms. The microbes can be stained to microscopically illuminate distinct features. Microorganisms can also be cultured *in vitro* for identification, but the results often take days or weeks. Phenotypic identification in culture can be based on colony size, color, and shape of the organisms. Once in culture, the susceptibility of the microorganism to different antimicrobial agents can also be determined. Genetic identification can also be performed using immunoassays.

Immunization Protocols

There are many immunizations recommended by the Centers for Disease Control and Prevention (CDC). While some vaccines can be administered with one dose, others require several boosters over time to ensure protection against the disease. The table below gives further detail about the immunization protocols recommended from birth through 18 years of age.

Vaccines	Birth	1 mo	2 mos	4 mos	6 mos	9 mos	12 mos	15 mos	18 mos	19-23 mos	2-3 yrs	4-6 yrs	7-10 yrs	11-12 yrs	13-15 yrs	16-18 yrs
Hepatitis B	1st dose	2nd dose			3rd dose											
Rotavirus			1st dose	2nd dose												
Diphtheria, tetanus, acellular pertussis (<7 yrs)			1st dose	2nd dose	3rd dose			4th dose				5th dose				
Diphtheria, tetanus, acellular pertussis (≥7 yrs)														(Tdap)		
Haemophilus influenza type b			1st dose	2nd dose	Possible 3rd dose		3rd or 4th dose									
Pneumococcal conjugate			1st dose	2nd dose	3rd dose		4th dose									
Inactivated Poliovirus			1st dose	2nd dose	3rd dose											
Influenza					Annual vaccination											
Measles, mumps, rubella							1st dose					2nd dose				
Varicella							1st dose					2nd dose				
Hepatitis A							2 dose series									
Human papillomavirus														3 dose series		
Meningococcal														1st dose		Booster

Cancer and Microbiology

While most microorganisms only cause infections or diseases, some cause more serious health problems like cancer. The bacteria *Helicobacter pylori* (*H pylori*) can cause ulcers in the stomach, as well as inflammation and damage to the inner stomach lining. Long-term infection with *H pylori* can lead to stomach cancer. The bacteria *Chlamydia trachomatis* can infect the female reproductive tract. When these bacteria encounter HPV, they can act together to promote growth of cancerous cells and cause cervical cancer.

Disease Transmission

Diseases can be transmitted from person to person either directly or indirectly. Direct transmission happens when an infected person exchanges bodily fluids with another person, either through direct contact or through droplet, including sneezing and coughing. Indirect transmission can occur through airborne transmission or touching contaminated objects, such as a doorknob, contaminated food or water, or insect bites. The most effective way to prevent disease transmission is through frequent hand-washing.

Host Defense Mechanisms

There are several ways a host can protect itself against infection. Natural barriers, such as skin and mucous membranes, are a physical barrier to the invasion of microorganisms. The respiratory tract has built-in filters against microorganisms. The acidic pH of the stomach does not allow for the growth of microorganisms. The immune system can send both nonspecific and specific immune responses to fight off pathogens. While nonspecific responses include cytokines that fight general microorganisms, the specific response includes antigens produced by vaccinations and other antibodies that target a specific pathogen.

Nosocomial Infections

A nosocomial infection is an infection contracted from a healthcare facility or hospital. The microorganisms that cause these infections are generally specific to these locations. Nosocomial infections occur up to 48 hours after a hospital admission, up to 3 days after hospital discharge, up to 30 days after an operation, or in a healthcare facility where the person was admitted for a different reason. These infections often occur because the person already has a compromised immune system, and therefore has increased susceptibility to acquire a new infection.

Immunity

The immune system is the body's defense against invading microorganisms (bacteria, viruses, fungi, and parasites) and other harmful, foreign substances. It is capable of limiting or preventing infection.

There are two general types of immunity: innate immunity and acquired immunity. Innate immunity uses physical and chemical barriers to block the entry of microorganisms into the body. The skin forms a physical barrier that blocks microorganisms from entering underlying tissues. Mucous membranes in the digestive, respiratory, and urinary systems secrete mucus to block and remove invading microorganisms. Saliva, tears, and stomach acids are examples of chemical barriers intended to block infection with microorganisms. In addition, macrophages and other white blood cells can recognize and eliminate foreign objects through phagocytosis or direct lysis.

Acquired immunity refers to a specific set of events used by the body to fight a particular infection. Essentially, the body accumulates and stores information about the nature of an invading microorganism. As a result, the body can mount a specific attack that is much more effective than innate immunity. It also provides a way for the body to prevent future infections by the same microorganism.

Acquired immunity is divided into a primary response and a secondary response. The primary immune response occurs the first time that a particular microorganism enters the body, where macrophages engulf the microorganism and travel to the lymph nodes. In the lymph nodes, macrophages present the invader to helper T lymphocytes, which then activate humoral and cellular immunity. Humoral immunity refers to immunity resulting from antibody production by B lymphocytes. After being activated by helper T lymphocytes, B lymphocytes multiply and divide into plasma cells and memory cells. Plasma cells are B lymphocytes that produce immune proteins called antibodies, or immunoglobulins. Antibodies then bind to the microorganism to flag it for destruction by other white blood cells. Cellular immunity refers to the immune response coordinated by T lymphocytes. After being activated by helper T lymphocytes, other T lymphocytes attack and kill cells that cause infection or disease.

The secondary immune response takes place during subsequent encounters with a known microorganism. Memory cells respond to the previously encountered microorganism by immediately producing antibodies. Memory cells are B lymphocytes that store information to produce antibodies. The secondary immune response is swift and powerful, because it eliminates the need for the time-consuming macrophage activation of the primary immune response. Suppressor T lymphocytes also take part to inhibit the immune response, as an overactive immune response could cause damage to healthy cells.

Active and Passive Immunity

Immunization is the process of inducing immunity. *Active immunization* refers to immunity gained by exposure to infectious microorganisms or viruses and can be *natural* or *artificial*. Natural immunization refers to an individual being exposed to an infectious organism as a part of daily life. For example, it was once common for parents to expose their children to childhood diseases such as measles or chicken pox. Artificial immunization refers to therapeutic exposure to an infectious organism as a way of protecting an individual from disease. Today, the medical community relies on artificial immunization as a way to induce immunity.

Vaccines are used for the development of active immunity. A vaccine contains a killed, weakened, or inactivated microorganism or virus that is administered through injection, by mouth, or by aerosol. Vaccinations are administered to prevent an infectious disease, but they do not always guarantee immunity.

Passive immunity refers to immunity gained by the introduction of antibodies. This introduction can be natural or artificial. The process occurs when antibodies from the mother's bloodstream are passed on to the bloodstream of the developing fetus. Breast milk can also transmit antibodies to a baby. Babies are born with passive immunity, which provides protection against general infection for approximately the first six months of life.

Human Anatomy and Physiology

Anatomy may be defined as the structural makeup of an organism. The study of anatomy may be divided into microscopic/fine anatomy and macroscopic/gross anatomy. Fine anatomy concerns itself with viewing the features of the body with the aid of a microscope, while gross anatomy concerns itself with viewing the features of the body with the naked eye. *Physiology* refers to the functions of an organism and it examines the chemical or physical functions that help the body function appropriately.

Cells

All the parts of the human body are built of individual units called *cells*. Groups of similar cells are arranged into *tissues,* different tissues are arranged into *organs,* and organs working together form entire *organ systems.* The human body has twelve organ systems that govern circulation, digestion, immunity, hormones, movement, support, coordination, urination and excretion, reproduction, respiration, and general protection.

Histology is the examination of specialized cells and cell groups that perform a specific function by working together. Although there are trillions of cells in the human body, there are only 200 different types of cells. Groups of cells form biological tissues, and tissues combine to form organs, such as the heart and kidney. Organs are structures that have many different functions that are vital to living creatures. There are four primary types of tissue: epithelial, connective, muscle, and neural. Each tissue type has specific characteristics that enable organs and organ systems to function properly.

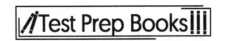

Mitosis and Meiosis

The human body is made of trillions of cells. Cell division and replication are responsible for growth of the body. There are many different types of cells in the body, and most undergo mitosis to divide and replicate. Mitosis also occurs to replenish damaged and dying cells. In mitosis, one cell replicates its own genetic material and splits into two identical daughter cells. It is an important part of both growth and the maintenance of homeostasis within the body.

Although the majority of cells undergo mitosis when replicating, gamete cells (reproductive cells) undergo a more complicated process, called meiosis. In the human body, the gametes are the egg and the sperm. Human reproduction happens by sexual reproduction, which means one gamete fertilizes another gamete. The resulting cell is not identical to either of its parent cells, which is in contrast to daughter cells produced by mitosis. Eggs and sperm cells contain twenty-three chromosomes each. They combine to form a diploid cell that contains all forty-six chromosomes. The diploid cell replicates its chromosomes and splits into two cells, each containing forty-six chromosomes. Those two cells split again to create four cells, each containing twenty-three chromosomes. None of the daughter gamete cells are identical to either of the parent gamete cells. During the process of meiosis, the chromosomes from each parent get mixed together, then split into the daughter gamete cells randomly. This process explains why children are not exactly identical to their parents, but instead have characteristics from each of them.

Tissues

Human tissues can be grouped into four categories:

Epithelial Tissue

Epithelial tissue covers the external surfaces of organs and lines many of the body's cavities. Epithelial tissue helps to protect the body from invasion by microbes (bacteria, viruses, parasites), fluid loss, and injury.

Epithelial cell shapes can be:

1. Squamous: cells with a flat shape
2. Cuboidal: cells with a cubed shape
3. Columnar: cells shaped like a column

Epithelial cells can be arranged in four patterns:

1. Simple: a type of epithelium composed solely from a single layer of cells
2. Stratified: a type of epithelium composed of multiple layers of cells
3. Pseudostratified: a type of epithelium that appears to be stratified but in reality, consists of only one layer of cells
4. Transitional: a type of epithelium noted for its ability to expand and contract

Connective Tissue

Connective tissue fills internal spaces and is not exposed to the outside of the body. It provides structural support for the body and stores energy. Fluid can be transported by connective tissue between different regions of the body. This type of tissue is also a protective barrier for delicate organs and for the body against microorganisms.

Muscle Tissue

Muscle tissue has characteristics that allow motion. Skeletal muscles are long fibers of actin and myosin that slide past each other to cause a contraction, which shortens the muscle. They are filled with mitochondria, because they expend a lot of energy. Smooth muscle tissue is structured differently, because its movement is in the form of peristalsis. For example, the esophagus moves food in a wave-like contraction, as opposed to a shortening of muscle to bring structures together. Smooth muscle tissues make up internal organs, with the exception of the heart, which is composed of thick, contracting muscle tissue called cardiac muscle.

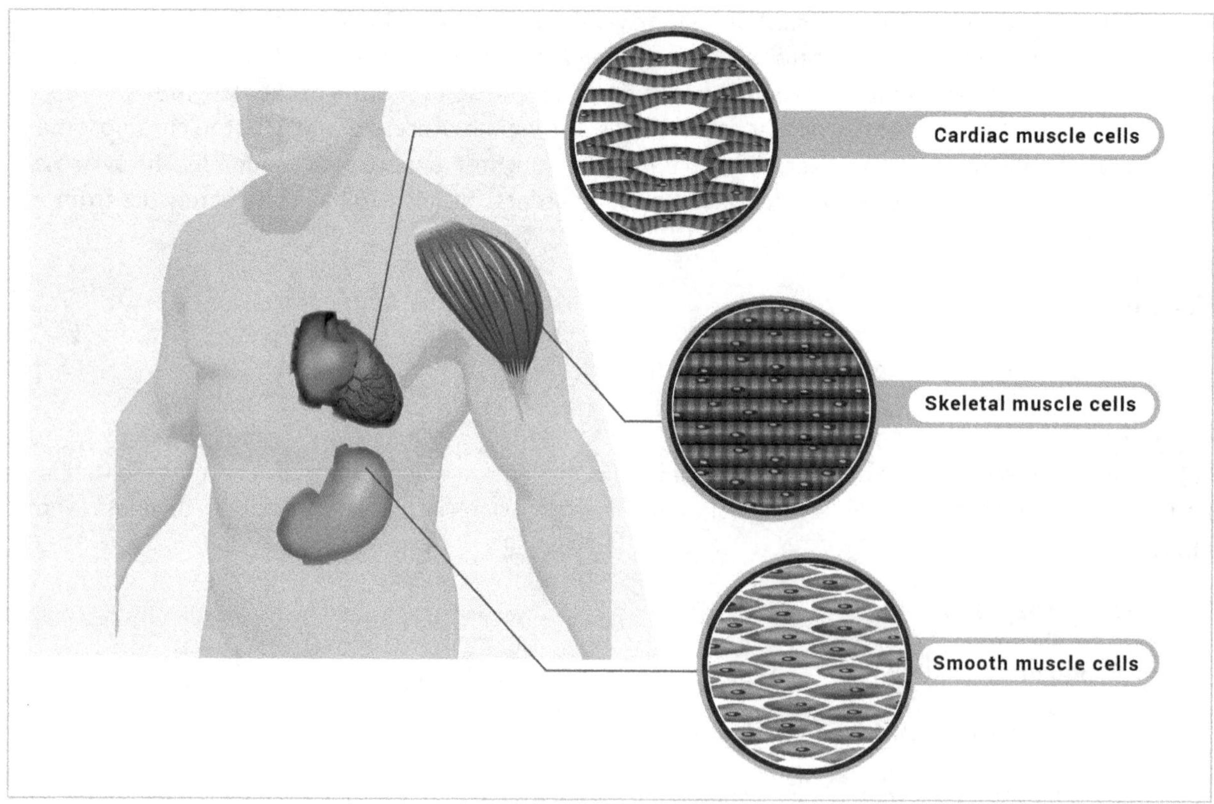

Neural Tissue

Neural tissue conducts electrical impulses, which help send information and instructions throughout the body. Most of it is concentrated in the brain and spinal cord. The changes in frequency and patterns of the impulse are important distinctions in the messages being sent. Its structure is composed of message-receiving projections called *dendrites* and a long, myelinated *axon*. The myelin sheath surrounds the axon to conduct the action potential, ultimately causing neurotransmitter release at the *synapse*, or the boundary between the axon of one cell and the dendrite of another.

Membranes

Membranes are formed by the combination of epithelia and connective tissues. They consist of an underlying connective tissue layer covered by an epithelial sheet, and together they cover and protect structures and tissues in the body. There are four types of membranes: mucous, serous, cutaneous, and synovial. Mucous membranes line cavities that connect with the exterior part of the body and form a barrier against pathogens. The epithelial layer is always moist with mucus or glandular secretions. The loose connective tissue layer is called the lamina propria, and it connects the epithelium to the underlying structures. Serous membranes consist of a mesothelium connected to loose connective tissue. These membranes line the subdivisions of the ventral body cavity. They are very thin and are firmly attached to both the body wall and the organs they are covering. Serous membranes are covered in fluid, called transudate, which helps minimize friction between the organs and the body wall and is the main function of the membrane. The cutaneous membrane is also known as skin. It consists of epithelium and an underlying layer of loose connective tissue that is reinforced by a layer of dense connective tissue and covers the entire surface of the body. It is a thick membrane and is usually dry. Synovial membranes consist of large areas of loose connective tissue bound by an incomplete layer of squamous or cuboidal cells. It is found between the joint capsule and joint cavity of synovial joints. Synovial fluid lubricates this area and distributes oxygen and nutrients. It also cushions impact and acts as a shock absorber at the joints.

Cartilage

Cartilage is a firm gel substance that contains complex polysaccharides, called chondroitin sulfates. It contains collagen fibers, which provide tensile strength, and chondrocytes, which are cartilage cells. It is an avascular material, because the chondrocytes do not allow blood vessels to form within the fibrous network. There are three types of cartilage: hyaline cartilage, elastic cartilage, and fibrocartilage. Hyaline cartilage is the body's most abundant cartilage, and is made of tightly-packed collagen fibers. It is tough and flexible, but is also the weakest type of cartilage. Elastic cartilage contains elastic fibers that make it very resilient and flexible. Fibrocartilage has densely woven collagen fibers that make it very durable and tough.

Organs

Glands

Glands are organs that synthesize and secrete chemical substances, such as hormones, for use inside the body or to be discharged outside the body. There are two types of glands: endocrine and exocrine. Endocrine glands secrete hormones into the bloodstream and are important in maintaining homeostasis within the body. They do not have a duct system. Examples of endocrine glands are the pancreas, the pineal gland, the thymus gland, the pituitary gland, the thyroid gland, and the adrenal glands. Exocrine glands have ducts that are used to secrete substances to the surface of the body and can be classified into three types: apocrine, holocrine, and merocrine. In apocrine glands, part of the cell's body is lost during secretion; in holocrine glands, the whole cell body disintegrates during secretion; and in merocrine glands, cells use exocytosis to secrete fluids. Exocytosis occurs when the chemical substance is carried in a vacuole across the cell membrane for release outside of the cell. The cells remain intact in merocrine glands.

Body Cavities

The body is partitioned into different hollow spaces that house organs. The human body contains the following cavities:

Cranial cavity: The cranial cavity is surrounded by the skull and contains organs such as the brain and pituitary gland.

Thoracic cavity: The thoracic cavity is encircled by the sternum (breastbone) and ribs. It contains organs such as the lungs, heart, trachea (windpipe), esophagus, and bronchial tubes.

Abdominal cavity: The abdominal cavity is separated from the thoracic cavity by the diaphragm. It contains organs such as the stomach, gallbladder, liver, small intestines, and large intestines. The abdominal organs are held in place by a membrane called the peritoneum.

Pelvic cavity: The pelvic cavity is enclosed by the pelvis, or bones of the hips. It contains organs such as the urinary bladder, urethra, ureters, anus, and rectum. It contains the reproductive organs as well. In females, the pelvic cavity also contains the uterus.

Spinal cavity: The spinal cavity is surrounded by the vertebral column. The vertebral column has five regions: cervical, thoracic, lumbar, sacral, and coccygeal. The spinal cord runs through the middle of the spinal cavity.

Systems

Skeletal System

The skeletal system consists of the 206 bones that make up the skeleton, as well as the cartilage, ligaments, and other connective tissues that stabilize them. Bone is made of collagen fibers and mineral salts (mainly calcium and phosphorous). The mineral salts are strong but brittle, and the collagen fibers are weak but flexible, but the combination in the bony matrix makes bone resistant to shattering.

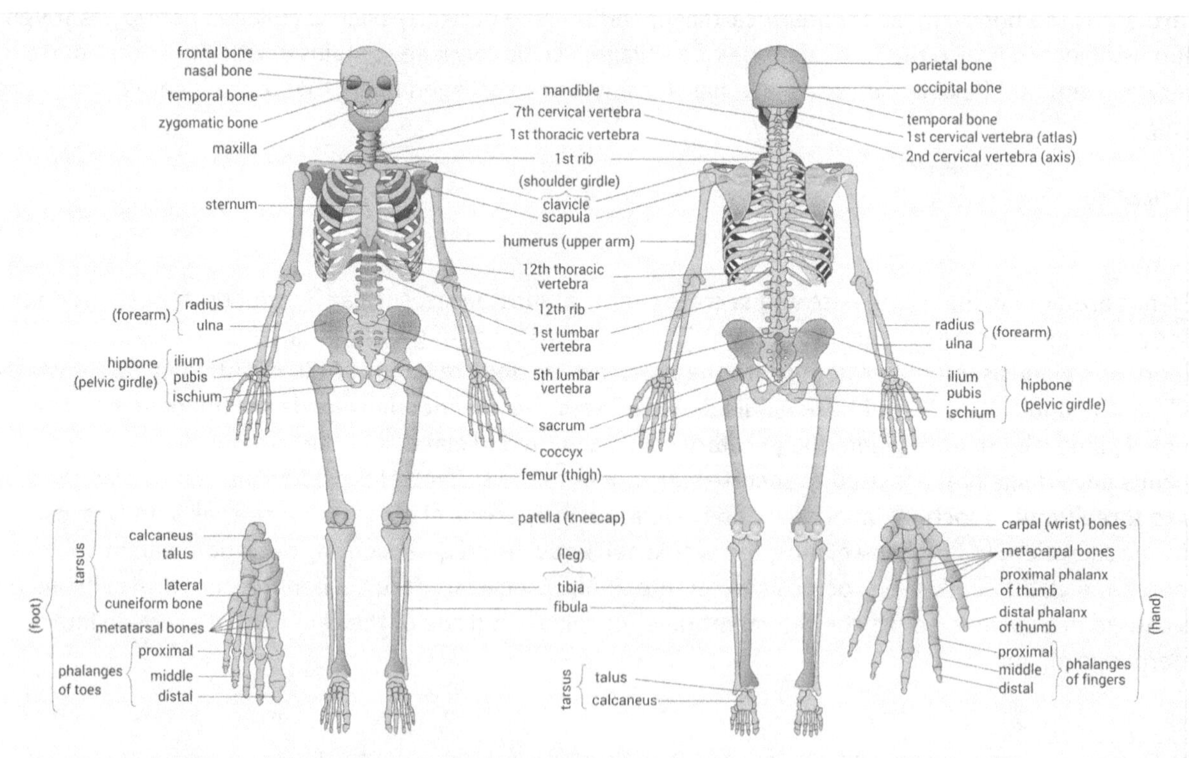

There are two types of bone: compact and spongy. *Compact bone* has a basic functional unit, called the *Haversian system*. Osteocytes, or bone cells, are arranged in concentric circles around a central canal, called the Haversian canal, which contains blood vessels. While Haversian canals run parallel to the surface of the bone, perforating canals, also known as the canals of Volkmann, run perpendicularly between the central canal and the surface of the bone. The concentric circles of bone tissue that surround the central canal within the Haversian system are called *lamellae*. The spaces that are found between the lamellae are called lacunae. The Haversian system is a reservoir for calcium and phosphorus for blood. Compact bone is also called cortical bone.

Spongy bone, in contrast to compact bone, is lightweight and porous. It covers the outside of the bone and it gives it a shiny, white appearance. It has a branching network of parallel lamellae, called *trabeculae*. Although spongy bone forms an open framework around the compact bone, it is still quite strong. Different bones have different ratios of compact-to-spongy bone, depending on their functions. Spongy bone is also called cancellous bone.

The outside of the bone is covered by a *periosteum*, which has four major functions. It isolates and protects bones from the surrounding tissue; provides a place for attachment of the circulatory and nervous system structures; participates in growth and repair of the bone; and attaches the bone to the deep fascia. An *endosteum* is found inside the bone, covers the trabeculae of the spongy bone, and lines the inner surfaces of the central canals.

One major function of the skeletal system is to provide structural support for the entire body. It provides a framework for the soft tissues and organs to attach to. The skeletal system also provides a reserve of important nutrients, such as calcium and lipids. Normal concentrations of calcium and phosphate in body fluids are partly maintained by the mineral salts stored in bone. Lipids that are stored in yellow bone marrow can be used as a source of energy. Red bone marrow produces red blood cells, white blood cells, and platelets that circulate in the blood. Certain groups of bones form protective barriers around delicate organs. The ribs, for example, protect the heart and lungs, the skull encloses the brain, and the vertebrae cover the spinal cord.

Muscular System

The muscular system is responsible for movement. There are approximately 700 muscles in the human body that are attached to the bones of the skeletal system and that make up half of the body's weight. Muscles are attached to the bones through tendons. Tendons are made up of dense bands of connective tissue and have collagen fibers that firmly attach to the bone on one side and the muscle on the other. Their fibers are actually woven into the coverings of the bone and muscle, so they can withstand the large forces that are put on them when muscles are moving. There are three types of muscle tissue in the body. Skeletal muscle tissue pulls on the bones of the skeleton and causes body movement, cardiac muscle tissue helps pump blood through veins and arteries, and smooth muscle tissue helps move fluids and solids along the digestive tract and contributes to movement in other body systems. All of these muscle tissues have four important properties in common. They are excitable, meaning they respond to stimuli; contractile, meaning they can shorten and pull on connective tissue; extensible, meaning they can be stretched repeatedly, but maintain the ability to contract; and elastic, meaning they rebound to their original length after a contraction.

Muscles begin at an *origin* and end at an *insertion*. Generally, the origin is proximal to the insertion and the origin remains stationary while the insertion moves. For example, when bending the elbow and moving the hand up toward the head, the part of the forearm that is closest to the wrist moves and the part closer to the elbow is stationary. Therefore, the muscle in the forearm has an origin at the elbow and an insertion at the wrist.

Body movements occur by muscle contraction. Each contraction causes a specific action. Muscles can be classified into one of three muscle groups based on the action they perform. *Primary movers*, or *agonists*, produce a specific movement, such as flexion of the elbow. *Synergists* are in charge of helping the primary movers complete their specific movements. They can help stabilize the point of origin or provide extra pull near the insertion. Some synergists can aid an agonist in preventing movement at a joint. *Antagonists* are muscles whose actions are the opposite of that of the agonist. If an agonist is contracting during a specific movement, the antagonist is stretched. During flexion of the elbow, the biceps brachii muscle contracts and acts as an agonist, while the triceps brachii muscle on the opposite side of the upper arm acts as an antagonist and stretches.

Skeletal muscle tissue has several important functions. It causes movement of the skeleton by pulling on tendons and moving the bones. It maintains body posture through the contraction of specific muscles responsible for the stability of the skeleton. Skeletal muscles help support the weight of internal organs and protect these organs from external injury. They also help to regulate body temperature within a normal range. Muscle contractions require energy and produce heat, which heats the body when cold.

Nervous System

The human nervous system coordinates the body's response to stimuli from inside and outside the body. There are two major types of nervous system cells: neurons and neuroglia. *Neurons* are the workhorses of the nervous system and form a complex communication network that transmits electrical impulses (termed *action potentials*), while *neuroglia* connect and support them.

Although some neurons monitor the senses, some control muscles, and some connect the brain to others, all neurons have four common characteristics:

1. Dendrites: These receive electrical signals from other neurons across small gaps called *synapses*.

2. Nerve cell body: This is the hub of processing and protein manufacture for the neuron.

3. Axon: This transmits the signal from the cell body to other neurons.

4. Terminals: These bridge the neuron to dendrites of other neurons and deliver the signal via chemical messengers called *neurotransmitters*.

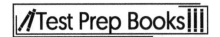

Here an illustration of a basic neuron:

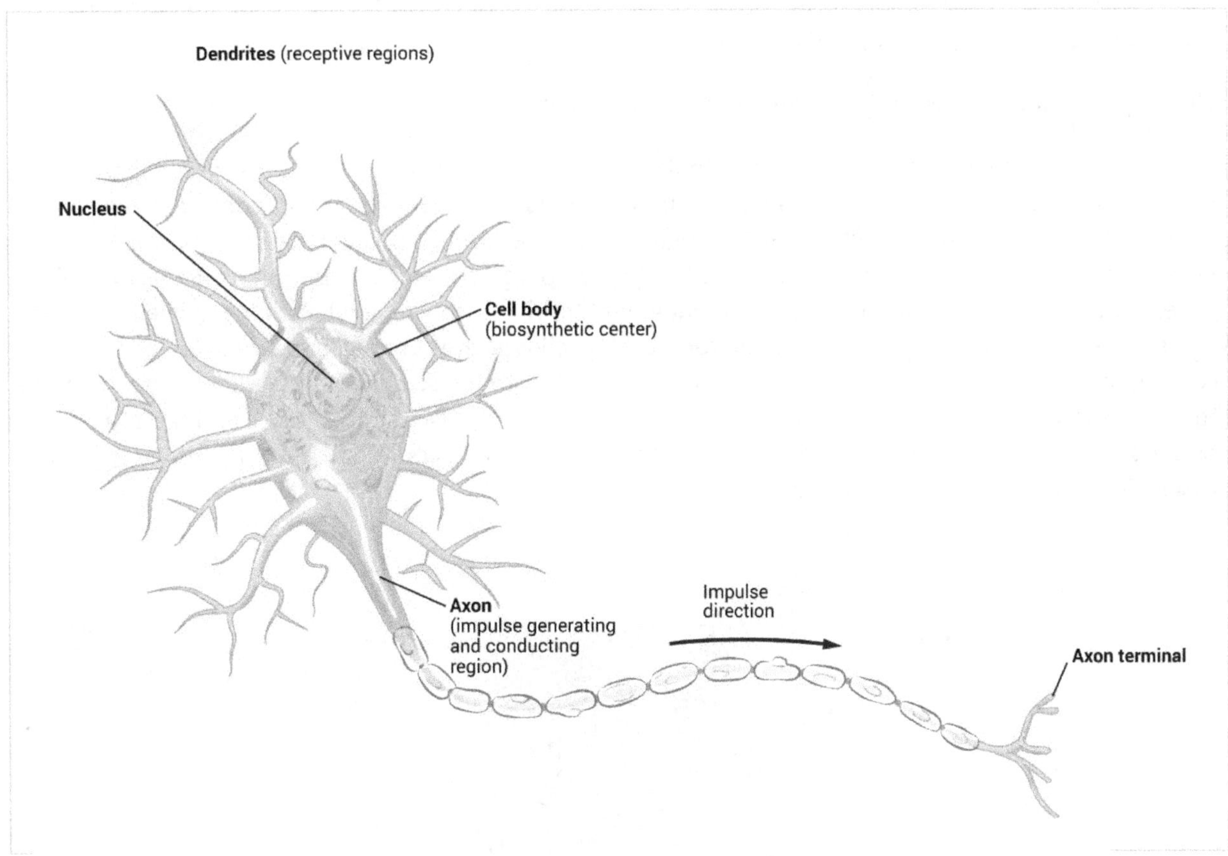

There are two major divisions of the nervous system: central and peripheral:

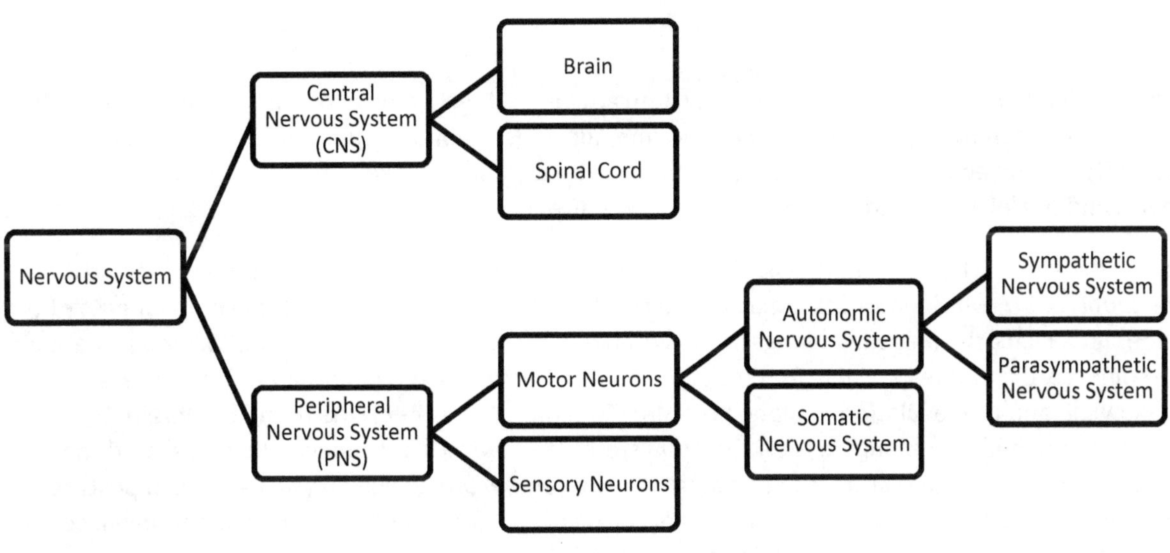

Central Nervous System

The central nervous system (CNS) consists of the brain and spinal cord. Three layers of membranes, called the *meninges,* cover and separate the CNS from the rest of the body.

The major divisions of the brain are the forebrain, the midbrain, and the hindbrain.

The forebrain consists of the cerebrum, the thalamus and hypothalamus, and the rest of the limbic system. The *cerebrum* is the largest part of the brain, and its most well-documented part is the outer cerebral cortex. The cerebrum is divided into right and left hemispheres, and each cerebral cortex hemisphere has four discrete areas, or lobes: frontal, temporal, parietal, and occipital. The frontal lobe governs duties such as voluntary movement, judgment, problem-solving, and planning, while the other lobes have more of a sensory function. The temporal lobe integrates hearing and language comprehension, the parietal lobe processes sensory input from the skin, and the occipital lobe functions to process visual input from the eyes. For completeness, the other two senses, smell and taste, are processed via the olfactory bulbs. The thalamus helps organize and coordinate all of this sensory input in a meaningful way for the brain to interpret.

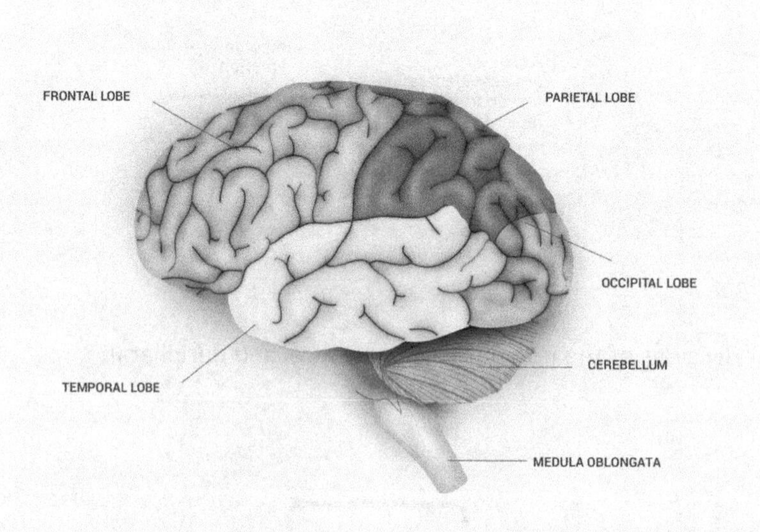

The *hypothalamus* controls the endocrine system and all of the hormones that govern long-term effects on the body. Each hemisphere of the *limbic system* includes a hippocampus (which plays a vital role in memory), an amygdala (which is involved with emotional responses like fear and anger), and other small bodies and nuclei associated with memory and pleasure.

The midbrain is in charge of alertness, sleep/wake cycles, and temperature regulation. It includes the *substantia nigra*, which produces melatonin to regulate sleep patterns. The notable components of the hindbrain include the medulla oblongata and cerebellum. The *medulla oblongata* is located just above the spinal cord and is responsible for crucial involuntary functions such as breathing, heart rate, swallowing, and the regulation of blood pressure. Together with other parts of the hindbrain, the midbrain and medulla oblongata form the brain stem. The *brain stem* connects the spinal cord to the rest of the brain. To the rear of the brain stem sits the *cerebellum,* which plays a key role in posture, balance, and muscular coordination. The spinal cord, encapsulated by its protective bony spinal column, carries sensory information to the brain and motor information to the body.

Peripheral Nervous System

The peripheral nervous system (PNS) includes all nervous tissue besides the brain and spinal cord. The PNS consists of the sets of cranial and spinal nerves and relays information between the CNS and the rest of the body. The PNS has two divisions: the autonomic nervous system and the somatic nervous system.

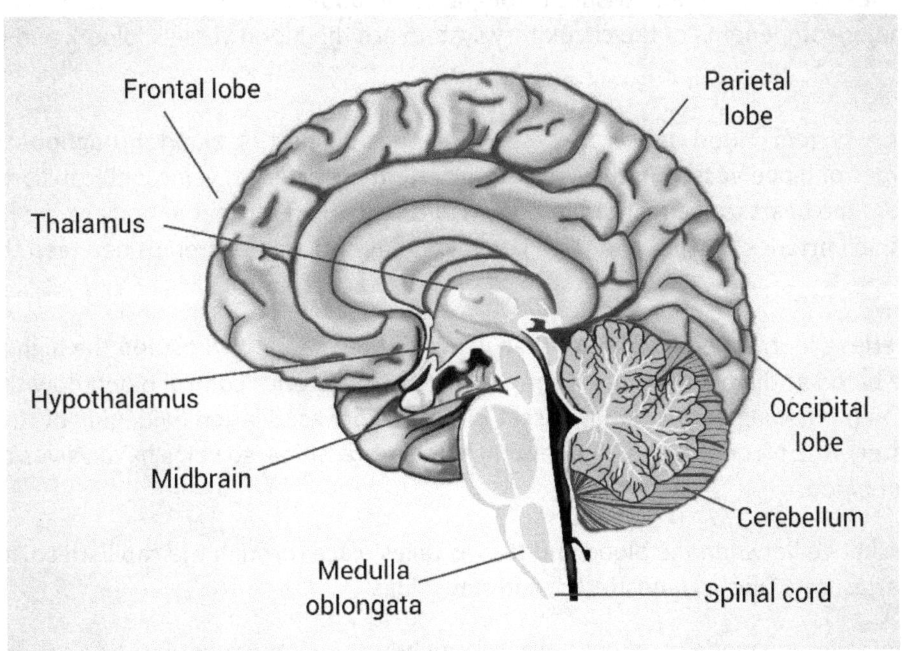

Autonomic Nervous System

The autonomic nervous system (ANS) governs involuntary, or reflexive, body functions. Ultimately, the autonomic nervous system controls functions such as breathing, heart rate, digestion, body temperature, and blood pressure.

The ANS is split between parasympathetic nerves and sympathetic nerves. These two nerve types are antagonistic, and have opposite effects on the body. *Parasympathetic* nerves typically are useful when resting or during safe conditions. They decrease heart rate and breath rate, prepare digestion, and allow urination and excretion. *Sympathetic* nerves, on the other hand, become active when a person is under stress or excited, and they increase heart rate and respiration rate, and inhibit digestion, urination, and excretion.

Somatic Nervous System and the Reflex Arc

The somatic nervous system (SNS) governs the conscious, or voluntary, control of skeletal muscles and their corresponding body movements. The SNS contains afferent and efferent neurons. Afferent neurons carry sensory messages from the skeletal muscles, skin, or sensory organs to the CNS. *Efferent neurons relay motor messages from the CNS to skeletal muscles, skin, or sensory organs.*

The SNS also has a role in involuntary movements called reflexes. A *reflex* is defined as an involuntary response to a stimulus. They are transmitted via what is termed a *reflex arc*, where a stimulus is sensed by an affector and its afferent neuron, interpreted and rerouted by an interneuron, and delivered to effector muscles by an efferent neuron, where the response to the initial stimulus is carried out. A reflex is able to bypass the brain by being rerouted through the spinal cord; the interneuron decides the proper course of action rather than the brain. The reflex arc results in an instantaneous, involuntary response. For example, a physician tapping on the knee produces an involuntary knee jerk referred to as the patellar tendon reflex.

Circulatory System

The circulatory system is a network of organs and tubes that transport blood, hormones, nutrients, oxygen, and other gases to cells and tissues throughout the body. It is also known as the cardiovascular system. The major components of the circulatory system are the blood vessels, blood, and heart.

Blood Vessels

In the circulatory system, blood vessels are responsible for transporting blood throughout the body. The three major types of blood vessels in the circulatory system are arteries, veins, and capillaries. *Arteries* carry blood from the heart to the rest of the body. *Veins* carry blood from the body to the heart. *Capillaries* connect arteries to veins and form networks that exchange materials between the blood and the cells.

In general, arteries are stronger and thicker than veins, as they need to withstand the high pressures exerted by the blood as the heart pumps it through the body. Arteries control blood flow through either vasoconstriction (narrowing of the blood vessel's diameter) or vasodilation (widening of the blood vessel's diameter). The blood in veins is under much lower pressures, so veins have valves to prevent the backflow of blood.

Most of the exchange between the blood and tissues takes place through the capillaries. There are three types of capillaries: continuous, fenestrated, and sinusoidal.

Continuous capillaries are made up of epithelial cells tightly connected together. As a result, they limit the types of substances that pass into and out of the blood. Continuous capillaries are the most common type of capillary. *Fenestrated capillaries* have openings that allow materials to be freely exchanged between the blood and tissues. They are commonly found in the digestive, endocrine, and urinary systems. *Sinusoidal capillaries* have larger openings and allow proteins and blood cells through. They are found primarily in the liver, bone marrow, and spleen.

Blood

Blood is vital to the human body. It is a liquid connective tissue that serves as a transport system for supplying cells with nutrients and carrying away their wastes. The average adult human has five to six quarts of blood circulating through their body. Approximately 55% of blood is plasma (the fluid portion), and the remaining 45% is composed of solid cells and cell parts. There are three major types of blood cells:

1. Red blood cells, or erythrocytes, transport oxygen throughout the body. They contain a protein called hemoglobin that allows them to carry oxygen. The iron in the hemoglobin gives the cells and the blood their red colors.

2. White blood cells, or leukocytes, are responsible for fighting infectious diseases and maintaining the immune system. There are five types of white blood cells: neutrophils, lymphocytes, eosinophils, monocytes, and basophils.

3. Platelets are cell fragments which play a central role in the blood clotting process.

All blood cells in adults are produced in the bone marrow—red blood cells from red marrow and white blood cells from yellow marrow.

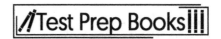

Heart

The heart is a two-part, muscular pump that forcefully pushes blood throughout the human body. The human heart has four chambers—two upper *atria* and two lower *ventricles*, a pair on the left and a pair on the right. Anatomically, *left* and *right* correspond to the sides of the body that the patient themselves would refer to as left and right.

Four valves help to section off the chambers from one another. Between the right atrium and ventricle, the three flaps of the *tricuspid valve* keep blood from backflowing from the ventricle to the atrium, similar to how the two flaps of the *mitral valve* work between the left atrium and ventricle. As these two valves lie between an atrium and a ventricle, they are referred to as *atrioventricular (AV) valves*. The other two valves are *semilunar (SL)*, and they control blood flow into the two great arteries leaving the ventricles. The pulmonary valve connects the right ventricle to the pulmonary artery while the aortic valve connects the left ventricle to the aorta.

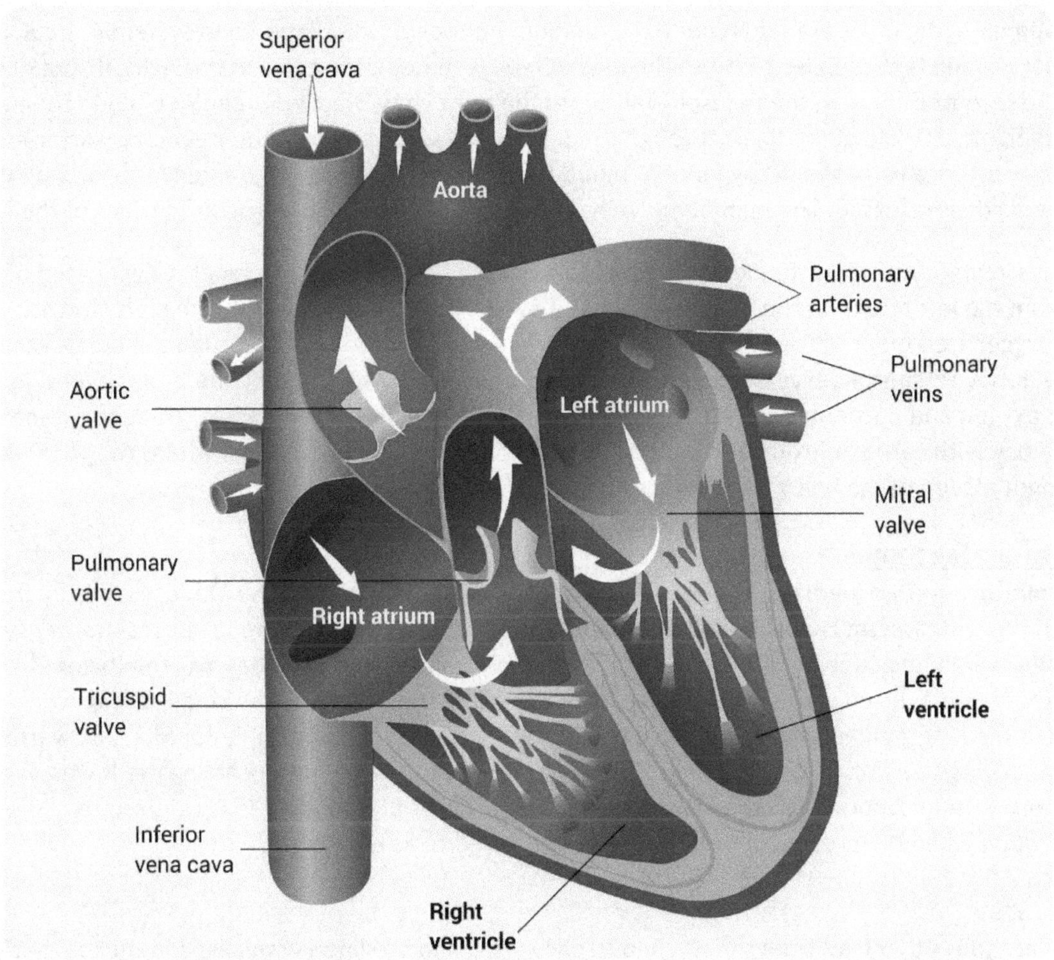

Cardiac Cycle

A cardiac cycle is one complete sequence of cardiac activity. The cardiac cycle represents the relaxation and contraction of the heart and can be divided into two phases: diastole and systole.

Diastole is the phase during which the heart relaxes and fills with blood. It gives rise to the diastolic blood pressure (DBP), which is the bottom number of a blood pressure reading. *Systole* is the phase during which the heart contracts and discharges blood. It gives rise to the systolic blood pressure (SBP), which is the top number of a blood pressure reading. The heart's electrical conduction system coordinates the cardiac cycle.

Types of Circulation

Five major blood vessels manage blood flow to and from the heart: the superior and inferior venae cava, the aorta, the pulmonary artery, and the pulmonary vein.

The superior vena cava is a large vein that drains blood from the head and the upper body. The inferior vena cava is a large vein that drains blood from the lower body. The aorta is the largest artery in the human body. It carries blood from the heart to body tissues. The pulmonary arteries carry blood from the heart to the lungs. The pulmonary veins transport blood from the lungs to the heart.

In the human body, there are two types of circulation: pulmonary circulation and systemic circulation. Pulmonary circulation supplies blood to the lungs. Deoxygenated blood enters the right atrium of the heart and is routed through the tricuspid valve into the right ventricle. Deoxygenated blood then travels from the right ventricle of the heart through the pulmonary valve and into the pulmonary arteries. The pulmonary arteries carry the deoxygenated blood to the lungs. In the lungs, oxygen is absorbed, and carbon dioxide is released. The pulmonary veins carry oxygenated blood to the left atrium of the heart.

Systemic circulation supplies blood to all other parts of the body, except the lungs. Oxygenated blood flows from the left atrium of the heart through the mitral, or bicuspid, valve into the left ventricle of the heart. Oxygenated blood is then routed from the left ventricle of the heart through the aortic valve and into the aorta. The aorta delivers blood to the systemic arteries, which supply the body tissues. In the tissues, oxygen and nutrients are exchanged for carbon dioxide and other wastes. The deoxygenated blood, along with carbon dioxide and waste products, enter the systemic veins, where they are returned to the right atrium of the heart via the superior and inferior vena cava.

Respiratory System

The respiratory system mediates the exchange of gas between the air and the blood, mainly by the act of breathing. This system is divided into the upper respiratory system and the lower respiratory system. The upper system includes the nose, the nasal cavity and sinuses, and the pharynx. The lower respiratory system includes the larynx (voice box), the trachea (windpipe), the small passageways leading to the lungs, and the lungs. The upper respiratory system is responsible for filtering, warming, and humidifying the air that gets passed to the lower respiratory system, protecting the lower respiratory system's more delicate tissue surfaces. The process of breathing in is referred to as *inspiration* while the process of breathing out is referred to as *expiration*.

The Lungs

Bronchi are tubes that lead from the trachea to each lung, and are lined with cilia and mucus that collect dust and germs along the way. The bronchi, which carry air into the lungs, branch into bronchioles and continue to divide into smaller and smaller passageways, until they become alveoli, which are the smallest passages. Most of the gas exchange in the lungs occurs between the blood-filled pulmonary capillaries and the air-filled alveoli. Within the lungs, oxygen and carbon dioxide are exchanged between the air in the alveoli and the blood in the pulmonary capillaries. Oxygen-rich blood returns to the heart and is pumped through the systemic circuit. Carbon dioxide-rich air is exhaled from the body. Together,

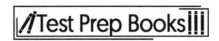

the lungs contain approximately 1,500 miles of airway passages, and this extremely large amount is due to the enormous amount of branching.

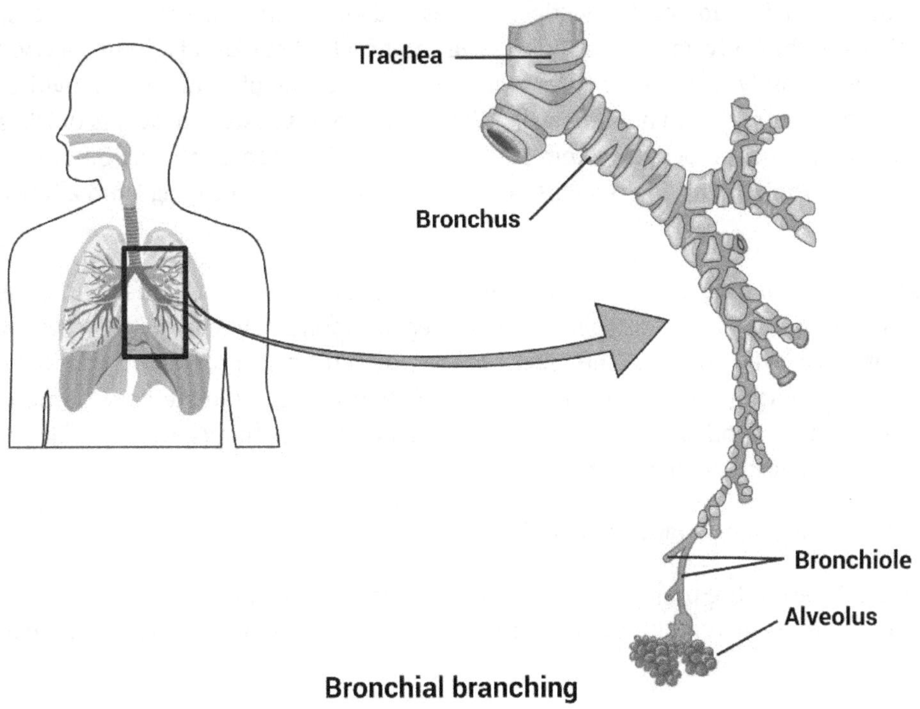

Bronchial branching

Breathing

When a breath of air is inhaled, oxygen enters the nose or mouth, and passes into the sinuses, where the temperature and humidity of the air are regulated. The air then passes into the trachea and is filtered. From there, the air travels into the bronchi and reaches the lungs. Bronchi are tubes that lead from the trachea to each lung, and are lined with cilia and mucus that collect dust and germs along the way. Within the lungs, oxygen and carbon dioxide are exchanged between the air in the alveoli and the blood in the pulmonary capillaries. Oxygen-rich blood returns to the heart and is pumped through the systemic circuit. Carbon dioxide-rich air is exhaled from the body.

Breathing is possible due to the muscular diaphragm contracting downward, which expands the space in the thoracic cavity. This allows the lungs to inhale, increasing their volume and decreasing their pressure. Air flows from the external high-pressure system to the low-pressure system inside the lungs. When breathing out, the diaphragm releases its pressure difference, decreases the lung volume, and forces the stale air back out.

Functions of the Respiratory System

The respiratory system has many functions. Most importantly, it provides a large area for gas exchange between the air and the circulating blood. It protects the delicate respiratory surfaces from environmental variations and defends them against pathogens. It is responsible for producing the sounds that the body makes for speaking and singing, as well as for non-verbal communication. It also helps regulate blood volume and blood pressure by releasing vasopressin, and it is a regulator of blood pH due to its control over carbon dioxide release, as the aqueous form of carbon dioxide is the chief buffering agent in blood.

Endocrine System

The endocrine system is made of the ductless tissues and glands that secrete hormones into the interstitial fluids of the body. Interstitial fluid is the solution that surrounds tissue cells within the body. This system works closely with the nervous system to regulate the physiological activities of the other systems of the body to maintain homeostasis. While the nervous system provides quick, short-term responses to stimuli, the endocrine system acts by releasing hormones into the bloodstream that get distributed to the whole body. The response is slow but long-lasting, ranging from a few hours to a few weeks.

Hormones are chemical substances that change the metabolic activity of tissues and organs. While regular metabolic reactions are controlled by enzymes, hormones can change the type, activity, or quantity of the enzymes involved in the reaction. They bind to specific cells and start a biochemical chain of events that changes the enzymatic activity. Hormones can regulate development and growth, digestive metabolism, mood, and body temperature, among other things. Often small amounts of hormone will lead to large changes in the body.

The following are the major endocrine glands:

Hypothalamus: A part of the brain, the hypothalamus connects the nervous system to the endocrine system via the pituitary gland. Although it is considered part of the nervous system, it plays a dual role in regulating endocrine organs.

Pituitary Gland: A pea-sized gland found at the bottom of the hypothalamus. It has two lobes, called the anterior and posterior lobes. It plays an important role in regulating the function of other endocrine glands. The hormones released control growth, blood pressure, certain functions of the sex organs, salt concentration of the kidneys, internal temperature regulation, and pain relief.

Thyroid Gland: This gland releases hormones, such as thyroxine, that are important for metabolism, growth and development, temperature regulation, and brain development during infancy and childhood. Thyroid hormones also monitor the amount of circulating calcium in the body.

Parathyroid Glands: These are four pea-sized glands located on the posterior surface of the thyroid. The main hormone secreted is called parathyroid hormone (PTH), which helps with the thyroid's regulation of calcium in the body.

Thymus Gland: The thymus is located in the chest cavity, embedded in connective tissue. It produces several hormones important for development and maintenance of normal immunological defenses. One hormone promotes the development and maturation of lymphocytes, which strengthens the immune system.

Adrenal Gland: One adrenal gland is attached to the top of each kidney. It produces adrenaline and is responsible for the "fight or flight" reactions in the face of danger or stress. The hormones epinephrine and norepinephrine cooperate to regulate states of arousal.

Pancreas: The pancreas is an organ that has both endocrine and exocrine functions. The endocrine functions are controlled by the pancreatic islets of Langerhans, which are groups of beta cells scattered throughout the gland that secrete insulin to lower blood sugar levels in the body. Neighboring alpha cells secrete glucagon to raise blood sugar.

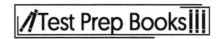

Pineal Gland: The pineal gland secretes melatonin, a hormone derived from the neurotransmitter serotonin. Melatonin can slow the maturation of sperm, oocytes, and reproductive organs. It also regulates the body's circadian rhythm, which is the natural awake/asleep cycle. It also serves an important role in protecting the CNS tissues from neural toxins.

Testes and Ovaries: These glands secrete testosterone and estrogen, respectively, and are responsible for secondary sex characteristics, as well as reproduction.

Digestive System

The human body relies completely on the digestive system to meet its nutritional needs. After food and drink are ingested, the digestive system breaks them down into their component nutrients and absorbs them so that the circulatory system can transport them to other cells to use for growth, energy, and cell repair. These nutrients may be classified as proteins, lipids, carbohydrates, vitamins, and minerals.

The digestive system is thought of chiefly in two parts: the digestive tract (also called the alimentary tract or gastrointestinal tract) and the accessory digestive organs. The digestive tract is the pathway in which food is ingested, digested, absorbed, and excreted. It is composed of the mouth, pharynx, esophagus, stomach, small and large intestines, rectum, and anus. *Peristalsis*, or wave-like contractions of smooth muscle, moves food and wastes through the digestive tract. The accessory digestive organs are the salivary glands, liver, gallbladder, and pancreas.

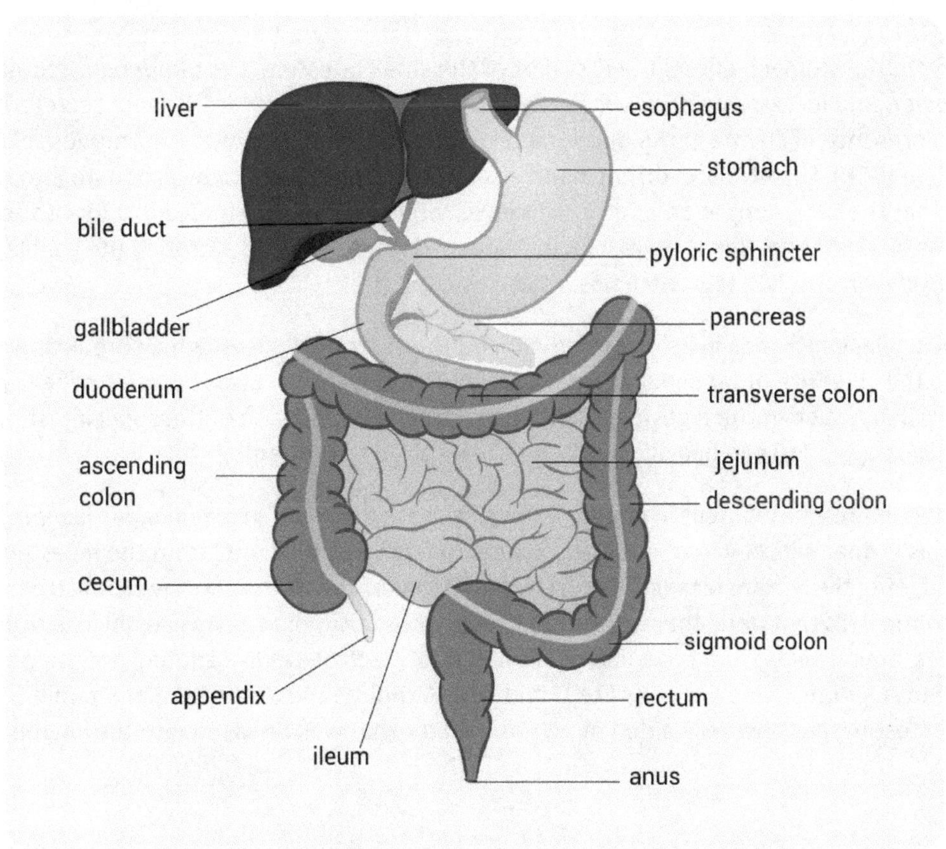

Mouth and Stomach

The mouth is the entrance to the digestive system. Here, the mechanical and chemical digestion of the ingested food begins. The food is chewed mechanically by the teeth and shaped into a *bolus* by the tongue so that it can be more easily swallowed by the esophagus. The food also becomes more watery and pliable with the addition of saliva secreted from the salivary glands, the largest of which are the parotid glands. The glands also secrete amylase in the saliva, an enzyme that begins chemical digestion and breakdown of the carbohydrates and sugars in the food.

The food then moves through the pharynx and down the muscular esophagus to the stomach.

The stomach is a large, muscular sac-like organ at the distal end of the esophagus. Here, the bolus is subjected to more mechanical and chemical digestion. As it passes through the stomach, it is physically squeezed and crushed while additional secretions turn it into a watery nutrient-filled liquid that exits into the small intestine as *chyme*.

The stomach secretes many substances into the *lumen* of the digestive tract. Some cells produce gastrin, a hormone that prompts other cells in the stomach to secrete a gastric acid composed mostly of hydrochloric acid (HCl). The HCl is at such a high concentration and low pH that it denatures most proteins and degrades a lot of organic matter. The stomach also secretes mucous to form a protective film that keeps the corrosive acid from dissolving its own cells. Gaps in this mucous layer can lead to peptic ulcers. Finally, the stomach also uses digestive enzymes like proteases and lipases to break down proteins and fats; although there are some gastric lipases here, the stomach is most known for breaking down proteins.

Small Intestine

The chyme from the stomach enters the first part of the small intestine, the *duodenum*, through the *pyloric sphincter*, and its extreme acidity is partly neutralized by sodium bicarbonate secreted along with mucous. The presence of chyme in the duodenum triggers the secretion of the hormones secretin and cholecystokinin (CCK). Secretin acts on the pancreas to dump more sodium bicarbonate into the small intestine so that the pH is kept at an appropriate level, while CCK acts on the gallbladder to release the *bile* that it has been storing. Bile is a substance produced by the liver and stored in the gallbladder which helps to *emulsify,* or dissolve, fats and lipids.

Because of the bile, which aids in lipid absorption, and the secreted lipases, which break down fats, the duodenum is the chief site of fat digestion in the body. The duodenum also represents the last major site of chemical digestion in the digestive tract, as the other two sections of the small intestine (the *jejunum* and *ileum*) are instead heavily involved in absorption of nutrients.

The small intestine reaches 40 feet in length, and its cells are arranged in small finger-like projections called *villi.* This is due to its key role in the absorption of nearly all nutrients from the ingested and digested food, effectively transferring them from the lumen of the GI tract to the bloodstream, where they travel to the cells that need them. These nutrients include simple sugars like glucose from carbohydrates, amino acids from proteins, emulsified fats, electrolytes like sodium and potassium, minerals like iron and zinc, and vitamins like D and B12. Although the absorption of vitamin B12 takes place in the intestines, it is actually aided by *intrinsic factor* that was released into the chyme back in the stomach.

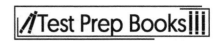

Large Intestine

The leftover parts of food that remain unabsorbed or undigested in the lumen of the small intestine next travel through the large intestine, which may also be referred to as the large bowel or colon. The large intestine is mainly responsible for water absorption. As the chyme at this stage no longer has anything useful that can be absorbed by the body, it is now referred to as *waste*, and it is stored in the large intestine until it can be excreted from the body. Removing the liquid from the waste transforms it from liquid to solid stool, or feces.

This waste first passes from the small intestine to the *cecum*, a pouch which forms the first part of the large intestine. In herbivores, it provides a place for bacteria to digest cellulose, but in humans most of it is vestigial and is known as the appendix. From the cecum, waste next travels up the ascending colon, across the transverse colon, down the descending colon, and through the sigmoid colon to the rectum. The rectum is responsible for the final storage of waste before being expelled through the anus. The anal canal is a small portion of the rectum leading through to the anus and the outside of the body.

Pancreas

The pancreas has endocrine and exocrine functions. The endocrine function involves releasing the hormones insulin, which decreases blood glucose levels, and glucagon, which increases blood glucose levels, directly into the bloodstream. Both hormones are produced in the islets of Langerhans—insulin in the beta cells and glucagon in the alpha cells.

The major part of the gland has an exocrine function, which consists of *acinar cells* secreting inactive digestive enzymes (zymogens) into the main pancreatic duct. The main pancreatic duct joins the common bile duct, which empties into the small intestine (specifically the duodenum). The digestive enzymes are then activated and take part in the digestion of carbohydrates, proteins, and fats within chyme (the mixture of partially digested food and digestive juices).

Integumentary System (Skin)

Skin consists of three layers: epidermis, dermis, and the hypodermis. There are four types of cells that make up the keratinized stratified squamous epithelium in the epidermis. They are keratinocytes, melanocytes, Merkel cells, and Langerhans cells. Skin is composed of many layers, starting with a basement membrane. On top of that sits the stratum germinativum, the stratum spinosum, the stratum granulosum, the stratum lucidum, and then the stratum corneum at the outer surface. Skin can be classified as thick or thin. These descriptions refer to the epidermis layer. Most of the body is covered with thin skin, but areas such as the palms are covered with thick skin. The dermis consists of a superficial papillary layer and a deeper reticular layer. The papillary layer is made of loose connective tissue, containing capillaries and the axons of sensory neurons. The reticular layer is a meshwork of tightly packed irregular connective tissue, containing blood vessels, hair follicles, nerves, sweat glands, and sebaceous glands. The hypodermis is a loose layer of fat and connective tissue. Since it is the third layer, if a burn reaches this third degree, it has caused serious damage.

Sweat glands and sebaceous glands are important exocrine glands found in the skin. Sweat glands regulate temperature, and remove bodily waste by secreting water, nitrogenous waste, and sodium salts to the surface of the body. Some sweat glands are classified as apocrine glands. Sebaceous glands are holocrine glands that secrete sebum, which is an oily mixture of lipids and proteins. Sebum protects the skin from water loss, as well as bacterial and fungal infections.

The three major functions of skin are protection, regulation, and sensation. Skin acts as a barrier and protects the body from mechanical impacts, variations in temperature, microorganisms, and chemicals.

It regulates body temperature, peripheral circulation, and fluid balance by secreting sweat. It also contains a large network of nerve cells that relay changes in the external environment to the body.

Immune System

The immune system is the body's defense against invading microorganisms (bacteria, viruses, fungi, and parasites) and other harmful, foreign substances. It is capable of limiting or preventing infection.

As mentioned, there are two general types of immunity: innate immunity and acquired immunity. Innate immunity uses physical and chemical barriers to block the entry of microorganisms into the body. Some of these barriers include the skin, mucous membranes, saliva, tears, stomach acid, and certain white blood cells.

Acquired immunity, which consists of a primary and secondary response, refers to a specific set of events used by the body to fight a particular infection after previously encountering it before.

Urinary System

The urinary system is made up of the kidneys, ureters, urinary bladder, and the urethra. It is the main system responsible for getting rid of the organic waste products, excess water and electrolytes are generated by the body's other systems. The kidneys are responsible for producing urine, which is a fluid waste product containing water, ions, and small soluble compounds. The urinary system has many important functions related to waste excretion. It regulates the concentrations of sodium, potassium, chloride, calcium, and other ions in the plasma by controlling the amount of each excreted in urine. This also contributes to the maintenance of blood pH. The urinary system also regulates blood volume and pressure by controlling the amount of water lost in the urine, and releasing erythropoietin and renin. It eliminates toxic substances, drugs, and organic waste products, such as urea and uric acid. It also synthesizes calcitriol, which is a hormone derivative of vitamin D3 that aids in calcium ion absorption by the intestinal epithelium.

The Kidneys

Under normal circumstances, humans have two functioning kidneys. They are the main organs that are responsible for filtering waste products out of the blood and transferring them to urine. Every day, the kidneys filter approximately 120 to 150 quarts of blood and produce one to two quarts of urine. Kidneys are made of millions of tiny filtering units, called nephrons. *Nephrons* have two parts: a glomerulus, which is the filter, and a tubule. As blood enters the kidneys, the glomerulus allows fluid and waste products to pass through it and enter the tubule. Blood cells and large molecules, such as proteins, do not pass through and remain in the blood. The filtered fluid and waste then pass through the tubule, where any final essential minerals are sent back to the bloodstream. The final product at the end of the tubule is called *urine*.

Waste Excretion

Once urine accumulates, it leaves the kidneys. The urine travels through the ureters into the urinary bladder, a muscular organ that is hollow and elastic. As more urine enters the urinary bladder, its walls stretch and become thinner so there is no significant difference in internal pressure. The urinary bladder stores the urine until the body is ready for urination, at which time, the muscles contract and force the urine through the urethra and out of the body.

Reproductive System

The reproductive system is responsible for producing, storing, nourishing, and transporting functional reproductive cells, or gametes, in the human body. It includes the reproductive organs, also known as gonads, the reproductive tract, the accessory glands and organs that secrete fluids into the reproductive tract, and the perineal structures, which are the external genitalia.

The Male System

The male gonads are called testes. The testes secrete androgens, mainly testosterone, and produce and store 500 million spermatocytes, which are the male gametes, each day. An androgen is a steroid hormone that controls the development and maintenance of male characteristics. Once the sperm are mature, they move through a duct system, where they mix with additional fluids secreted by accessory glands, forming a mixture called semen.

The Female System

The female gonads are the ovaries. Ovaries generally produce one immature gamete, or oocyte, per month. They are also responsible for secreting the hormones estrogen and progesterone. When the oocyte is released from the ovary, it travels along the uterine tubes, or Fallopian tubes, and then into the uterus. The uterus opens into the vagina. When sperm cells enter the vagina, they swim through the uterus and may fertilize the oocyte in the Fallopian tubes. The resulting zygote travels down the tube and implants into the uterine wall. The uterus protects and nourishes the developing embryo for nine months until it is ready for the outside environment. If the oocyte is not fertilized, it is released in the uterine, or menstrual, cycle. The menstrual cycle occurs monthly and involves the shedding of the functional part of the uterine lining.

Mammary glands are a specialized accessory organ of the female reproductive system. The mammary glands are located in the breast tissue, and during pregnancy, they begin to grow, and the cells proliferate in preparation for lactation. After pregnancy, the cells begin to secrete nutrient-filled milk, which is transferred into a duct system and out through the nipple for nourishment of the baby.

Human Reproduction

Humans procreate through sexual reproduction. Sexual reproduction involves the fusion of gametes, one from each parent, through a process called fertilization. Gametes are created by the human reproductive systems. In women, the ovaries produce on average one mature egg per month, which is referred to as the menstrual cycle. The release of an egg from the ovaries is termed *ovulation*. The female menstrual cycle is under the control of hormones such as luteinizing hormone (LH), follicle stimulating hormone (FSH), estrogen, and progesterone. In men, the testes produce sperm, the male gamete, and they produce millions of sperm at a time. The hormones LH and testosterone regulate the production of sperm in the testes. Leydig cells in the testes produce testosterone, while sperm is manufactured in the seminiferous tubules of the testes.

The fusion of the gametes (egg and sperm) is termed *fertilization*, and the resulting fusion creates a *zygote*. The zygote takes approximately seven days to travel through the fallopian tube and implant itself into the uterus. Upon implantation, it has developed into a *blastocyst* and will next grow into a *gastrula*. It is during this stage that the embryological germ layers are formed. The three germ layers are the ectoderm (outer layer), mesoderm (middle layer), and endoderm (inner layer). All of the human body systems develop from one or more of the germ layers. The gastrula further develops into an *embryo,* which then matures into a fetus. The entire process takes approximately nine months and culminates in labor and birth.

Practice Questions

1. What is the theory that certain physical and behavioral survival traits give a species an evolutionary advantage called?
   a. Gradualism
   b. Evolutionary Advantage
   c. Punctuated Equilibrium
   d. Natural Selection

2. How can microorganisms be genetically identified in the laboratory?
   a. Light microscopy
   b. Immunoassay
   c. In culture
   d. Fluorescent staining

3. What is a metabolic reaction that releases energy called?
   a. Catabolic
   b. Thermodynamic
   c. Anabolic
   d. Endothermic

4. What organic compounds facilitate chemical reactions by lowering activation energy?
   a. Carbohydrates
   b. Lipids
   c. Enzymes
   d. Nucleotides

5. Which structure is exclusively in eukaryotic cells?
   a. Cell wall
   b. Nucleus
   c. Cell membrane
   d. Vacuole

6. Which of these is NOT found in the cell nucleus?
   a. Golgi complex
   b. Chromosomes
   c. Nucleolus
   d. Chromatin

7. Which of the following is the cellular organelle used for digestion to recycle materials?
   a. Golgi apparatus
   b. Lysosome
   c. Centriole
   d. Mitochondria

8. What are the energy-generating structures of the cell called?
    a. Nucleoplasms
    b. Mitochondria
    c. Golgi Apparatus
    d. Ribosomes

9. Which of the following is a component of plant cells NOT found in animal cells?
    a. Nucleus
    b. Plastid
    c. Cell membrane
    d. Cytoplasm

10. Diffusion and osmosis are examples of what type of transport mechanism?
    a. Active
    b. Passive
    c. Extracellular
    d. Intracellular

11. The combination of alleles of an organism, when expressed, manifests as the organism's what?
    a. Genotype
    b. Phenotype
    c. Genes
    d. Karyotype

12. Which of the choices below are the reproductive cells produced by meiosis?
    a. Genes
    b. Alleles
    c. Chromatids
    d. Gametes

13. What is the process of cell division in somatic (most body) cells called?
    a. Mitosis
    b. Meiosis
    c. Respiration
    d. Cytogenesis

14. When human cells divide by meiosis, how many chromosomes do the resulting cells contain?
    a. 96
    b. 54
    c. 46
    d. 23

15. Which choice is a consequence of tetrad formation in meiosis?
    a. Causes diversity
    b. Determines gender
    c. Causes non-disjunction
    d. Causes transcription

16. What is an alteration in the normal gene sequence called?
 a. DNA mutation
 b. Gene migration
 c. Polygenetic inheritance
 d. Incomplete dominance

17. Blood type is a trait determined by multiple alleles, and two of them are co-dominant: I^A codes for A blood and I^B codes for B blood. i codes for O blood and is recessive to both. If an A heterozygote individual and an O individual have a child, what is the probability that the child will have type A blood?
 a. 25%
 b. 50%
 c. 75%
 d. 100%

18. What are the building blocks of DNA referred to as?
 a. Helices
 b. Proteins
 c. Genes
 d. Nucleotides

19. Which statement is NOT true about RNA?
 a. It contains uracil.
 b. It has ribose sugar.
 c. It has uracil.
 d. It only exists in three forms.

20. What do microbiological tests detect when used as part of food-production supply chains?
 a. Artificial colors
 b. Germ content
 c. Radiation
 d. Temperature

21. What is the term used for the set of metabolic reactions that convert chemical bonds to energy in the form of ATP?
 a. Photosynthesis
 b. Reproduction
 c. Active transport
 d. Cellular respiration

22. What's the greatest concern when an individual contracts a GI infection?
 a. Fatigue
 b. Dehydration
 c. Rash
 d. Pain

23. What food preservation technique uses microorganisms to convert starch and sugar to alcohol?
 a. Vacuum packing
 b. Pasteurization
 c. Irradiation
 d. Fermentation

24. How do microorganisms function as a carbon sink?
   a. They take CO_2 from the atmosphere and store it underground.
   b. They convert N_2 to NH_3.
   c. They release carbon from underground sources into the atmosphere.
   d. They metabolize methane.

25. What is the cell structure responsible for protein synthesis called?
   a. DNA
   b. Golgi Apparatus
   c. Nucleus
   d. Ribosome

26. At which stage does an infection progress to a disease?
   a. The microorganism attaches to a target site in the body.
   b. The microorganism multiplies itself.
   c. The microorganism starts to cause damage to an individual's vital functions and systems.
   d. The microorganism obtains nutrients from the host.

27. Which type of vaccine is made from a fragment of a whole microorganism?
   a. Toxoid
   b. Inactivated
   c. Subunit
   d. DNA

28. Which statement is true?
   a. Ligaments attach skeletal muscles to bone.
   b. Tendons connect bones at joints.
   c. Cartilage adds mechanical support to joints.
   d. Most veins deliver oxygenated blood to cells.

29. Which layer of skin contains sensory receptors and blood vessels?
   a. Epidermis
   b. Dermis
   c. Hypodermis
   d. Subcutaneous

30. What locations in the digestive system are sites of chemical digestion?
   I. Mouth
   II. Stomach
   III. Small Intestine
   a. II only
   b. III only
   c. II and III only
   d. I, II, and III

31. The radius and ulna are to the humerus as the tibia and fibula are to which bone?
   a. Mandible
   b. Femur
   c. Scapula
   d. Carpal

32. What are concentric circles of bone tissue called?
   a. Lacunae
   b. Lamellae
   c. Trabeculae
   d. Diaphysis

33. When de-oxygenated blood first enters the heart, which of the following choices is in the correct order for its journey to the aorta?
   I. Tricuspid valve → Lungs → Mitral valve
   II. Mitral valve → Lungs → Tricuspid valve
   III. Right ventricle → Lungs → Left atrium
   IV. Left ventricle → Lungs → Right atrium
   a. I and III only
   b. I and IV only
   c. II and III only
   d. II and IV only

34. Which characteristics are true for skeletal muscle?
   I. Contain sarcomeres
   II. Have multiple nuclei
   III. Are branched
   a. I only
   b. I and II only
   c. I, II, and III only
   d. II and III only

35. Which is the simplest nerve pathway that bypasses the brain?
   a. Autonomic
   b. Reflex arc
   c. Somatic
   d. Sympathetic

36. What is the order of filtration in the nephron?
   a. Collecting Duct → Proximal tubule → Loop of Henle
   b. Proximal tubule → Loop of Henle → Collecting duct
   c. Loop of Henle → Collecting duct → Proximal tubule
   d. Loop of Henle → Proximal tubule → Collecting duct

37. Which function below corresponds to the parasympathetic nervous system?
   a. Stimulates the fight-or-flight response
   b. Increases heart rate
   c. Stimulates digestion
   d. Increases bronchiole dilation

38. Which of the following neurons transmit signals from the CNS to effector tissues and organs?
   a. Motor
   b. Sensory
   c. Interneuron
   d. Reflex

39. Which statement is NOT true regarding brain structure?
  a. The corpus collosum connects the hemispheres.
  b. Broca and Wernicke's areas are associated with speech and language.
  c. The cerebellum is important for long-term memory storage.
  d. The brainstem is responsible for involuntary movement.

40. Which is NOT a function of the pancreas?
  a. Secretes the hormone insulin in response to growth hormone stimulation
  b. Secretes bicarbonate into the small intestine to raise the pH from stomach secretions
  c. Secretes enzymes used by the small intestine to digest fats, sugars, and proteins
  d. Secretes hormones from its endocrine portion in order to regulate blood sugar levels

41. Which organ is NOT a component of the lymphatic system?
  a. Thymus
  b. Spleen
  c. Tonsil
  d. Gall bladder

42. Which action is unrelated to blood pH?
  a. Exhalation of carbon dioxide
  b. Kidney reabsorption of bicarbonate
  c. ADH secretion
  d. Nephron secretion of ammonia

43. Which gland regulates calcium levels?
  a. Thyroid
  b. Pineal
  c. Adrenal
  d. Parathyroid

44. What are the functions of the hypothalamus?
    I. Regulate body temperature
    II. Send stimulatory and inhibitory instructions to the pituitary gland
    III. Receive sensory information from the brain
  a. I and II
  b. I and III
  c. II and III
  d. I, II, and III

45. Which muscle system is unlike the others?
  a. Biceps : Triceps
  b. Quadriceps : Hamstrings
  c. Gluteus maximus : Gluteus minimus
  d. Trapezius/Rhomboids : Pectoralis major

46. Which blood component is chiefly responsible for clotting?
  a. Platelets
  b. Red blood cells
  c. Antigens
  d. Plasma cells

47. Which is the first event to happen in a primary immune response?
    a. Macrophages phagocytose pathogens and present their antigens.
    b. Neutrophils aggregate and act as cytotoxic, nonspecific killers of pathogens.
    c. B lymphocytes make pathogen-specific antibodies.
    d. Helper T cells secrete interleukins to activate pathogen-fighting cells.

48. Where does sperm maturation take place in the male reproductive system?
    a. Seminal vesicles
    b. Prostate gland
    c. Epididymis
    d. Vas Deferens

49. Which hormone in the female reproductive system is responsible for progesterone production?
    a. FSH
    b. LH
    c. hCG
    d. Estrogen

50. Which epithelial tissue comprises the cell layer found in a capillary bed?
    a. Squamous
    b. Cuboidal
    c. Columnar
    d. Stratified

51. What type of archaeal species uses inorganic compounds as an energy source?
    a. Lithotrophs
    b. Organotrophs
    c. Phototrophs
    d. Eukaryotes

52. How are bacteria beneficial to the environment?
    a. They act as parasites and spread disease.
    b. They multiply rapidly.
    c. They turn nitrogen from the air into organic compounds that plants use as energy.
    d. They prevent the decay of landfill materials.

53. How do bacteria reproduce?
    a. Meiosis
    b. Binary fission
    c. Absorbing another microorganism
    d. Mitosis

54. How does serology help with identification of infection diseases?
    a. The number of red blood cells can be determined.
    b. It can help determine if a disease was contracted directly or indirectly.
    c. It involves disinfecting the blood.
    d. Antibodies within the blood serum can be identified.

55. Which does NOT describe how an antimicrobial agent works?
    a. They disrupt the inside of the microorganism.
    b. They inhibit microbial growth.
    c. They attack the host.
    d. They inhibit microbial reproduction.

Answer Explanations

1. D: The theory that certain physical and behavioral traits give a species an evolutionary advantage is called natural selection. Charles Darwin developed the theory of natural selection, which explains the evolutionary process. He postulated that heritable genetic differences could aid an organism's chance of survival in its environment. The organisms with favorable traits pass genes to their offspring, and because they have more reproductive success than those that do not carry the adaptation, the favorable gene spreads throughout the population. Those that do not contain the adaptation often perish prematurely; thus, their genes are not passed on. In this way, nature "selects" for the organisms that have more fitness in their environment. Birds with bright colored feathers and cacti with spines are examples of "fit" organisms.

2. B: Genetic identification of microorganisms can happen by immunoassay, which looks at the nucleic acid structure of the microbes. Light microscopy and fluorescent staining illuminate the appearance and physical characteristics of different strains. Culturing microorganisms allows microbiologists to see the growth patterns of the microbes.

3. A: Catabolic reactions release energy and are exothermic. Catabolism breaks down complex molecules into simpler molecules. Anabolic reactions are just the opposite—they absorb energy in order to form complex molecules from simpler ones. Proteins, carbohydrates (polysaccharides), lipids, and nucleic acids are complex organic molecules synthesized by anabolic metabolism. The monomers of these organic compounds are amino acids, monosaccharides, triglycerides, and nucleotides.

4. C: Metabolic reactions utilize enzymes to decrease their activation energy. Enzymes that drive these reactions are proteins catalysts. Their mechanism is sometimes referred to as the "lock-and-key" model. "Lock and key" references the fact that enzymes have exact specificity with their substrate (reactant) like a lock does to a key. The substrate binds to the enzyme snugly, the enzyme facilitates the reaction, and then product is formed while the enzyme is unchanged and ready to be reused.

5. B: The structure exclusively found in eukaryotic cells is the nucleus. Animal, plant, fungi, and protist cells are all eukaryotic. DNA is contained within the nucleus of eukaryotic cells, and they also have membrane-bound organelles that perform complex intracellular metabolic activities. Prokaryotic cells (archaea and bacteria) do not have a nucleus or other membrane-bound organelles and are less complex than eukaryotic cells.

6. A: The Golgi complex, also known as the Golgi apparatus, is not found in the nucleus. Chromosomes, the nucleolus, and chromatin are all found within the nucleus of the cell. The Golgi apparatus is found in the cytoplasm and is responsible for protein maturation, the process of proteins folding into their secondary, tertiary, and quaternary configurations. The structure appears folded in membranous layers and is easily visible with microscopy. The Golgi apparatus packages proteins in vesicles for export out of the cell or to their cellular destination.

7. B: The cell structure responsible for cellular storage, digestion, and waste removal is the lysosome. Lysosomes are like recycle bins. They are filled with digestive enzymes that facilitate catabolic reactions to regenerate monomers.

8. B: The mitochondria are cellular energy generators and the "powerhouses" of the cell. They provide cellular energy in the form of adenosine triphosphate (ATP). This process, called aerobic respiration, uses oxygen plus sugars, proteins, and fats to produce ATP, carbon dioxide, and water. Mitochondria contain their own DNA and ribosomes, which is significant because according to endosymbiotic theory, these structures provide evidence that they used to be independently-functioning prokaryotes.

9. B: Plastids are the photosynthesizing organelles of plants that are not found in animal cells. Plants have the ability to generate their own sugars through photosynthesis, a process where they use pigments to capture the sun's light energy. Chloroplasts are the most prevalent plastid, and chlorophyll is the light-absorbing pigment that absorbs all energy carried in photons except that of green light. This explains why the photosynthesizing parts of plants, predominantly leaves, appear green.

10. B: Diffusion and osmosis are examples of passive transport. Unlike active transport, passive transport does not require cellular energy. Diffusion is the movement of particles, such as ions, nutrients, or waste, from high concentration to low ones. Osmosis is the spontaneous movement of water from an area of high concentration to one of low concentration. Facilitated diffusion is another type of passive transport where particles move from high concentration to low concentration via a protein channel.

11. B: Phenotypes are observable traits, such as eye color, hair color, blood type, etc. They can also be biochemical or have physiological or behavioral traits. A genotype is the collective gene representation of an individual, whether the genes are expressed or not. Alleles are different forms of the same gene that code for specific traits, like blue eyes or brown eyes. In simple genetics, there are two forms of a gene: dominant and recessive. More complex genetics involves co-dominance, multiple alleles and sex-linked genes. The other answer choices are incorrect because gender is determined by the presence of an entire chromosome, the Y chromosome, and a karyotype is an image of all of individual's chromosomes.

12. D: Reproductive cells are referred to as gametes: egg (female) and sperm (male). These cells have only one set of 23 chromosomes and are haploid so that when they combine during fertilization, the zygote has the correct diploid number, 46. Reproductive cell division is called meiosis, which is different from mitosis, the type of division process for body (somatic) cells.

13. A: The process of cell division in somatic is mitosis. In interphase, which precedes mitosis, cells prepare for division by copying their DNA. Once mitotic machinery has been assembled in interphase, mitosis occurs, which has five distinct phases: prophase, prometaphase, metaphase, anaphase, and telophase, followed by cytokinesis, which is the final splitting of the cytoplasm. The two diploid daughter cells are genetically identical to the parent cell.

14. D: Human gametes each contain 23 chromosomes. This is referred to as haploid—half the number of the original germ cell (46). Germ cells are diploid precursors of the haploid egg and sperm. Meiosis has two major phases, each of which is characterized by sub-phases similar to mitosis. In Meiosis I, the DNA of the parent cell is duplicated in interphase, just like in mitosis. Starting with prophase I, things become a little different. Two homologous chromosomes form a tetrad, cross over, and exchange genetic content. Each shuffled chromosome of the tetrad migrates to the cell's poles, and two haploid daughter cells are formed. In Meiosis II, each daughter undergoes another division more similar to mitosis (with the exception of the fact that there is no interphase), resulting in four genetically-different cells, each with only half of the chromosomal material of the original germ cell.

15. A: The crossing over, or rearrangement of chromosomal sections in tetrads during meiosis, results in each gamete having a different combination of alleles than other gametes. Choice *B* is incorrect because the presence of a Y chromosome determines gender. Choice *C* is incorrect because it is improper separation in anaphase, not recombination, that causes non-disjunction. Choice *D* is incorrect because transcription is an entirely different process involved in protein expression.

16. A: An alteration in the normal gene sequence is called a DNA point mutation. Mutations can be harmful, neutral, or even beneficial. Sometimes, as seen in natural selection, a genetic mutation can improve fitness, providing an adaptation that will aid in survival. DNA mutations can happen as a result of environmental damage, for example, from radiation or chemicals. Mutations can also happen during cell replication, as a result of incorrect pairing of complementary nucleotides by DNA polymerase. There are also chromosomal mutations as well, where entire segments of chromosomes can be deleted, inverted, duplicated, or sent or received from a different chromosome.

17. B: 50%. According to the Punnett square, the child has a 2 out of 4 chance of having A-type blood, since the dominant allele I^A is present in two of the four possible offspring. The O-type blood allele is masked by the A-type blood allele since it is recessive.

I^A i	ii
I^A i	ii

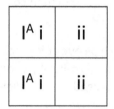

18. D: The building blocks of DNA are nucleotides. A nucleotide is a five-carbon sugar with a phosphate group and a nitrogenous base (Adenine, Guanine, Cytosine, and Thymine). DNA is a double helix and looks like a spiral ladder. Each side has a sugar/phosphate backbone, and the rungs of the ladder that connect the sides are the nitrogenous bases. Adenine always pairs with thymine via two hydrogen bonds, and cytosine always pairs with guanine via three hydrogen bonds. The weak hydrogen bonds are important because they allow DNA to easily be opened for replication and transcription.

19. D: There are actually many different types of RNA. The three involved in protein synthesis are messenger RNA (mRNA), ribosomal RNA (rRNA), and transfer RNA (tRNA). Others, including small interfering RNA, micro RNA, and piwi associated RNA, are being investigated. Their known functions include gene regulation, facilitating chromosome wrapping, and unwrapping. RNA can be single stranded (such as mRNA), and unlike DNA, has a ribose sugar (rather than deoxyribose in DNA), and contains uracil (in place of thymine).

20. B: Microbiological tests are an important part of food production. They help to ensure that food products are safe to consume and free of microorganisms. These tests detect germ content, yeasts, and spoilage organisms. They don't solely test temperature or look for artificial colors. Irradiation is a method to preserve food.

21. D: Cellular respiration is the term used for the set of metabolic reactions that convert chemical bonds to energy in the form of ATP. All respiration starts with glycolysis in the cytoplasm, and in the presence of oxygen, the process will continue to the mitochondria. In a series of oxidation/reduction reactions, primarily glucose will be broken down so that the energy contained within its bonds can be transferred to the smaller ATP molecules. It's like having a $100 bill (glucose) as opposed to having one hundred $1 bills. This is beneficial to the organism because it allows energy to be distributed throughout the cell very easily in smaller packets of energy.

When glucose is broken down, its electrons and hydrogen atoms are involved in oxidative phosphorylation in order to make ATP, while its carbon and oxygen atoms are released as carbon dioxide. Anaerobic respiration does not occur frequently in humans, but during rigorous exercise, lack of available oxygen in the muscles can lead to anaerobic ATP production in a process called lactic acid fermentation. Alcohol fermentation is another type of anaerobic respiration that occurs in yeast. Anaerobic respiration is much less efficient than aerobic respiration, as it has a net yield of 2ATP, while aerobic respiration's net yield exceeds 30 ATP.

22. B: The largest worry with GI infections is dehydration. When a virus, bacteria, or parasite attacks the GI system, it is often hard for the host to retain food or water. They lack nutrient intake along with hydration. Without adequate hydration, many of the body's systems may stop functioning properly. Rashes aren't common with GI infections. Pain and fatigue may be other side effects of a GI infection.

23. D: Fermentation is the process of using microorganisms to convert starch and sugar to alcohol. This creates an environment that's toxic to all microorganisms, including those used for the conversion of starch and sugar, so that nothing can live or multiply in the food product. Vacuum packing involves sealing packages of food without any air in them. Pasteurization involves heating food to a certain temperature and for a certain period in order to kill pathogenic bacteria. Irradiation involves the application of ionizing radiation to food products in order to kill microorganisms.

24. A: Microorganisms function as a carbon sink by taking CO_2 from the atmosphere and storing it underground for long periods of time. Reducing the amount of carbon in the air is beneficial to the environment by reducing the greenhouse gases trapped inside the Earth's atmosphere. The process of turning gaseous nitrogen to ammonia is called nitrogen fixation. While methane metabolism is an important process that microorganisms help with, it's not part of the carbon sink process.

25. D: Ribosomes are the structures responsible for protein synthesis using amino acids delivered by tRNA molecules. They are numerous within the cell and can take up as much as 25% of the cell. Ribosomes are found free-floating in the cytoplasm and also attached to the rough endoplasmic reticulum, which resides alongside the nucleus. Ribosomes translate messenger RNA into chains of amino acids that become proteins. Ribosomes themselves are made of protein, as well as rRNA. Choice *B* might be an attractive choice, since the Golgi apparatus is the site of protein maturation; however, it is not where proteins are synthesized. Choice *A* might be an attractive choice as well because DNA provides the instructions for proteins to be made, but DNA does not make the protein itself.

26. C: Infections begin with a microorganism entering the body and reaching its target site. The microorganism then multiplies and begins to use the host's resources for nutrition. Once the individual's vital functions and systems start to get affected by the infection, it progresses to a disease state. Each disease has a specific set of symptoms that are the result of that microorganism attacking that location in the body.

27. C: A subunit vaccine is made from a fragment of a whole microorganism that is still large enough to cause an effective immune response to develop immunity from the disease. A toxoid vaccine is developed from an inactive, toxic compound, not from a microorganism. An inactivated vaccine is developed from an inactive microorganism that causes disease. A DNA vaccine is a genetically-engineered strand of DNA that can be injected into an individual and causes the individual's cells to produce a specific antigen.

28. C: Cartilage adds mechanical support to joints. It provides a flexible cushion that aids in mobility while offering support. The first two choices are switched—it is ligaments that connect bones at joints and tendons that attach skeletal muscles to bones. Choice *D* is incorrect because arteries, not veins, deliver oxygenated blood.

29. B: The dermis is the skin layer that contains nerves, blood vessels, hair follicles, and glands. These structures are called skin appendages. These appendages are scattered throughout the connective tissue (elastin and collagen), and the connective tissue provides support to the outer layer, the epidermis. The epidermal surface is a thin layer (except feet and palms where it is thick) of continually-regenerating cells that do not have a blood supply of their own, which explains why superficial cuts do not bleed. The hypodermis is the subcutaneous layer underneath the dermis, and it is composed primarily of fat in order to provide insulation.

30. D: Mechanical digestion is physical digestion of food and tearing it into smaller pieces using force. This occurs in the stomach and mouth. Chemical digestion involves chemically changing the food and breaking it down into small organic compounds that can be utilized by the cell to build molecules. The salivary glands in the mouth secrete amylase that breaks down starch, which begins chemical digestion. The stomach contains enzymes such as pepsinogen/pepsin and gastric lipase, which chemically digest protein and fats, respectively. The small intestine continues to digest protein using the enzymes trypsin and chymotrypsin. It also digests fats with the help of bile from the liver and lipase from the pancreas. These organs act as exocrine glands because they secrete substances through a duct. Carbohydrates are digested in the small intestine with the help of pancreatic amylase, gut bacterial flora and fauna, and brush border enzymes, like lactase. Brush border enzymes are contained in the towel-like microvilli in the small intestine that soak up nutrients.

31. B: The radius and ulna are the bones from the elbow to the wrist, and the humerus is the bone between the elbow and the shoulder. The tibia and fibula are the bones from the knee to the ankle, and the femur is the bone from the knee to the hip. The other choices are bones in the body as well, just not limb bones. The mandible is the jaw, the scapula is the shoulder blade, and the carpal bones are in the wrist.

32. B: In the Haversian system found in compact bone, concentric layers of bone cells are called lamellae. Between the lamellae are lacunae, which are gaps filled with osteocytes. The Haversian canals on the outer regions of the bone contain capillaries and nerve fibers. Spongy (cancellous) bone is on the extremities of long bones, which makes sense because the ends are softer due to the motion at joints (providing flexibility and cushion). The middle of the bone between the two spongy regions is called the diaphysis region. Spongy bone is highly vascular and is the site of red bone marrow (the marrow that makes red blood cells). Long bones, on the other hand, are long, weight-bearing bones like the tibia or femur that contain yellow marrow in adulthood. Trabeculae is a dense, collagenous, rod-shaped tissue that add mechanical support to the spongy regions of bone. Muscular trabeculae can be found in the heart and are similar in that they offer physical reinforcement.

33. A: Carbon dioxide rich blood is delivered and collected in the right atrium and moved to the right ventricle. The tricuspid valve prevents backflow between the two chambers. From there, the pulmonary artery takes blood to the lungs where diffusion causes gas exchange. Then, blood collects in the left atrium and moves to the left ventricle. The mitral valve prevents the backflow of blood from the ventricle to the atrium. Finally, blood is pumped to the body and released in the aorta.

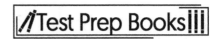

34. B: Smooth, skeletal, and cardiac muscle have defining characteristics, due to their vastly different functions. All have actin and myosin microfilaments that slide past each other to contract.

Skeletal muscles have long fibers made of clearly defined sarcomeres, which make them appear striated. Sarcomeres consist of alternating dark A bands (thick myosin) and light I bands (thin actin). Upon muscle contraction, fibers slide past each. Skeletal muscles are attached to bone via tendons and are responsible for voluntary movement; their contraction brings bones together. They contain multiple nuclei, due to their bundling into fibers.

Cardiac muscles also contain sarcomeres and appear striated, but are branched cells with a single nucleus. Branching allows each cell to connect with several others, forming a huge network that has more strength (the whole is greater than the sum of its parts).

Smooth muscles are non-striated and are responsible for involuntary movement (such as digestion). They do not form cylindrical fibers like skeletal muscles. Their lack of striations is because they have no sarcomeres, and the filaments are randomly arranged.

35. B: The reflex arc is the simplest nerve pathway. The stimulus bypasses the brain, going from sensory receptors through an afferent (incoming) neuron to the spinal cord. It synapses with an efferent (outgoing) neuron in the spinal cord and is transmitted directly to muscle. There is no interneuron involved in a reflex arc. The classic example of a reflex arc is the knee jerk response. Tapping on the patellar tendon of the knee stretches the quadriceps muscle of the thigh, resulting in contraction of the muscle and extension of the knee.

36. B: Proximal tubule → Loop of Henle → Collecting duct is correct. Kidneys filter blood using nephrons that span the outer renal cortex and inner renal medulla. The inner kidneys are composed of the renal pelvis, which collects urine and sends it to the bladder via the ureters. Filtrate first enters the filtering tube of the nephron via the glomerulus, a bundle of capillaries where blood fluid (but not cells) diffuses into the Bowman's capsule, the entryway into the kidney filtration canal. Bowman's capsule collects fluid, but the nephron actually starts filtering blood in the proximal tubule where necessary ions, nutrients, wastes, and (depending on blood osmolarity) water are absorbed or released. Also, blood pH is regulated here, as the proximal tubule fine-tunes pH by utilizing the blood buffering system, adjusting the amounts of hydrogen ions, bicarbonate, and ammonia in the filtrate. Down the loop of Henle in the renal medulla, the filtrate becomes more concentrated as water exits, while on the way back up the loop of Henle, ion concentration is regulated with ion channels. The distal tubule continues to regulate ion and water concentrations, and the collecting duct delivers the filtrate to the renal pelvis.

37. C: The sympathetic nervous system initiates the "fight-or-flight" response and is responsible for body changes that direct all available energy towards survival. Digestion is completely sacrificed so that energy can be used to increased heart rate and breathing (thus bronchiole dilation). The liver is stimulated to release glycogen (a carbohydrate-based starch) to provide available energy. The parasympathetic system is the one responsible for stimulating every-day activities like digestion.

38. A: Motor neurons transmit signals from the CNS to effector tissues and organs, such as skeletal muscles and glands. Sensory neurons carry impulses from receptors in the extremities to the CNS. Interneurons relay impulses from neuron to neuron.

39. C: The cerebellum is important for balance and motor coordination. Aside from the brainstem and cerebellum, the outside portion of the brain is the cerebrum, which is the advanced operating system of the brain and is responsible for learning, emotion, memory, perception, and voluntary movement. The amygdala (involved in emotions), language areas, and corpus collosum all exist within the cerebrum.

40. A: The exocrine portion of the pancreas (the majority of it) is an accessory organ to the digestive system (meaning that food never touches it—it is not part of the alimentary canal). It secretes bicarbonate to neutralize stomach acid and enzymes to aid in digestion. It also regulates blood sugar levels through the complementary actions of insulin and glucagon, which are located in the Islets of Langerhan (endocrine portion). Choice *A* is incorrect because it is not growth hormone that stimulates insulin secretion, but rather blood sugar levels.

41. D: The lymphatic system is composed of one-way vessels, lymph, and organs. It filters pathogens and debris from the blood, returns nutrients that have leaked from the blood, and maintains, and even stimulates, the immune system, if necessary. It also circulates lymph, a clear fluid filled with blood plasma that has leaked from capillary beds. The lymphatic system delivers lymph—a clear, colorless fluid, to the neck. It has several organs:

1. Lymph nodes, which remove debris from lymph and form lymphocytes
2. The thymus, which develops lymphocytes
3. The spleen, which removes pathogens from blood and makes lymphocytes
4. Tonsils, which collect debris

The lymphatic system also absorbs lipids and fat-soluble vitamins from the gut and returns them to the circulatory system.

42. C: ADH secretion is correct. Antidiuretic hormone controls water reabsorption. In its presence, water is reabsorbed, and urine is more concentrated. When absent, water is excreted, and urine is dilute. It is a regulator of blood volume, not pH. The other choices do affect blood pH.

$$H_2O + CO_2 \leftrightarrow H_2CO_3 \leftrightarrow H^+ + HCO_3^-$$

This chemical reaction can be fine-tuned in order to tweak the pH. It is helpful to notice the hydrogen ion on the product side of the equation. The more hydrogen ions there are, the more acidic the blood is. Carbonic acid, the "middle-man," regulates blood by being a buffer. Exhaling releases carbon dioxide. This pushes the reaction to the left, which will decrease hydrogen ions and make blood less acidic. Kidney regulation of bicarbonate will also shift the reaction to the left or right, raising or lowering pH as necessary.

Ammonia secreted by the proximal tubule of the nephron also regulates pH, since it will trap hydrogen ions and convert into ammonium ions. Reduced hydrogen ions make blood less acidic.

$$NH_3 + H^+ \leftrightarrow NH_4^+$$

43. D: The gland that regulates blood calcium levels is the parathyroid gland. Humans have four parathyroid glands located by the thyroid on each side of the neck, just below the larynx. Typical with the endocrine system, the parathyroid glands operate via feedback loops. If calcium in the blood is low, the parathyroid glands produce parathyroid hormone, which circulates to the bones and removes calcium. If calcium is high, they turn off parathyroid hormone production.

44. D: The hypothalamus is the link between the nervous and endocrine systems. It receives information from the brain and sends signals to the pituitary gland, instructing it to release or inhibit the release of hormones. Aside from its endocrine function, it controls body temperature, hunger, sleep, circadian rhythms, and is part of the limbic system.

45. C: When skeletal muscles contract, they pull bones together. They cannot push apart though, so they work in antagonistic pairs where they are on opposite sides of the bone.

When the biceps brachii contracts, the arm bends, and the triceps brachii is relaxed; on the other hand, when the triceps brachii contracts, the arm opens, and the biceps brachii relaxes.

The quadriceps on the thigh straighten the knee; the hamstrings behind the thigh bend the knee.

The trapezius, rhomboid major, and rhomboid minor are muscles on the upper back that pull the shoulders back. The pectoralis major and minor (pecs) are on the chest and allow movement of the shoulder (throwing, lifting, rotating).

The gluteus maximus is the buttocks muscle and extends to the hip. It is the major muscle of the gluts and is responsible for large movements like jumping. The gluteus medius and minimus stabilize the pelvis. The antagonist muscle to the gluteus maximus is the iliopsoas, the flexor muscles. Therefore, Choice *C* is correct, since the gluts are not antagonistic muscles.

46. A: Platelets are the blood components responsible for clotting. There are between 150,000 and 450,000 platelets in healthy blood. When a clot forms, platelets adhere to the injured area of the vessel and promote a molecular cascade that results in adherence of more platelets. Ultimately, the platelet aggregation results in recruitment of a protein called fibrin, which adds structure to the clot. Too many platelets can cause clotting disorders, while too few can cause bleeding disorders.

47. A: Choice *B* might be an attractive answer choice, but neutrophils are part of the innate immune system and are not considered part of the primary immune response. The first event that happens in a primary immune response is that macrophages ingest pathogens and display their antigens. Then, they secrete interleukin 1 to recruit helper T cells. Once helper T cells are activated, they secrete interleukin 2 to simulate plasma B cell and killer T cell production. Only then can plasma B cells make the pathogen-specific antibodies.

48. C: The epididymis stores sperm and is a coiled tube located near the testes. The immature sperm that enters the epididymis from the testes migrates through the 20-foot long epididymis tube in about two weeks, where viable sperm are concentrated at the end. The vas deferens is a tube that transports mature sperm from the epididymis to the urethra. Seminal vesicles are pouches attached that add fructose to the ejaculate to provide energy for sperm. The prostate gland excretes fluid that makes up about a third of semen released during ejaculation. The fluid reduces semen viscosity and contains enzymes that aid in sperm functioning; both effects increase sperm motility and ultimate success.

49. C: The female reproductive system is a symphony of different hormones that work together in order to propagate the species. FSH stimulates the ovaries to develop mature follicles, LH stimulates the release of the egg from the follicle, while hCG stimulates progesterone production.

50. A: Epithelial cells line cavities and surfaces of body organs and glands, and the three main shapes are squamous, columnar, and cuboidal. Epithelial cells contain no blood vessels, and their functions involve absorption, protection, transport, secretion, and sensing. Simple squamous epithelial are flat cells that are present in lungs and line the heart and vessels. Their flat shape aids in their function, which is diffusion of materials. The tunica intima, the inner layer of blood vessels, is lined with simple squamous epithelial tissue that sits on the basement membrane. Simple cuboidal epithelium is found in ducts, and simple columnar epithelium is found in tubes with projections (uterus, villi, bronchi). Any of these types of epithelial cells can be stacked, and then they are called stratified, not simple.

51. A: There are three types of archaeal species. Each uses a different source of energy. Lithotrophs use inorganic compounds for energy, phototrophs use sunlight for energy, and organotrophs use organic compounds for energy. All archaeal species are single-celled prokaryotes, not eukaryotic organisms.

52. C: Bacteria have several properties that make them beneficial to the environment. Gaseous nitrogen cannot be used by plants. Bacteria convert the gaseous nitrogen into a form that plants can use for energy. Bacteria also help with the decay of landfill materials and other debris. Spreading disease is not one of the beneficial traits of bacteria.

53. B: Bacteria reproduce by binary fission. They grow to twice their normal size and then split into two equally-sized daughter cells. This produces exact replicas of the original bacterium. They do not reproduce by meiosis, which is sexual reproduction, by mitosis, or by ingesting another microorganism.

54. D: Serology is the study of the blood serum. Identifying the antibodies present in blood serum can help determine what type of infection is attacking the body. This information allows for a treatment plan to be made against the infectious disease. Red blood cells are not included in the blood serum.

55. C: Antimicrobial agents are specifically toxic to the microorganism and not the individual host. The therapeutic index of antimicrobial agents indicates how toxic the agent is to the individual compared to the microorganism. These agents attack the cell wall of the microorganism and disrupt the internal cell contents. They do not allow the microorganism to continue growing or reproducing within the host.

Chemical Processes

General Chemistry

Atomic Structure

Atoms are made up of three subatomic particles: protons, neutrons, and electrons. The protons have a positive charge and are located in the nucleus of the atom. Neutrons have a neutral charge and are also located in the nucleus. Electrons have a negative charge, are the smallest of the three particles, and are located in orbitals that surround the nucleus. An atom is neutral if it has an equal number of electrons and protons. If an atom does not have an equal number of electrons and protons, it is an *ion*. When there are fewer electrons than protons, leaving it with a positive charge, it is termed a *cation*. When there are more electrons than protons, leaving a negative charge, it is an *anion*.

There are many levels of orbitals that surround the nucleus and house electrons. Each orbital has a distinct shape and three quantum numbers that characterize it: n, l, and m_l. The n is the principal quantum number and is always a positive integer, or whole number. As n increases, the size of the orbital increases and the electrons are less tightly bound to the nucleus. The angular momentum quantum number is represented by l and defines the shape of the orbital. There are four numerical values of l that correspond to four letter representations of the orbital: 0 or s, 1 or p, 2 or d, and 3 or f. Lastly, m_l represents the magnetic quantum number and describes the orientation of the orbital in space. It has a value in between $-l$ and l, including zero.

Electrons exist outside the nucleus in energy levels, and with each increasing period, there is an additional energy level. Hydrogen and helium are the only elements that have only one energy level, which is an s orbital that can only hold two electrons. Their relative electron configurations are $1s^1$ and $1s^2$, respectively. Each orbital holds two electrons with opposite spins.

The second energy level can hold a total of eight electrons: two in the *s* orbital, and six in the *p* orbital, of which there are three, since electrons pair up: $p_xp_yp_z$. All alkali metals and alkali Earth metals have an electron configuration that ends in either s^1 or s^2. For example, magnesium ends in $3s^s$ and cesium ends in $6s^1$. Groups 3A to 8A all end in the Xp^y configuration, with X representing the energy level and y representing how for inland it is. For example, oxygen is $2p^4$. The third energy level has s, p, and d orbitals, and together can hold 18 electrons, since d can hold 10. D orbitals start with the transition metals, and even though it appears that they are in the fourth energy level, they actually are on the third. The energy level for the whole d block is actually the period number minus one.

Example:

Mn: $1s^2 2s^2 2p^6 3s^2 3p^6 4s^2 3d^5$

The f block, which can hold 14 electrons, has a similar pattern for its preceding number, except two are subtracted from the period number.

Structure

Atoms are the most basic portion of an element that still retains its properties. All of the elements known to man are catalogued in the periodic table, a chart of elements arranged by increasing atomic number. The atomic number refers to the number of protons in an atom's nucleus. It can be found either in the upper left-hand corner of the box or directly above an element's chemical symbol on the periodic table. For example, the atomic number for hydrogen (H) is 1. The term "atomic mass" refers to the sum of protons and neutrons in an atom's nucleus. The atomic mass can be found beneath an element's abbreviation on the periodic table. For example, the average atomic mass of hydrogen (H) is 1.008. Because protons have a positive charge and neutrons have a neutral charge, an atom's nucleus typically has a positive electrical charge. Electrons orbiting the nucleus have a negative charge. As a result, elements with equal numbers of protons and electrons have no net charge.

Atomic Radii

Atomic radius refers to the size of an atom. Going down a group, because each level represents an energy level, atomic radii increase. For example, when comparing lithium and potassium, potassium will have a greater atomic radius because it has two more energy levels.

Contrary to what might be predicted, when going from left to right on the periodic table across a period, atomic radius actually decreases. This is due to proton pull. As each element gains a proton in its nucleus, it is like gaining a positive magnet in the middle. The more magnets in the middle, the stronger they will suck in any outer electrons. Comparing carbon and fluorine, fluorine has a smaller atomic radius due to more (stronger) proton pull of the nucleus.

Ionic radius is a bit different. When sodium forms a cation, it loses an electron, losing an entire energy level. Thus, the ionic radii of cations are smaller than their elemental form. Anions, however, have a larger radius than their elemental form. This is because an extra electron is like adding a negative magnet to seven other negative magnets, resulting in a repulsive force that pushes them apart.

When atoms collide, in solutions, for example, they touch each other and then ricochet apart. The closest they come to each other is the combined length of each of their radii. This radius is known as *van der Waals radius* for each atom. When atoms bond with each other, however, they must come closer together than they would if they were just colliding. Their attraction also draws them closer together. The bonding atomic radius, or the *covalent radius*, is equal to one-half of the distance between the two atoms when they are bonded together. Within each group in the periodic table, the covalent radius increases from top to bottom. Within each period, the covalent radius decreases from left to right.

Ions

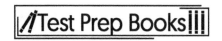

Atoms that have gained or lost electrons wind up having a net electrical charge and are termed ions. The following are the main ions related to human health:

Bicarbonate	HCO^{3-}	A major buffer in blood. The lungs and kidneys regulate its concentration.
Chloride	Cl^-	Important in stomach acid and usually ingested as the salts sodium chloride (NaCl) and potassium chloride (KCl)
Calcium	Ca^{2+}	Important in muscle contraction and bone construction
Copper	Cu	Specialized chemical reactions in the cell
Iodine	I	Specialized chemical reactions in the cell
Iron	Fe	Important in hemoglobin for transport of oxygen, and also part of the electron transport chain
Magnesium	Mg^{2+}	Important in chlorophyll and animal energy production as well as a constituent of bone
Phosphate	PO_4^{3-}	A minor intracellular pH buffer that is regulated by the kidneys and is an important factor in bone
Potassium	K^+	The most plentiful mineral inside of cells and is important for nerve and muscle function
Sodium	Na^+	The most common mineral outside of cells and is important for water and osmolarity regulation as well as nerve and muscle function
Sulfate	SO_4^{2-}	A minor pH buffer for body fluids

For the majority of light atoms, the number of protons is similar to the number of neutrons. An isotope is a variation of an element having the same number of protons, but a different number of neutrons. For example, all isotopes of carbon (C) have six protons. Nevertheless, C-12 has six neutrons, C-13 has seven neutrons, and C-14 has eight neutrons.

Some isotopes are radioactive and result in nuclear decay. Not all radioactive isotopes are harmful, and some are even useful to scientists and physicians. For example, C-14 is radioactive and can be used in the process of radiocarbon dating, which can be used to determine the age of organic remains. A radioactive isotope of gold (Au-198) can be utilized to treat ovarian, prostate, and brain cancer.

Periodicity

Periodicity refers to the repeating patterns, or trends, in the properties of elements. The atomic number and atomic structure are the key determinants of the properties of elements. During the mid-1800s, the Russian chemist Dmitri Mendeleev utilized the principal of periodicity to arrange elements in a manner similar to the modern periodic table. Mendeleev's periodic table was arranged in rows according to increasing atomic mass and in columns according to similar chemical behavior. The modern periodic table is arranged in order of increasing atomic number, which is defined as the number of protons in an atom's nucleus. Elements near each other are more similar than elements that are distant on the periodic table.

Periodic Table

Periodic Table of the Elements

1A	2A	3B	4B	5B	6B	7B	8B			11B	12B	3A	4A	5A	6A	7A	8A
1 H hydrogen 1.008																	2 He helium 4.003
3 Li lithium 6.94	4 Be beryllium 9.012											5 B boron 10.81	6 C carbon 12.01	7 N nitrogen 14.01	8 O oxygen 16.00	9 F fluorine 19.00	10 Ne neon 20.18
11 Na sodium 22.99	12 Mg magnesium 24.31											13 Al aluminum 26.98	14 Si silicon 28.09	15 P phosphorus 30.97	16 S sulfur 32.06	17 Cl chlorine 35.45	18 Ar argon 39.95
19 K potassium 39.10	20 Ca calcium 40.08	21 Sc scandium 44.96	22 Ti titanium 47.88	23 V vanadium 50.94	24 Cr chromium 52.00	25 Mn manganese 54.94	26 Fe iron 55.85	27 Co cobalt 58.93	28 Ni nickel 58.69	29 Cu copper 63.55	30 Zn zinc 65.39	31 Ga gallium 69.72	32 Ge germanium 72.64	33 As arsenic 74.92	34 Se selenium 78.96	35 Br bromine 79.90	36 Kr krypton 83.79
37 Rb rubidium 85.47	38 Sr strontium 87.62	39 Y yttrium 88.91	40 Zr zirconium 91.22	41 Nb niobium 92.91	42 Mo molybdenum 95.96	43 Tc technetium (98)	44 Ru ruthenium 101.1	45 Rh rhodium 102.9	46 Pd palladium 106.4	47 Ag silver 107.9	48 Cd cadmium 112.4	49 In indium 114.8	50 Sn tin 118.7	51 Sb antimony 121.8	52 Te tellurium 127.6	53 I iodine 126.9	54 Xe xenon 131.3
55 Cs cesium 132.9	56 Ba barium 137.3	57-71	72 Hf hafnium 178.5	73 Ta tantalum 180.9	74 W tungsten 183.9	75 Re rhenium 186.2	76 Os osmium 190.2	77 Ir iridium 192.2	78 Pt platinum 195.1	79 Au gold 197.0	80 Hg mercury 200.5	81 Tl thallium 204.4	82 Pb lead 207.2	83 Bi bismuth 209.0	84 Po polonium (209)	85 At astatine (210)	86 Rn radon (222)
87 Fr francium (223)	88 Ra radium (226)	89-103	104 Rf rutherfordium (265)	105 Db dubnium (268)	106 Sg seaborgium (271)	107 Bh bohrium (270)	108 Hs hassium (277)	109 Mt meitnerium (276)	110 Ds darmstadtium (281)	111 Rg roentgenium (280)	112 Cn copernicium (285)	113 Uut ununtrium (284)	114 Fl flerovium (289)	115 Uup ununpentium (288)	116 Lv livermorium (293)	117 Uus ununseptium (294)	118 Uuo ununoctium (294)

Lanthanide Series	57 La lanthanum 138.9	58 Ce cerium 140.1	59 Pr praseodymium 140.9	60 Nd neodymium 144.2	61 Pm promethium (145)	62 Sm samarium 150.4	63 Eu europium 152.0	64 Gd gadolinium 157.2	65 Tb terbium 158.9	66 Dy dysprosium 162.5	67 Ho holmium 164.9	68 Er erbium 167.3	69 Tm thulium 168.9	70 Yb ytterbium 173.0	71 Lu lutetium 175.0
Actinide Series	89 Ac actinium (227)	90 Th thorium 232	91 Pa protactinium 231	92 U uranium 238	93 Np neptunium (237)	94 Pu plutonium (244)	95 Am americium (243)	96 Cm curium (247)	97 Bk berkelium (247)	98 Cf californium (251)	99 Es einsteinium (252)	100 Fm fermium (257)	101 Md mendelevium (258)	102 No nobelium (259)	103 Lr lawrencium (262)

Alkaline Metal	Alkaline Earth	Transition Metal	Basic Metal	Semimetal	Nonmetal	Halogen	Noble Gas	Lanthanide	Actinide

The periodic table is a chart of all 118 known elements. The elements are organized according to their quantity of protons, also known as their *atomic number*, their electron configurations, and their chemical properties. The rows are called *periods* and the columns are called *groups*. Groups have similar chemical behavior. For example, Group 8A is the noble gases, and because their outer electron shell is full, they are non-reactive. The closer the element is to having a full set of valence electrons, the more reactive it is. Group 1, the alkali metals, and Group 7, the halogens, are both highly reactive for that reason. The alkali metals form cations and lose their lone electron while halogens pick up an electron.

In each box in the period table, an element's symbol is the abbreviation in the center and its full name is located directly below that. The number in the top left corner is the atomic number and the atomic mass of the element is the number underneath. The *atomic mass* of the element is noted in atomic mass units, or amu, which represents the number of protons and neutrons combined. The number of protons defines the element, but the mass number can be different due to the existence of elements with a different number of neutrons, also called isotopes. The amu shown on the periodic table is a weighted mass (based on abundance) of all known isotopes of a particular element.

Ionization Energy and Electron Affinity

Energy is required to remove an electron from an atom or ion while it is in its ground state, usually as a gas. *Ionization energy* applies to all elements; it is just greater for those on the right side of the table. The ionization energy of an atom or ion is the minimum amount of energy required to do so. The greater the ionization energy, the harder it is to remove the electron. The energy required for the first electron is noted as I_1, the second as I_2, and then continues consecutively numbered for each successive electron. With each electron that is removed, the ionization energy of the element increases. I_1 increases in elements across the periods and moving down the columns of the period table. In contrast to ionization energy, energy is released from an atom when an electron is added. This negative change in energy is known as *electron affinity*. Ionization energies are always positive, because atoms require more energy to let go of an electron than to add one.

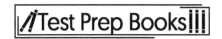

Looking at the periodic table, elements on the left, the alkali metals and alkali earth metals, have a low ionization energy. It takes little energy to peel off of their electron, because they have the least (weakest) proton pull in their period. Elements on the right, like halogens (gases), have an extremely high ionization energy, because they have a very strong proton pull pulling electrons in, so it would require even more energy to peel off an electron. Noble gases have an extremely high ionization energy.

Going down a group, as energy levels increase, proton pull becomes weaker, so ionization energy decreases.

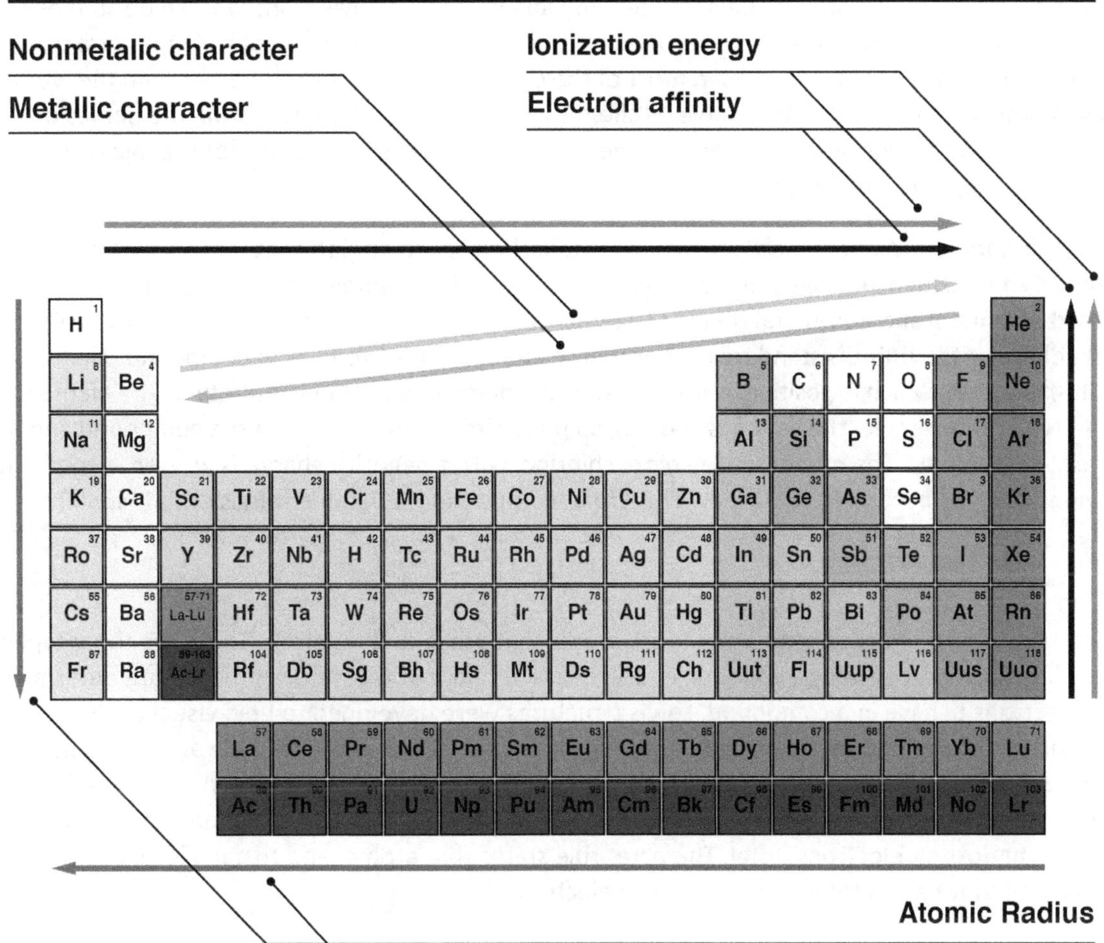

Molecular Weight

Elements can exist alone or combine to form compounds and molecules. Using the atomic mass, or atomic weights, that are noted on the periodic table, the molecular weight of a substance can be found by multiplying the subscript of each element by the atomic mass of that element and then adding together the weights of all of the elements in the molecule together. For example, to find the molecular weight of one glucose molecule, $C_6H_{12}O_6$, the atomic mass of carbon is multiplied by six, the atomic mass of hydrogen is multiplied by twelve, the atomic mass of oxygen is multiplied by six and then the three resulting numbers are added together. The answer is one glucose molecule has a molecular weight of 180 amu.

Chemical Bonding

Nomenclature and Formulas

Chemical *nomenclature* refers to how compounds and substances are named, and the formulas are how they are written. Inorganic substances do not contain carbon, while organic ones do. Some common compounds have "household names," like water, ammonia, and table salt in addition to their chemical formulas, whereas others are strictly referred to by their official nomenclature.

There are a variety of conventions or standards by which chemists derive the names for chemical compounds. These systematic rules help create unity and establish conventions worldwide so that a given substance is referred to the same way around the world. The International Union of Pure and Applied Chemistry (IUPAC) has developed most of the chemical nomenclature used around the world and has published "color books" that serve as chemical dictionaries in a sense, listing the names of compounds based on their type. For example, the *Blue Book* contains the names for organic compounds, while the *Red Book* lists inorganic ones.

For inorganic compounds, nomenclature may be established based on different factors such as the substance's composition, arrangement, and type of bonding. For example, ionic compounds, which are composed of a metal and non-metal bonded together (e.g., NaCl, sodium chloride, and Ca_3N_2, calcium nitride) adhere to the IUPAC's standard conventions established for this type of compound. The monoatomic cation, which is positive, is listed first in the name and formula and retains the element's name. In NaCl, for example, the cation is sodium, so it is written and said first in the compound and is simply called "sodium." The monoatomic anion, chlorine, with a negative charge is written second and is given the suffix *-ide,* becoming "chloride." Therefore, compound NaCl, table salt, is called "sodium chloride."

Bonding

Chemical bonding occurs between two or more atoms that are joined together. There are three types of chemical bonds: ionic, covalent, and metallic. The characteristics of the different bonds are determined by how electrons behave in a compound. Lewis structures were developed to help visualize the electrons in molecules; they are a method of writing a compound structure formula and including its electron composition. A Lewis symbol for an element consists of the element symbol and a dot for each valence electron. The dots are located on all four sides of the symbol, with a maximum of two dots per side, and eight dots, or electrons, total. The octet rule states that atoms tend to gain, lose, or share electrons until they have a total of eight valence electrons.

Ionic Bonds

Ionic bonds are formed from the electrostatic attractions between oppositely charged atoms. They result from the transfer of electrons from a metal on the left side of the periodic table to a nonmetal on the right side. The metallic substance often has low ionization energy and will transfer an electron easily to the nonmetal, which has a high electron affinity. An example of this is the compound NaCl, which is sodium chloride, or table salt, where the Na atom transfers an electron to the Cl atom.

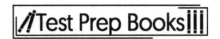

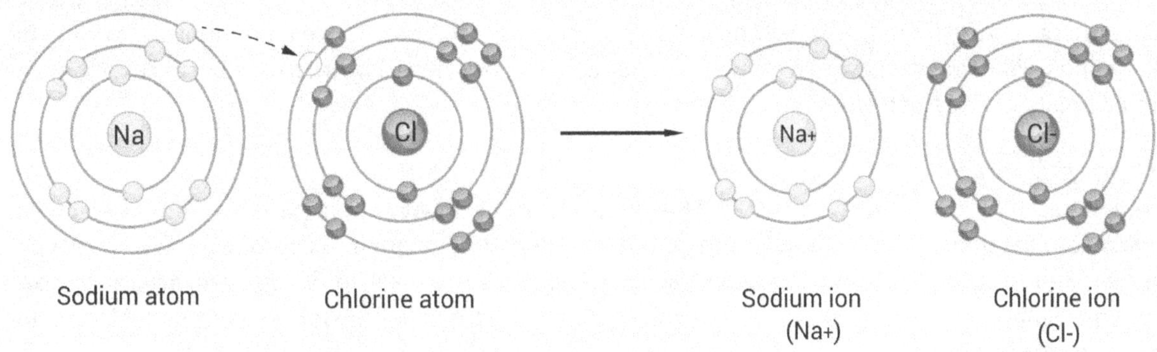

Due to strong bonding, ionic compounds have several distinct characteristics. They have high melting and boiling points, and are brittle and crystalline. They are arranged in rigid, well-defined structures, which allow them to break apart along smooth, flat surfaces. The formation of ionic bonds is a reaction that is exothermic. In the opposite scenario, the energy it takes to break up a one mole quantity of an ionic compound is referred to as *lattice energy*, which is generally endothermic. The Lewis structure for NaCl is written as follows:

$$Na + \cdot\ddot{\underset{\cdot\cdot}{Cl}}: \rightarrow Na^{+} + :\ddot{\underset{\cdot\cdot}{Cl}}:^{-}$$

Covalent Bonds

Covalent bonds are formed when two atoms share electrons, instead of transferring them as in ionic compounds. The atoms in covalent compounds have a balance of attraction and repulsion between their protons and electrons, which keeps them bonded together. Two atoms can be joined by single, double, or even triple covalent bonds. As the number of electrons that are shared increases, the length of the bond decreases. Covalent substances have low melting and boiling points, and are poor conductors of heat and electricity.

The Lewis structure for Cl_2 is written as follows:

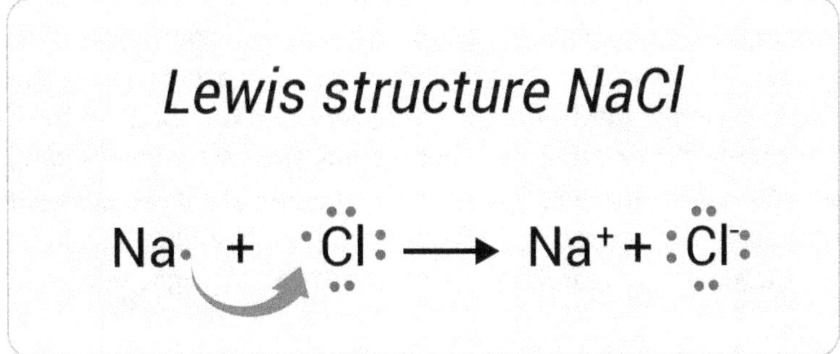

Metallic Bonds

Metallic bonds are formed by electrons that move freely through metal. They are the product of the force of attraction between electrons and metal ions. The electrons are shared by many metal cations and act like glue that holds the metallic substance together, similar to the attraction between oppositely-charged atoms in ionic substances, except the electrons are more fluid and float around the bonded metals and form a sea of electrons. Metallic compounds have characteristic properties that include strength, conduction of heat and electricity, and malleability. They can conduct electricity by passing energy through the freely moving electrons, creating a current. These compounds also have high melting and boiling points. Lewis structures are not common for metallic structures because of the free-roaming ability of the electrons.

Hydrogen Bonding

Hydrogen bonds are temporary and weak. They typically occur between two partial, opposite electrical charges. For example, hydrogen bonds form when a hydrogen (H) atom is in the vicinity of nitrogen (N), fluorine (F), or oxygen (O) atoms. These partial electrical charges are called *dipoles,* and are caused by the unequal sharing of electrons between covalent bonds. Water is the most prevalent molecule that forms hydrogen bonds.

Hydrogen bonds contribute to the adhesiveness and cohesiveness properties of molecules like water. Adhesiveness confers glue-like properties to molecules which ensure they stick or connect more easily with other molecules, similar to wetting a suction cup before sticking it to a surface. Cohesiveness refers to a molecule's ability to form hydrogen bonds with itself. For example, the cohesiveness of water is the reason why it has a high boiling point, which is a physical property.

Reactions and Reaction Mechanisms

Chemical reactions are represented by chemical equations. The equations help to explain how the molecules change during the reaction. For example, when hydrogen gas (H_2) combines with oxygen gas (O_2), two molecules of water are formed. The equation is written as follows, where the "+" sign means *reacts with* and the "→" means *produces*:

$$2\ H_2 + O_2 \rightarrow 2\ H_2O$$

Two hydrogen molecules react with an oxygen molecule to produce two water molecules. In all chemical equations, the quantity of each element on the reactant side of the equation should equal the quantity of the same element on the product side of the equation due to the law of conservation of matter. If this is true, the equation is described as *balanced*. To figure out how many of each element there is on each side of the equation, the coefficient of the element should be multiplied by the subscript next to the element. Coefficients and subscripts are noted for quantities larger than one. The coefficient is the number located directly to the left of the element. The subscript is the small-sized number directly to the right of the element. In the equation above, on the left side, the coefficient of the hydrogen is two and the subscript is also two, which makes a total of four hydrogen atoms. Using the same method, there are two oxygen atoms. On the right side, the coefficient two is multiplied by the subscript in each element of the water molecule, making four hydrogen atoms and two oxygen atoms. This equation is balanced because there are four hydrogen atoms and two oxygen atoms on each side. The states of the reactants and products can also be written in the equation: gas (g), liquid (l), solid (s), and dissolved in water (aq). If they are included, they are noted in parentheses on the right side of each molecule in the equation.

Types of Chemical Reactions

Chemical reactions are characterized by a chemical change in which the starting substances, or reactants, differ from the substances formed, or products. Chemical reactions may involve a change in color, the production of gas, the formation of a precipitate, or changes in heat content. The following are the five basic types of chemical reactions:

Reaction Type	Definition	Example
Decomposition	A compound is broken down into two or more smaller elements or compounds.	$2H_2O \rightarrow 2H_2+O_2$
Synthesis	Two or more elements or compounds are joined together.	$2H_2+O_2 \rightarrow 2H_2O$
Single Displacement	A single element or ion takes the place of another in a compound. Also known as a substitution reaction.	$Zn+2HCl \rightarrow ZnCl_2+H_2$
Double Displacement	Two elements or ions exchange a single atom each to form two different compounds, resulting in different combinations of cations and anions in the final compounds. Also known as a metathesis reaction.	$H_2SO_4+2NaOH \rightarrow Na_2So_4+2H_2O$
Oxidation-Reduction	Elements undergo a change in oxidation number. Also known as a redox reaction.	$2S_2O_3^{2-}(aq)+I_2(aq) \rightarrow S_4O_6^{2-}(aq)+2I^-(aq)$
Acid-Base	Involves a reaction between an acid and a base, which usually produces a salt and water	$HBr+NaOH \rightarrow NaBr+H_2O$
Combustion	A hydrocarbon (a compound composed of only hydrogen and carbon) reacts with oxygen to form carbon dioxide and water.	$CH_4+2O_2 \rightarrow CO_2+2H_2O$

Oxidation-Reduction Reactions

Oxidation-reduction reactions, or *redox reactions*, are chemical reactions in which electrons are transferred from one compound to another. A helpful mnemonic device to remember the basic properties of redox reactions is "LEO the lion says GER", in which "LEO" means Lose Electrons Oxidation and "GER" stands for Gain Electrons Reduction. A *reducing agent* is an electron donor and an *oxidizing agent* is an electron acceptor.

An example of an oxidation-reduction reaction is the electrochemical cell, which is the basis for batteries. The electrochemical cell comprises two different cells, each equipped with a separate conductor, and a salt bridge. The salt bridge isolates reactants, but maintains the electric current. The cathode is the electrode that is reduced, and the anode is the electrode that is oxidized. Anions and cations carry electrical current within the cell and electrons carry current within the electrodes.

Balancing Chemical Reactions

Chemical reactions are conveyed using chemical equations. As mentioned, chemical equations must be balanced with equivalent numbers of atoms for each type of element on each side of the equation. Antoine Lavoisier, a French chemist, was the first to propose the Law of Conservation of Mass for the purpose of balancing a chemical equation. The law states, "Matter is neither created nor destroyed during a chemical reaction."

The reactants are located on the left side of the arrow, while the products are located on the right side of the arrow. Coefficients are the numbers in front of the chemical formulas. Subscripts are the numbers to the lower right of chemical symbols in a formula. To tally atoms, one should multiply the formula's coefficient by the subscript of each chemical symbol. For example, the chemical equation

$$2\ H_2 + O_2 \rightarrow 2H_2O$$

is balanced. For H, the coefficient of 2 multiplied by the subscript 2 = 4 hydrogen atoms. For O, the coefficient of 1 multiplied by the subscript 2 = 2 oxygen atoms. Coefficients and subscripts of 1 are understood and never written. When known, the form of the substance is noted with (g) for gas, (s) for solid, (l) for liquid, or (aq) for aqueous.

Balancing Redox Reactions

Keep track of oxidation states or oxidation numbers to ensure the chemical equation is balanced. Oxidation numbers are assigned to each atom in a neutral substance or ion. For ions made up of a single atom, the oxidation number is equal to the charge of the ion. For atoms in their original elemental form, the oxidation number is always zero. Each hydrogen atom in an H_2 molecule, for example, has an oxidation number of zero. The sum of the oxidation numbers in a molecule should be equal to the overall charge of the molecule. If the molecule is a positively-charged ion, the sum of the oxidation number should be equal to overall positive charge of the molecule. In ionic compounds that have a cation and anion joined, the sum of the oxidation numbers should equal zero.

All chemical equations must have the same number of elements on each side of the equation to be balanced. Redox reactions have an extra step of counting the electrons on both sides of the equation to be balanced. Separating redox reactions into oxidation reactions and reduction reactions is a simple way to account for all of the electrons involved. The individual equations are known as half-reactions. The number of electrons lost in the oxidation reaction must be equal to the number of electrons gained in the reduction reaction for the redox reaction to be balanced. The oxidation of tin (Sn) by iron (Fe) can be balanced by the following half-reactions:

Oxidation: $Sn^{2+} \rightarrow Sn^{4+} + 2e^-$

Reduction: $2Fe^{3+} + 2e^- \rightarrow 2Fe^{2+}$

Complete redox reaction: $Sn^{2+} + 2Fe^{3+} \rightarrow Sn^{4+} + 2Fe^{2+}$

Equilibrium and Reaction Rates

Reaction Rates

The rate of a reaction is the measure of the change in concentration of the reactants or products over a certain period of time. Many factors affect how quickly or slowly a reaction occurs, such as concentration, pressure, or temperature. As the concentration of a reactant increases, the rate of the reaction also increases, because the frequency of collisions between elements increases. High-pressure situations for reactants that are gases cause the gas to compress and increase the frequency of gas molecule collisions, similar to solutions with higher concentrations. Reactions rates are then increased with the higher frequency of gas molecule collisions. Higher temperatures usually increase the rate of the reaction, adding more energy to the system with heat, and increasing the frequency of molecular collisions.

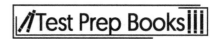

Equilibrium

Equilibrium is described as the state of a system when no net changes occur. Chemical equilibrium occurs when opposing reactions occur at equal rates. In other words, the rate of reactants forming products is equal to the rate of the products breaking down into the reactants—the concentration of reactants and products in the system does not change. Although the concentrations are not changing, the forward and reverse reactions are likely still occurring. This type of equilibrium is called a *dynamic equilibrium*. In situations where all reactions have ceased, a static equilibrium is reached. Chemical equilibriums are also described as homogeneous or heterogeneous. Homogeneous equilibrium involves substances that are all in the same phase, while heterogeneous equilibrium means the substances are in different phases when equilibrium is reached.

When a reaction reaches equilibrium, the conditions of the equilibrium are described by the following equation, based on the chemical equation aA + bB ↔ cC + dD:

$$K_c = \frac{[C]^c[D]^d}{[A]^a[B]^b}$$

This equation describes the law of mass action. It explains how the reactants and products react during dynamic equilibrium. K_c is the equilibrium constant and it is obtained when molarity values are put into the equation for the reactants and products. It is important to note that K_c is only dependent on the stoichiometry of the equation. If K_c is greater than 1, the equilibrium occurs when there are more products generated; the equilibrium lies to the right. If K_c is less than 1, the equilibrium occurs when there are more reactants generated and the equilibrium is to the left.

Similar to finding K_c, the quantity of reactants and products, as well as the direction of the reaction, can be determined at any point of time by finding Q, the reaction quotient. Q_c is substituted for the K_c in the equation above. If Q is less than K, the concentration of the reactants is too large and the concentration of the products is too small, so the reaction must move from left to right to achieve equilibrium. If Q is equal to K, the system is at equilibrium. If Q is greater than K, the concentration of the products is too large and the concentration of the reactants is too small; the reaction must move from right to left to reach equilibrium.

Catalysts

Catalysts are substances that accelerate the speed of a chemical reaction. A catalyst remains unchanged throughout the course of a chemical reaction. In most cases, only small amounts of a catalyst are needed. Catalysts increase the rate of a chemical reaction by providing an alternate path that requires less activation energy. Activation energy refers to the amount of energy necessary for the initiation of a chemical reaction.

Catalysts can be homogeneous or heterogeneous. Catalysts in the same phase of matter as its reactants are homogeneous, while catalysts in a different phase than the reactants are heterogeneous. It is important to remember catalysts are selective. They do not accelerate the speed of all chemical reactions, but catalysts do accelerate specific chemical reactions.

Enzymes

Enzymes are a class of catalysts instrumental in biochemical reactions, and in most, if not all, instances, they are proteins. Like all catalysts, enzymes increase the rate of a chemical reaction by providing an alternate path that requires less activation energy. Enzymes catalyze thousands of chemical reactions in the human body. Enzymes possess an active site, which is the part of the molecule that binds the reacting molecule, or *substrate*. The "lock and key" analogy is used to describe the substrate key fitting precisely into the active site of the enzyme lock to form an enzyme-substrate complex.

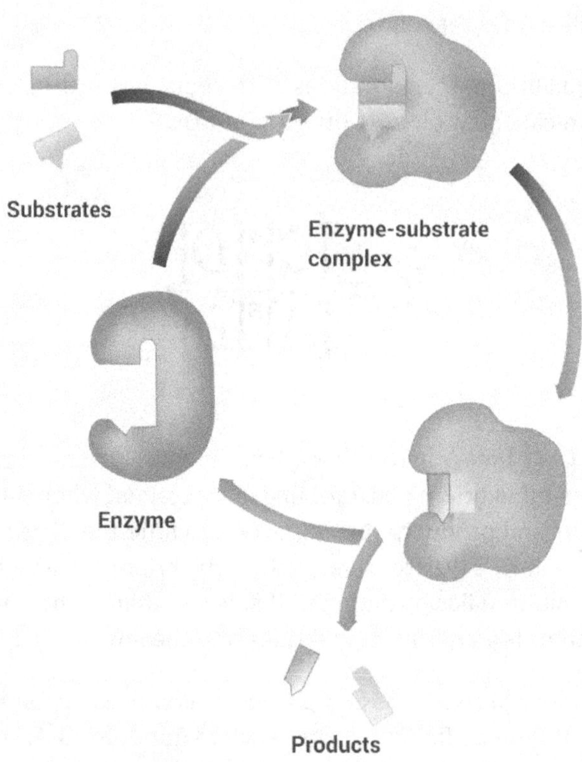

Many enzymes work in tandem with cofactors or coenzymes to catalyze chemical reactions. *Cofactors* can be either inorganic (not containing carbon) or organic (containing carbon). Organic cofactors can be either coenzymes or prosthetic groups tightly bound to an enzyme. *Coenzymes* transport chemical groups from one enzyme to another. Within a cell, coenzymes are continuously regenerating, and their concentrations are held at a steady state.

Several factors—including temperature, pH, and concentrations of the enzyme and substrate—can affect the catalytic activity of an enzyme. For humans, the optimal temperature for peak enzyme activity is approximately body temperature at 98.6 ^{0}F, while the optimal pH for peak enzyme activity is approximately 7-8. Increasing the concentrations of either the enzyme or substrate will also increase the rate of reaction, up to a certain point.

The activity of enzymes can be regulated. One common type of enzyme regulation is termed *feedback inhibition*, which involves the product of the pathway inhibiting the catalytic activity of the enzyme involved in its manufacture.

Stoichiometry

Stoichiometry investigates the quantities of chemicals that are consumed and produced in chemical reactions. Chemical equations are made up of reactants and products; stoichiometry helps elucidate how the changes from reactants to products occur, as well as how to ensure the equation is balanced.

Limiting Reactants

Chemical reactions are limited by the amount of starting material—or reactants—available to drive the process forward. The reactant that is present in the smallest quantity in a reaction is called the limiting reactant. The limiting reactant is completely consumed by the end of the reaction. The other reactants are called excess reactants. For example, gasoline is used in a combustion reaction to make a car move and is the limiting reactant of the reaction. If the gasoline runs out, the combustion reaction can no longer take place, and the car stops.

Reaction Yield

The quantity of product that should be produced after using up all of the limiting reactant can be calculated, and is called the *theoretical yield* of the reaction. Since the reactants do not always act as they should, the actual amount of resulting product is called the *actual yield*. The actual yield is divided by the theoretical yield and then multiplied by 100 to find the percent yield for the reaction.

Solution Stoichiometry

Solution stoichiometry deals with quantities of solutes in chemical reactions that occur in solutions. The quantity of a solute in a solution can be calculated by multiplying the molarity of the solution by the volume. Similar to chemical equations involving simple elements, the number of moles of the elements that make up the solute should be equivalent on both sides of the equation.

Sample Titration Curve

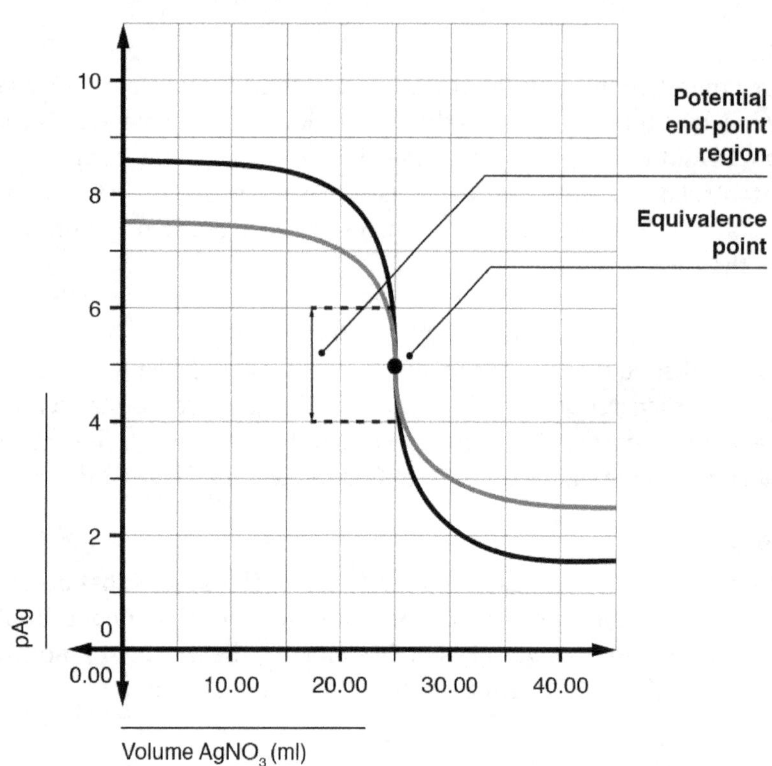

When the concentration of a particular solute in a solution is unknown, a titration is used to determine that concentration. In a titration, the solution with the unknown solute is combined with a standard solution, which is a solution with a known solute concentration. The point at which the unknown solute has completely reacted with the known solute is called the *equivalence point*. Using the known information about the standard solution, including the concentration and volume, and the volume of the unknown solution, the concentration of the unknown solute is determined in a balanced equation. For example, in the case of combining acids and bases, the equivalence point is reached when the resulting solution is neutral. HCl, an acid, combines with NaOH, a base, to form water, which is neutral, and a solution of Cl^- ions and Na^+ ions. Before the equivalence point, there is an unequal number of cations and anions and the solution is not neutral.

Kinetic Theory

The *Kinetic Theory of Matter* states that matter is composed of a large number of small particles (specifically, atoms and molecules) that are in constant motion. The distance between the separations in these particles determines the state of the matter: solid, liquid, or gas. In gases, the particles have a large separation and no attractive forces. In liquids, there is moderate separation between particles and some attractive forces to form a loose shape. Solids have almost no separation between their particles, which gives them a defined, set shape. The constant movement of particles causes them to bump into each other, thus allowing the particles to transfer energy among one another. This bumping and transferring of energy helps explain the transfer of heat and the relationship between pressure, volume, and temperature.

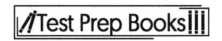

According to kinetic molecular theory:

- Gas particles have Brownian, or random, motion (consistent with the second law of thermodynamics).
- Gas particles travel in a straight line until they hit another object and change direction.
- The volume of a gas particle is virtually zero.
- There are no attractive or repulsive forces between gas particles, and there are no unaccounted chemical or physical interactions between particles.
- There are elastic collisions between the gas and its container and other particles; particles do not slow down, and they are constantly moving.
- Movement, or kinetic energy, is a function of temperature. As temperature increases, kinetic energy increases. Average kinetic energy is equal to temperature in Kelvin.

Collision theory is closely related to kinetic molecular theory. Based on the fact that as temperature increases, movement increases, the premise of collision theory is that reactions happen faster as temperature increases due to the increases in reactant collisions with each other and with catalysts. Of note, from a biological perspective, there is a limit to this temperature increase because, if it is a reaction involving biological protein catalysts (enzymes), the enzyme will eventually denature, "cook," and lose functionality.

States of Matter

Chemistry is the study of matter, including its properties and behavior. *Matter* is the material that the universe is made of; it is any object that occupies space and has mass. Despite the diversity of items found in the universe, matter is comprised of only about 100 substances, known as elements. Elements cannot be broken down into simpler substances. Hydrogen and oxygen are two examples of elements. When different elements join together, they form compounds. Water is a compound made from hydrogen and oxygen. Atoms and molecules are among the smallest forms of matter.

Matter can be found in three different states: gas, liquid, or solid. Gas is a state that does not have a fixed volume or shape. It can expand to fill large containers or compress to fill smaller ones. Gas molecules are far apart from each other and float around at high speeds. They collide with each other and the container they are in, filling the container uniformly. When the gas is compressed, the space between the molecules decreases and the frequency of collisions between them increases. A liquid has an exact volume. It molds to the shape of the container that holds it. Liquid molecules are close together but still move rapidly. They cannot be compressed and slide over each other easily when liquids are poured. Solids have a definitive shape and volume. Similar to liquids, solids cannot be compressed. The molecules are packed together tightly in a specific arrangement that does not allow for much movement.

The physical and chemical properties of matter can help distinguish different substances. Physical properties include color, odor, density, and hardness. These are properties that can be observed without changing the substance's identity or composition. When a substance undergoes a physical change, its physical appearance changes but its composition remains the same. Chemical properties are those that describe the way a substance might change to form another substance. Examples of chemical properties are flammability, toxicity, and ability to oxidize. These properties are observed by changing the environment of the substance and seeing how the substance reacts. A substance's composition is changed when it undergoes a chemical change.

Many properties of matter can be measured quantitatively, meaning the measurement is associated with a number. When a property of matter is represented by a number, it is important to include the unit of measure, otherwise the number is meaningless. For example, saying a pencil measures 10 is meaningless. It could be referring to 10 of something very short or 10 of something very long. The correct measurement notation would be 10 centimeters, because a centimeter has a designated length. Other examples of properties of matter that can be measured quantitatively are mass, time, and temperature, among others.

Gas Laws

The *Ideal Gas Law* states that pressure, volume, and temperature are all related through the equation: $PV = nRT$, where P is pressure, V is volume, n is the amount of the substance in moles, R is the gas constant, and T is temperature.

Through this relationship, volume and pressure are both proportional to temperature, but pressure is inversely proportional to volume. Therefore, if the equation is balanced and the volume decreases in the system, pressure needs to increase proportionally to keep both sides of the equation balanced. In contrast, if the equation is unbalanced and the pressure increases, then the temperature would also increase, since pressure and temperature are directly proportional.

Causes and Effects of Changes in State

When environmental changes occur, such as temperature or pressure changes, one state of matter can convert to another. States of matter are able to undergo phase transitions. Vaporization refers to the transformation of a solid or liquid into a gas. There are two types of vaporization—evaporation and boiling. Evaporation is a surface phenomenon and involves the conversion of a liquid into a gas below the boiling temperature at a given pressure. Evaporation is also an important component of the water cycle. Boiling occurs below the surface and involves the conversion of liquid into a gas at or above the boiling temperature. Condensation represents the conversion of a gas into a liquid. It is the reverse of evaporation and an important process in the water cycle. It is a crucial component of distillation. There is one other state of matter called *plasma*, which is seen in lightning, television screens, and neon lights. Plasma is most commonly converted from the gas state at extremely high temperatures.

The amount of energy needed to change matter from one state to another is labeled by the terms for phase changes. For example, the temperature needed to supply enough energy for matter to change from a liquid to a gas is called the *heat of vaporization*. When heat is added to matter in order to cause a change in state, there will be an increase in temperature until the matter is about to change its state. During its transition, all of the added heat is used by the matter to change its state, so there is no increase in temperature. Once the transition is complete, then the added heat will again yield an increase in temperature.

Each state of matter is considered to be a phase, and changes between phases are represented by phase diagrams. These diagrams show the effects of changes in pressure and temperature on matter. The states of matter fall into areas on these charts called *heating curves*.

Solutions

Concentration (pH)

One mole is the amount of matter contained in 6.02 x 10^{23} of any object, such as atoms, ions, or molecules. It is a useful unit of measure for items in large quantities. This number is also known as Avogadro's number. One mole of ^{12}C atoms is equivalent to 6.02 x 10^{23} ^{12}C atoms. Avogadro's number is often written as an inverse mole, or as 6.02 x 10^{23}/mol.

Molar Mass

A mole is always the same number, equivalent to Avogadro's number. The molar mass of a substance is the mass in grams of one mole of molecules of that substance. It is numerically equivalent to the molecular weight of the substance. The molecular weight of glucose ($C_6H_{12}O_6$) is 180 amu. Therefore, the molar mass of glucose is 180 grams per mole, written as 180 g/mol. In other words, one mole of glucose, or 6.02 x 10^{23} molecules of glucose, has a mass of 180 grams. Two substances with different molecular weights will have two different molar masses. Compared to glucose, O_2 has a molecular weight of 32 amu, which is less than that of glucose. So, the molar mass of O_2 is 32 g/mol. One mole of O_2 has an equivalent number of molecules as one mole of glucose, but it weighs less.

A simple calculation can determine how many moles are in a certain number of grams of a substance. The amount of substance in grams is divided by the molar mass of that substance and the result is the number of moles of the substance. Similarly, to convert the number of moles of a substance to the number of grams, multiply the number of moles by the molar mass of the substance. The result is the number of grams of the substance.

It is also possible to calculate the number of molecules in a certain number of grams of substance using Avogadro's number and the molar mass. The number of known grams is divided by the molar mass and then multiplied by Avogadro's number. The result is the number of molecules in the starting number of grams.

Molarity

Molarity is the concentration of a solution. It is based on the number of moles of solute in one liter of solution and is written as the capital letter M. A 1.0 molar solution, or 1.0 M solution, has one mole of solute per liter of solution. The molarity of a solution can be determined by calculating the number of moles of the solute and dividing it by the volume of the solution in liters. The resulting number is the mol/L or M for molarity of the solution.

Ionic solutions can also be described by molarity values. Since ionic compounds dissolve in solution, the chemical formula of the compound can be used to determine the relative concentrations of the ions in the solution. For example, in a 1.0 M solution of NaCl, there is 1.0 M Na^+ ions and 1.0 M Cl^- ions. In a 1.0 M solution of Na_2SO_4, there are two Na^+ ions (2.0 M) for each individual SO_4^{2-} ion (1.0 M).

pH Scale

pH refers to the power or potential of hydrogen atoms and is used as a scale for a substance's acidity. In chemistry, pH represents the hydrogen ion concentration (written as $[H^+]$) in an aqueous, or watery, solution. The hydrogen ion concentration, $[H^+]$, is measured in moles of H^+ per liter of solution.

The pH scale is a logarithmic scale used to quantify how acidic or basic a substance is. pH is the negative logarithm of the hydrogen ion concentration: pH = -log $[H^+]$. A one-unit change in pH correlates with a ten-fold change in hydrogen ion concentration. The pH scale typically ranges from 0 to 14, although it is possible to have pHs outside of this range. Pure water has a pH of 7, which is considered neutral. pH values less than 7 are considered acidic, while pH values greater than 7 are considered basic, or alkaline.

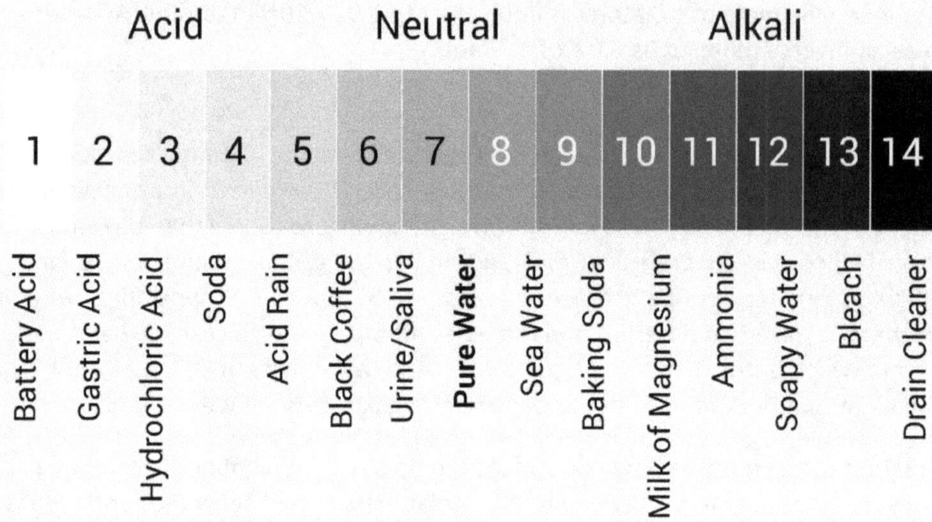

Generally speaking, an acid is a substance capable of donating hydrogen ions, while a base is a substance capable of accepting a hydrogen ion. A buffer is a molecule that can act as either a hydrogen ion donor or acceptor. Buffers are crucial in the blood and body fluids, and prevent the body's pH from fluctuating into dangerous territory. pH can be measured using a pH meter, test paper, or indicator sticks.

Solubility

A *solution* is a homogenous mixture of more than one substance. A *solute* is another substance that can be dissolved into a substance called a *solvent*. If only a small amount of solute is dissolved in a solvent, the solution formed is said to be *diluted*. If a large amount of solute is dissolved into the solvent, then the solution is said to be *concentrated*. For example, water from a typical, unfiltered household tap is diluted because it contains other minerals in very small amounts.

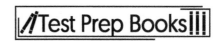

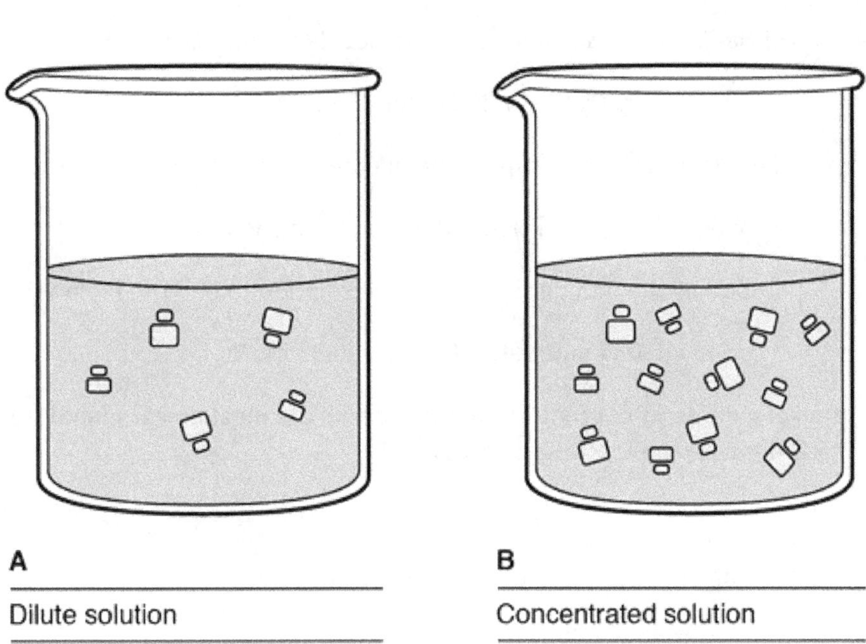

If more solute is being added to a solvent, but not dissolving, the solution is called *saturated*. For example, when hummingbirds eat sugar-water from feeders, they prefer it as sweet as possible. When trying to dissolve enough sugar (solute) into the water (solvent), there will be a point where the sugar crystals will no longer dissolve into the solution and will remain as whole pieces floating in the water. At this point, the solution is considered saturated and cannot accept more sugar. This level, at which a solvent cannot accept and dissolve any more solute, is called its *saturation point*. In some cases, it is possible to force more solute to be dissolved into a solvent, but this will result in crystallization. The state of a solution on the verge of crystallization, or in the process of crystallization, is called a *supersaturated* solution. This can also occur in a solution that seems stable, but if it is disturbed, the change can begin the crystallization process.

Although the terms *dilute*, *concentrated*, *saturated*, and *supersaturated* give qualitative descriptions of solutions, a more precise quantitative description needs to be established for the use of chemicals. This holds true especially for mixing strong acids or bases. The method for calculating the concentration of a solution is done through finding its molarity. In some instances, such as environmental reporting, molarity is measured in parts per million (ppm). Parts per million, is the number of milligrams of a substance dissolved in one liter of water. To find the *molarity*, or the amount of solute per unit volume of solution, for a solution, the following formula is used:

$$c = \frac{n}{V}$$

In this formula, *c* is the molarity (or unit moles of solute per volume of solution), *n* is the amount of solute measured in moles, and *V* is the volume of the solution, measured in liters.

Example:

What is the molarity of a solution made by dissolving 2.0 grams of NaCl into enough water to make 100 mL of solution?

To solve this, the number of moles of NaCl needs to be calculated:

First, to find the mass of NaCl, the mass of each of the molecule's atoms is added together as follows:

23.0g (Na) + 35.5g (Cl) = 58.5g NaCl

Next, the given mass of the substance is multiplied by one mole per total mass of the substance:

2.0g NaCl × (1 mol NaCl/58.5g NaCl) = 0.034 mol NaCl

Finally, the moles are divided by the number of liters of the solution to find the molarity:

(0.034 mol NaCl)/(0.100L) = 0.34 M NaCl

To prepare a solution of a different concentration, the *mass solute* must be calculated from the molarity of the solution. This is done via the following process:

Example:

How would you prepare 600.0 mL of 1.20 M solution of sodium chloride?

To solve this, the given information needs to be set up:

1.20 M NaCl = 1.20 mol NaCl/1.00 L of solution

0.600 L solution × (1.20 mol NaCl/1.00 L of solution) = 0.72 moles NaCl

0.72 moles NaCl × (58.5g NaCl/1 mol NaCl) = 42.12 g NaCl

This means that one must dissolve 42.12 g NaCl in enough water to make 600.0 L of solution.

Factors Affecting the Solubility of Substances and the Dissolving Process

Certain factors can affect the rate in dissolving processes. These include temperature, pressure, particle size, and agitation (stirring). As mentioned, the *ideal gas law* states that $PV = nRT$, where P equals pressure, V equals volume, and T equals temperature. If the pressure, volume, or temperature are affected in a system, it will affect the entire system. Specifically, if there is an increase in temperature, there will be an increase in the dissolving rate. An increase in the pressure can also increase the dissolving rate. Particle size and agitation can also influence the dissolving rate, since all of these factors contribute to the breaking of intermolecular forces that hold solute particles together. Once these forces are broken, the solute particles can link to particles in the solvent, thus dissolving the solute.

A *solubility curve* shows the relationship between the mass of solute that a solvent holds at a given temperature. If a reading is on the solubility curve, the solvent is *full* (*saturated*) and cannot hold anymore solute. If a reading is above the curve, the solvent is *unstable* (*supersaturated*) from holding more solute than it should. If a reading is below the curve, the solvent is *unsaturated* and could hold more solute.

If a solvent has different electronegativities, or partial charges, it is considered to be *polar*. Water is an example of a polar solvent. If a solvent has similar electronegativities, or lacking partial charges, it is considered to be *non-polar*. Benzene is an example of a non-polar solvent. Polarity status is important when attempting to dissolve solutes. The phrase "like dissolves like" is the key to remembering what will happen when attempting to dissolve a solute in a solvent. A polar solute will dissolve in a like, or polar solvent. Similarly, a non-polar solute will dissolve in a non-polar solvent. When a reaction produces a solid, the solid is called a *precipitate.* A precipitation reaction can be used for removing a salt (an ionic compound that results from a neutralization reaction) from a solvent, such as water. For water, this process is called *ionization*.

When a solute is added to a solvent to lower the freezing point of the solvent, it is called *freezing point depression*. This is a useful process, especially when applied in colder temperatures. For example, the addition of salt to ice in winter allows the ice to melt at a much lower temperature, thus creating safer road conditions for driving. Unfortunately, the freezing point depression from salt can only lower the melting point of ice so far and is ineffectual when temperatures are too low. This same process, with a mix of ethylene glycol and water, is also used to keep the radiator fluid (antifreeze) in an automobile from freezing during the winter.

Acids-Base Theories

Acids and bases are defined in many different ways. An acid can be described as a substance that increases the concentration of H^+ ions when it is dissolved in water, as a proton donor in a chemical equation, or as an electron-pair acceptor. A base can be a substance that increases the concentration of OH^- ions when it is dissolved in water, accepts a proton in a chemical reaction, or is an electron-pair donor.

Water can act as either an acid or a base. When mixed with an acid, water can accept a proton and become an H_3O^+ ion. When mixed with a base, water can donate a proton and become an OH^- ion. Sometimes water molecules donate and accept protons from each other; this process is called *autoionization*. The chemical equation is written as follows: $H_2O + H_2O \rightarrow OH^- + H_3O^+$.

Strength of Acids and Bases

Acids and bases are characterized as strong, weak, or somewhere in between. Strong acids and bases completely or almost completely ionize in aqueous solution. The chemical reaction is driven completely forward, to the right side of the equation, where the acidic or basic ions are formed. Weak acids and bases do not completely disassociate in aqueous solution. They only partially ionize, and the solution becomes a mixture of the acid or base, water, and the acidic or basic ions. Strong acids are complemented by weak bases, and vice versa. A conjugate acid is an ion that forms when its base pair gains a proton. For example, the conjugate acid NH_4^+ is formed from the base NH_3. The conjugate base that pairs with an acid is the ion that is formed when an acid loses a proton. NO_2^- is the conjugate base of the acid HNO_2.

Nuclear Chemistry: Radioisotopes

Nuclear chemistry is the study of reactions in which the nuclei of atoms are transformed and their identities are changed. These reactions can involve large changes in energy—much larger than the energy changes that occur when chemical bonds between atoms are made or broken. Nuclear chemistry is also used to create electricity.

Nuclear reactions are described by nuclear equations, which have different notations than regular chemical equations. Nuclear equations are written as follows, with the superscript being the mass number and the subscript being the atomic number for each element:

$$^{238}_{92}U \rightarrow \, ^{234}_{90}Th + \, ^{4}_{2}He$$

The equation describes the spontaneous decomposition of uranium into thorium and helium via alpha decay. When this happens, the process is referred to as nuclear decay. Similar to chemical equations, nuclear equations must be balanced on each side; the sum of the mass numbers and the sum of the atomic numbers should be equal on both sides of the equation.

In some cases, the nucleus of an atom is unstable and constantly emits particles due to this instability. These atoms are described as radioactive and the isotopes are referred to as *radioisotopes*. There are three types of radioactive decay that occur most frequently: alpha (α), beta (β), and gamma (γ). Alpha radiation is emitted when a nucleus releases a stream of alpha particles, which are helium-4 nuclei. Beta radiation occurs when a stream of high-speed electrons is emitted by an unstable nucleus. The beta particles are often noted as β^-. Gamma radiation occurs when the nucleus emits high-energy photons. In gamma radiation, the atomic number and the mass remain the same for the unstable nucleus. This type of radiation represents a rearrangement of an unstable nucleus into a more stable one and often accompanies other types of radioactive emission. Radioactive decay is often described in terms of its half-life, which is the time that it takes for half of the radioactive substance to react. For example, the radioisotope strontium-90 has a half-life of 28.8 years. If there are 10 grams of strontium-90 to start with, after 28.8 years, there would be 5 grams left.

There are two distinct types of nuclear reactions: fission and fusion reactions. Both involve a large energy release. In *fission* reactions, a large atom is split into two or more smaller atoms. The nucleus absorbs slow-moving neutrons, resulting in a larger nucleus that is unstable. The unstable nucleus then undergoes fission. Nuclear power plants depend on nuclear fission reactions for energy. *Fusion* reactions involve the combination of two or more lighter atoms into a larger atom. Fusion reactions do not occur in Earth's nature due to the extreme temperature and pressure conditions required to make them happen. Fusion products are generally not radioactive. Fusion reactions are responsible for the energy that is created by the Sun.

Organic Chemistry

Organic chemistry is a branch of chemistry that involves the study of the structures, properties, and reactions of organic compounds. *Organic compounds* are molecules that have carbon as the backbone molecule. Organic chemistry studies range from understanding the nature of various molecules to describing chemical reactions in laboratories and living organisms.

Structures and Properties

Organic compounds are carbon-based compounds, meaning the carbon (C) atoms form the skeleton or backbone of the molecule. In organic compounds, the C atoms bind to other atoms, mostly hydrogen

(H), oxygen (O), and nitrogen (N). Organic molecules can also contain other atoms, including sulfur (S), phosphorus (P), and halogens (X) such as fluorine (F), chlorine (Cl), bromine (Br), and iodine (I). *Functional groups* are the different atoms and how they are bonded together. Functional groups give the organic compound its molecular properties and reactivity.

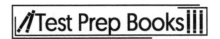

In organic chemistry, functional groups help predict the chemical behavior of an organic compound because molecules possessing the same function groups undergo similar patterns of chemical reactions. Adjacent functional groups may also influence this reactivity. Functional groups are used to classify organic compounds into different chemical classes. An example of this is *alcohols*. The molecular and structural formula of an *alcohol* is shown below. The functional group is the –OH group.

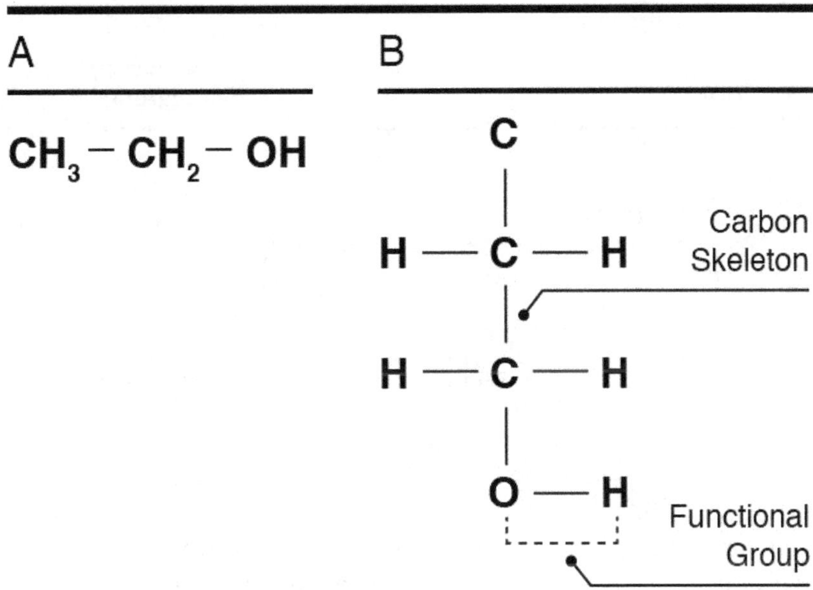

Structural Formulas and Bonding

Hydrocarbons are organic compounds that consist of only H and C atoms. They are classified into two major categories: aliphatic hydrocarbons (open chain) or cyclic hydrocarbons (closed chain). These groups are further divided. The overall classification of hydrocarbons is illustrated in the chart below:

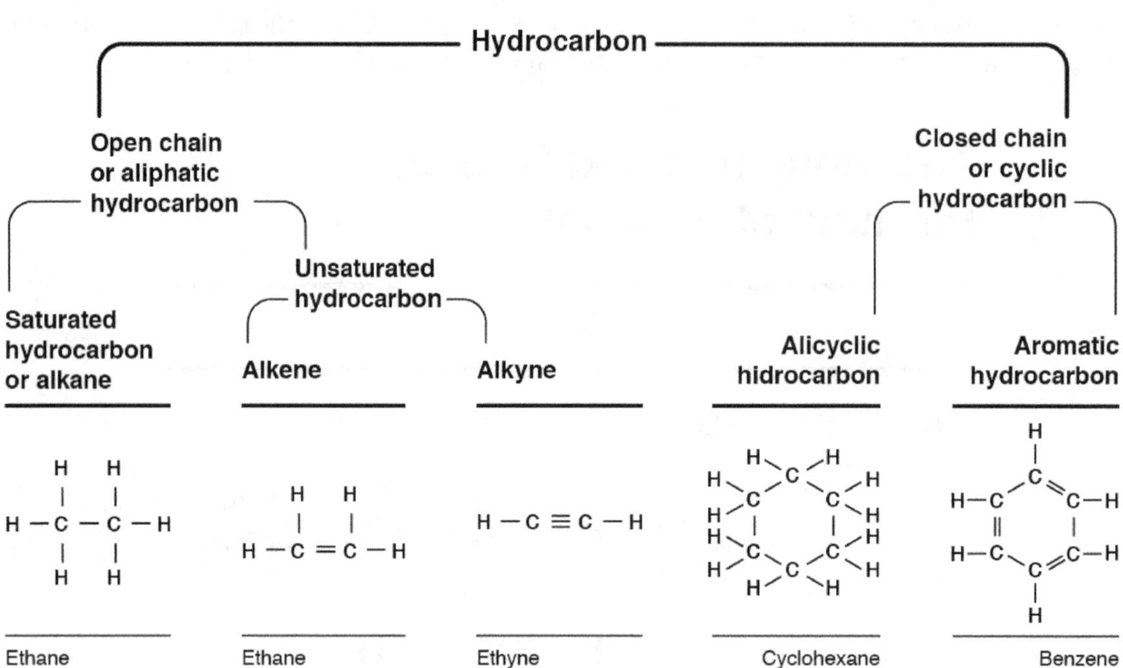

Aliphatic Hydrocarbons (Open Chain)

Aliphatic hydrocarbons have two open ends, meaning the C atoms at two terminals of the chain do not connect together. Because an aliphatic hydrocarbon chain has an open structure, it is often called an open chain hydrocarbon. Aliphatic hydrocarbons can contain single, double and/or triple C-C bonds. These different types of bonds classify aliphatic hydrocarbons into saturated hydrocarbons and unsaturated hydrocarbons.

Saturated hydrocarbons are the simplest form of hydrocarbons, and a type of aliphatic hydrocarbons. They contain only single bonds and are called alkanes. The single bonds are σ-bonds. Therefore, saturated hydrocarbons are more stable (or less susceptible to chemical reactions) than unsaturated hydrocarbons, and there is full rotation between all C-C bonds. In these molecules, the carbon bonds have the maximum number of H atoms possible, and are fully saturated with H atoms. Saturated hydrocarbons can have a linear or branched structure. In a linear structure, all of the carbon atoms form one single line. In a branched structure, the carbon chain splits off, creating multiple "branches" of carbon chains. The general molecular formula of saturated hydrocarbons (or alkanes) is C_nH_{2n+2}, where *n* is the number of C atoms in the chain. Below are examples of short-chain saturated hydrocarbons.

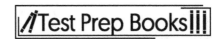

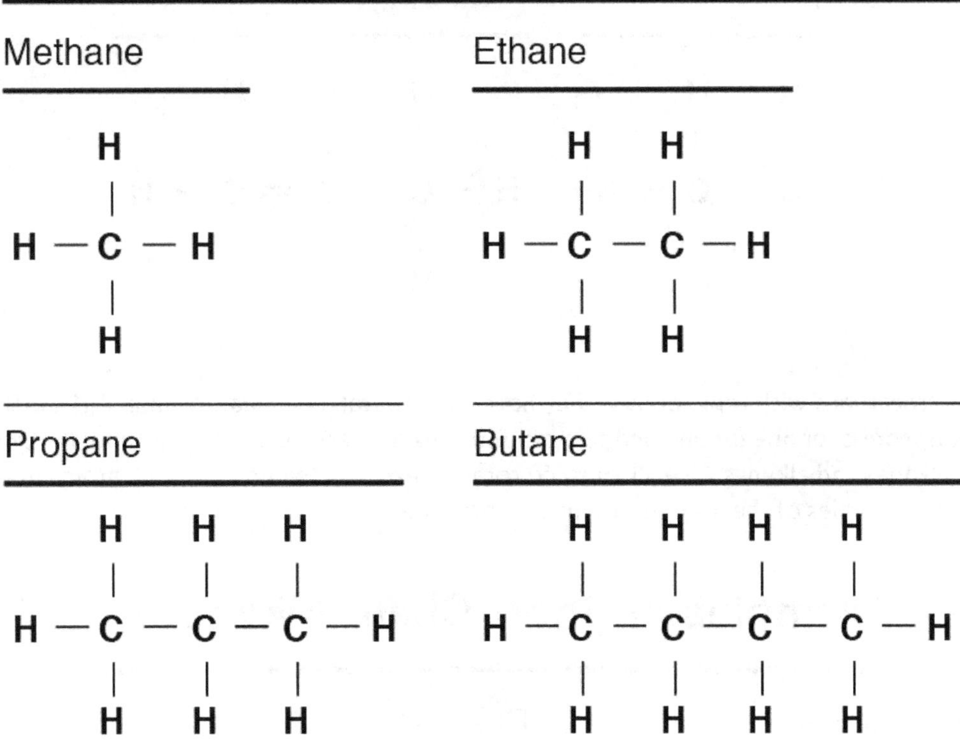

Unsaturated hydrocarbons are hydrocarbons that contain one or more double or triple bonds between C atoms in the hydrocarbon chain. They are further categorized into two groups: alkenes and alkynes.

Alkenes are hydrocarbons with double bonds. They have the general molecular formula of C_nH_{2n}. In their double bonds, one bond is a σ-bond and the other is a π-bond. Because of the presence of π-bonds, alkenes are more chemically reactive than saturated hydrocarbons. Additionally, there is no rotation between the two C atoms in a double bond. Below are examples of the short-chain alkenes ethene and propene:

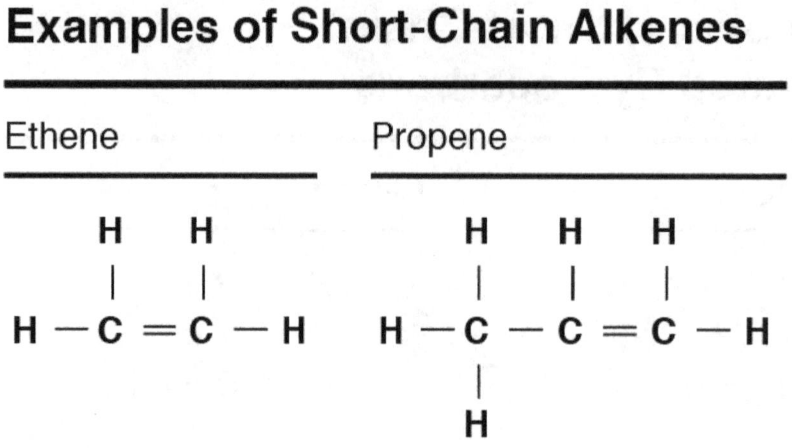

Examples of Short-Chain Alkenes

Ethene	Propene

```
    H   H           H   H   H
    |   |           |   |   |
H — C = C — H   H — C — C = C — H
                    |
                    H
```

Alkynes are hydrocarbons with triple bonds. They have the general molecular formula C_nH_{2n-2}. The triple bonds in alkynes consist of one σ-bond and two π-bonds. Alkynes are quite unstable and are more reactive than alkanes and alkenes. Like alkenes, no rotation exists between the two C atoms in a triple bond. Below are examples of the alkynes ethyne and propyne:

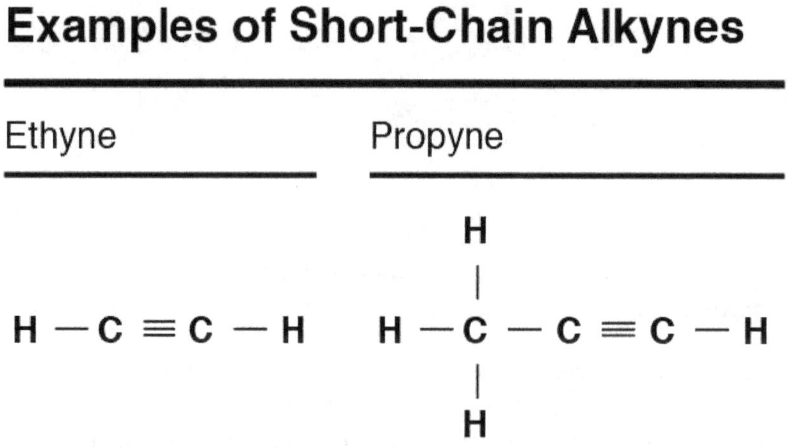

Examples of Short-Chain Alkynes

Ethyne	Propyne

```
                    H
                    |
H — C ≡ C — H   H — C — C ≡ C — H
                    |
                    H
```

Cyclic Hydrocarbons (Closed Chain)

Cyclic hydrocarbons have the terminal C atoms connected to each other, forming a closed, cyclic structure. Therefore, they are closed chain hydrocarbons. These hydrocarbons might have single, double, or triple bonds. Cyclic hydrocarbons are classified into alicyclic hydrocarbons and aromatic hydrocarbons.

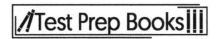

Alicyclic hydrocarbons have one or more carbon rings and can contain either saturated or unsaturated bonds. They have similar properties to aliphatic hydrocarbons. Below are examples of alicyclic hydrocarbons:

Examples of Alicyclic Hydrocarbons

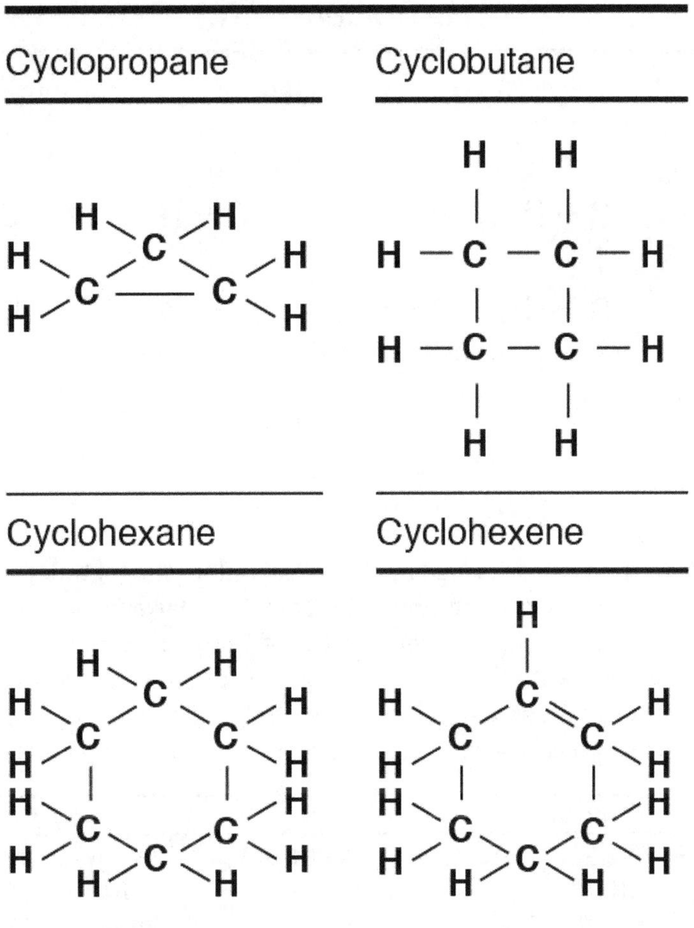

Cyclopropane

Cyclobutane

Cyclohexane

Cyclohexene

Aromatic hydrocarbons are cyclic hydrocarbons with σ-bonds and delocalized π-electrons between the carbon atoms that form the ring. Delocalized π-electrons are the result of a structure with resonance. This structure is often written as a molecule with a double bond between every other carbon atom, but this description is not entirely accurate. The double bonds are "shared" between all of the carbon atoms in the ring. This creates a very stable, unreactive structure. The geometry of these rings is flat and rigid. These compounds are also called arene, or aryl, hydrocarbons. Benzene is the simplest aromatic hydrocarbon. Historically, individuals thought that aromatic hydrocarbons contained a pleasant odor, resulting in the descriptive name. Aromatic hydrocarbons constitute a major part of crude oil and are highly flammable in nature.

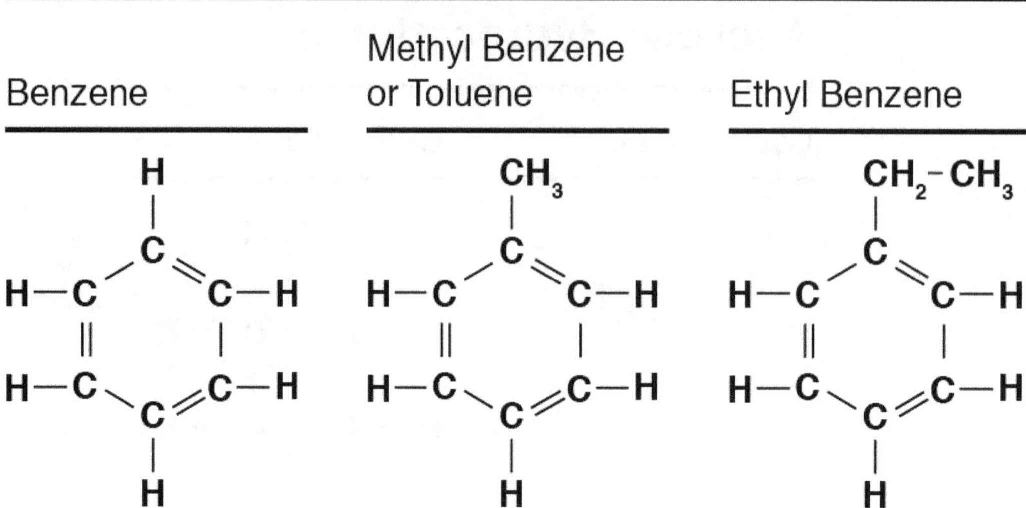

Naming of Hydrocarbons

The naming of hydrocarbons is performed by the IUPAC (International Union of Pure and Applied Chemistry). According to this system, saturated hydrocarbons (alkane) are named by adding "ane" to the end of the prefix that corresponds to the number of C atoms present in the chain. An "alkyl" group is the name for a hydrocarbon with one H atom removed. These often serve as functional groups, and their name corresponds to the name of the alkane with the same number of C atoms. The table below lists alkanes and corresponding alkyl groups based on the number of C atoms in the chain.

C atoms	Prefix	Structure	Name	Alkyl Group	
C_1	Meth-	CH_4	Methane	Methyl	$-CH_3$
C_2	Eth-	CH_3-CH_3	Ethane	Ethyl	CH_3-CH_2-
C_3	Prop-	CH_3-CH_2-CH_3	Propane	Propyl	CH_3-CH_2- CH_2-
C_4	But-	CH_3-$(CH_2)_2$-CH_3	Butane	Butyl	CH_3-$(CH_2)_2$-CH_2 -
C_5	Pent-	CH_3-$(CH_2)_3$-CH_3	Pentane	Pentyl	CH_3-$(CH_2)_3$-CH_2 -
C_6	Hex-	CH_3-$(CH_2)_4$-CH_3	Hexane	Hexyl	CH_3-$(CH_2)_4$-CH_2 -
C_7	Hept-	CH_3-$(CH_2)_5$-CH_3	Heptane	Heptyl	CH_3-$(CH_2)_5$-CH_2 -
C_8	Oct-	CH_3-$(CH_2)_6$-CH_3	Octane	Octyl	CH_3-$(CH_2)_6$-CH_2 -
C_9	Non-	CH_3-$(CH_2)_7$-CH_3	Nonane	Nonyl	CH_3-$(CH_2)_7$-CH_2 -
C_{10}	Dec-	CH_3-$(CH_2)_8$-CH_3	Decane	Decyl	CH_3-$(CH_2)_8$-CH_2 -

When alkanes are branched chains, the following rules are followed:

1. Find the longest chain of C atoms. This is the parent hydrocarbon. Name the alkane by using the rules listed above.

2. Identify all of the alkyl groups attached to the parent chain.

3. Number the parent chain so the first alkyl group is located closest to the number 1. If there are different alkyl groups equidistant from each terminal C atom, assign the lowest number to the one with the most substitutions or the one that that will come first in the name.

4. Name each substitution, starting with the number of the C atom, denoting its location and the name of the alkyl group. If more than one of the same alkyl group exists, list them all with commas separating the C atom number. In some cases, they may be on the same C atom.

Please note this is a simplified version of the rules. More rules exist for side chain priority.

Naming Saturated Hydrocarbons

a.	b.
2, 2, 4 - trimethyl pentane	**2, 4, 4 - trimethyl pentane**
Correct naming	*Incorrect naming*

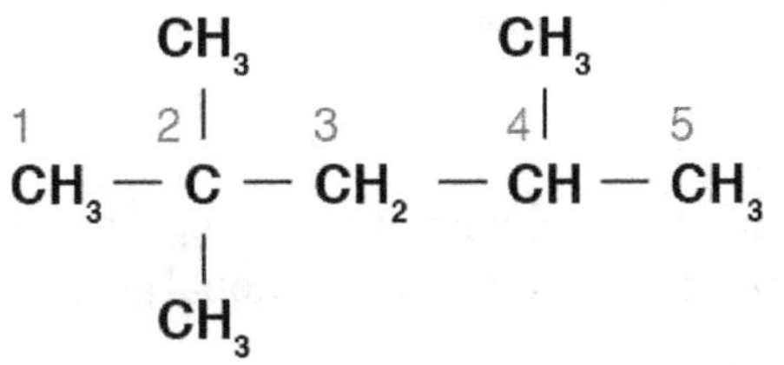

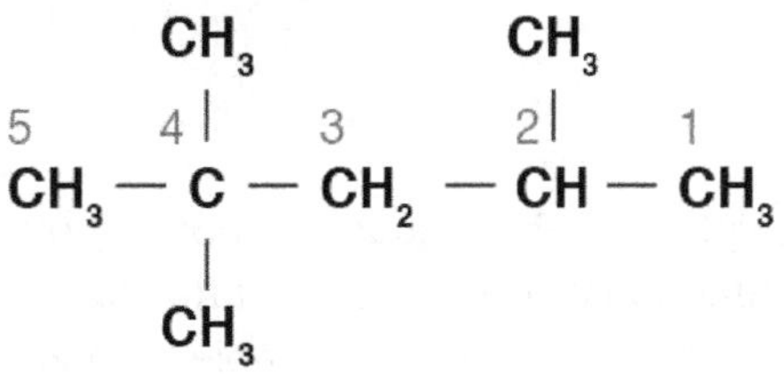

a.

$$\overset{1}{CH_3} - \overset{2}{\underset{CH_3}{\overset{CH_3}{C}}} - \overset{3}{CH_2} - \overset{4}{\overset{CH_3}{CH}} - \overset{5}{CH_3}$$

b.

$$\overset{5}{CH_3} - \overset{4}{\underset{CH_3}{\overset{CH_3}{C}}} - \overset{3}{CH_2} - \overset{2}{\overset{CH_3}{CH}} - \overset{1}{CH_3}$$

Similar to saturated hydrocarbons, unsaturated hydrocarbons are named using the longest C chain, but with adding "ene" (double bond) and "yne" (triple bond) to the end. The number of the C atom containing the double bond is added to the end of the name. The terminal C atom closest to the unsaturated bond is numbered 1. Below are examples of unsaturated hydrocarbons:

Naming Unsaturated Hydrocarbons

a.	b.
4 - methyl pentene - 2	**5 - methyl hexyne - 1**

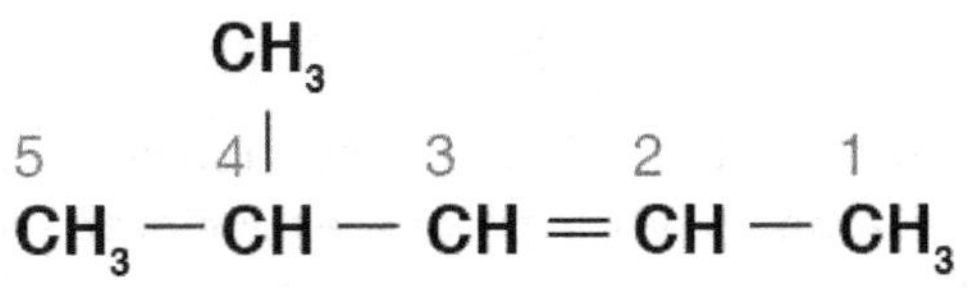

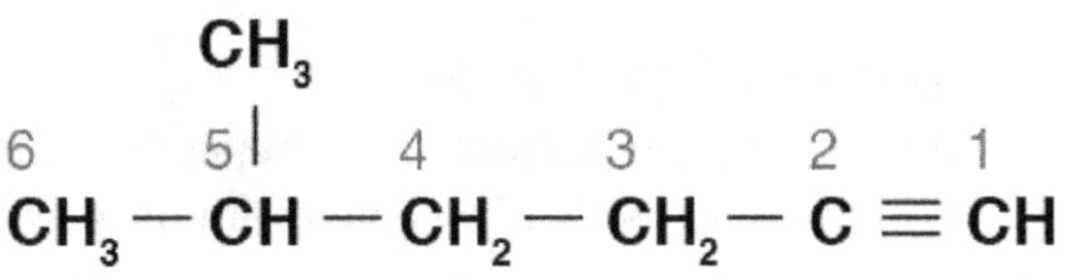

a.

$$\overset{5}{CH_3} - \overset{4}{\overset{CH_3}{CH}} - \overset{3}{CH} = \overset{2}{CH} - \overset{1}{CH_3}$$

b.

$$\overset{6}{CH_3} - \overset{5}{\overset{CH_3}{CH}} - \overset{4}{CH_2} - \overset{3}{CH_2} - \overset{2}{C} \equiv \overset{1}{CH}$$

If the hydrocarbon chain contains two or three double bonds, then they are called "alka-di-ene" and "alka-tri-ene," respectively. Similarly, the unsaturated chains containing two or three triple bonds are called "alka-di-yne" and "alka-tri-yne," respectively.

Naming Unsaturated Hydrocarbons that Contain Two or Three Double Bonds

a.	b.
2 - methyl - 1, penta-di-ene	**5 - methyl - 1, 3 - hexa-di-yne**
CH_3 on C2; 1 2 3 4 5: $CH_2=C-CH=CH-CH_3$	CH_3 on C5; 6 5 4 3 2 1: $CH_3-CH-C\equiv C-C\equiv CH$

The C chain might contain various functional group(s), and they are named accordingly by adding the name of the functional group to that of the parent carbon chain. Common functional groups found in organic compounds are listed in the table below:

Name	Functional Group	Example
Alkyl	$-(CH_2)_n-CH_3$ (n=0, 1, 2,...)	$CH_3CH_2CH_3$ (propane)
Alkenyl	-CH=CH-	$CH_3-CH=CH_2$ (propene)
Amine	$-NH_2$	CH_3NH_2 (methyl amine)
Ether	-O-	CH_3OCH_3 (dimethyl ether)
Aldehyde	-CHO	CH_3CHO (acetaldehyde)
Ketone	-CO-	CH_3COCH_3 (acetone)
Carboxylic Acid	-COOH	CH_3COOH (acetic acid)
Ester	$-CO_2R$ (R=alkyl group)	$CH_3CO_2CH_3$ (methyl acetate)
Acyl Chloride	-COCl	CH_3COCl (acetyl chloride)
Amide	$-CONH_2$	CH_3CONH_2 (acetamide)
Hydroxyl	-OH	CH_3CH_2OH (ethanol)
Halide	-F, -Cl, -Br and –I	CH_3Br (methyl bromide)

Isomers and their Classifications

Isomers are two or more molecules with the same molecular formula, but with different arrangements of atoms in the molecule, which can give them different chemical and physical properties. For example, ethanol (CH_3-CH_2-OH) and dimethyl ether (CH_3-O-CH_3) have the same molecular formula, C_2H_6O. However, they have different physical and chemical properties, due to the variation in their structural formula.

Isomerism is divided into two major categories: structural (constitutional) isomerism and stereoisomerism (spatial isomerism).

Structural isomerism is a type of isomerism in which the isomers have identical molecular formula, but the atoms in the molecules have different arrangements. There are four types of structural isomerisms: chain isomerism, position isomerism, functional group isomerism, and tautomerism.

1. *Chain isomerism* is also called skeletal isomerism. *Chain isomerism* occurs when the backbone atoms (usually C atoms) have different arrangements, such as straight or branch structures. Using the figure below as an example, butane and 2-methyl propane (isobutene) have the same molecular formula, C_4H_{10}, but different chain structures. This results in different physical and chemical properties.

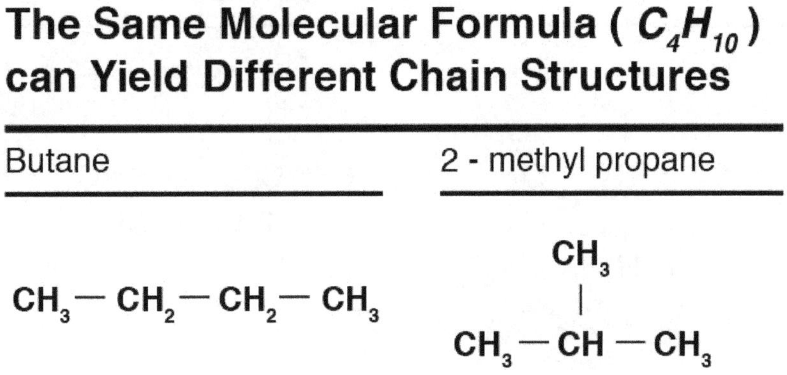

The Same Molecular Formula (C_4H_{10}) can Yield Different Chain Structures

Butane	2 - methyl propane
$CH_3 - CH_2 - CH_2 - CH_3$	$CH_3 - CH(CH_3) - CH_3$

2. *Position isomerism*, also termed regioisomerism, occurs when unsaturated (double or triple) bonds or functional groups have different locations in the chain. For example, 1-butene and 2-butene are position isomers because they have the same molecular formula (C_4H_8), but the double bonds are located at different positions. The same is true for 1-propanol and 2-propanol (isopropyl alcohol), where the functional group (-OH) is located on different C atoms. Position isomerism is also possible in aromatic compounds, based on the relative positions of the substituent atoms/groups in the benzene-ring structure.

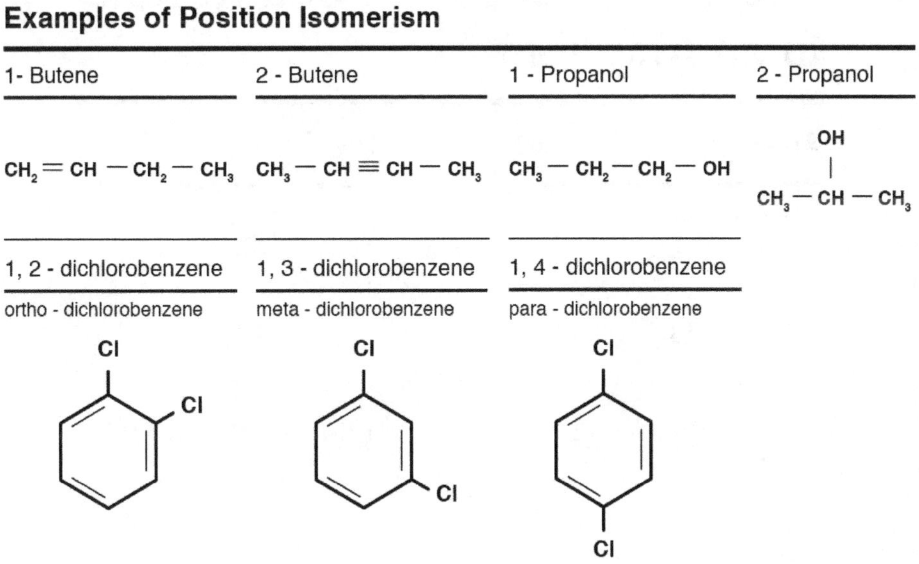

Examples of Position Isomerism

1- Butene	2 - Butene	1 - Propanol	2 - Propanol
$CH_2 = CH - CH_2 - CH_3$	$CH_3 - CH \equiv CH - CH_3$	$CH_3 - CH_2 - CH_2 - OH$	$CH_3 - CH(OH) - CH_3$

1, 2 - dichlorobenzene	1, 3 - dichlorobenzene	1, 4 - dichlorobenzene
ortho - dichlorobenzene	meta - dichlorobenzene	para - dichlorobenzene
Cl, Cl	Cl, Cl	Cl, Cl

3. *Functional group isomerism* refers to isomers that have the same molecular formula but different functional groups. For example, ethanol (CH_3-CH_2-OH) and dimethyl ether (CH_3-O-CH_3) are functional isomers because they have same molecular formula (C_2H_6O), but have different functional groups—hydroxyl (-OH) and ether (-O-) groups.

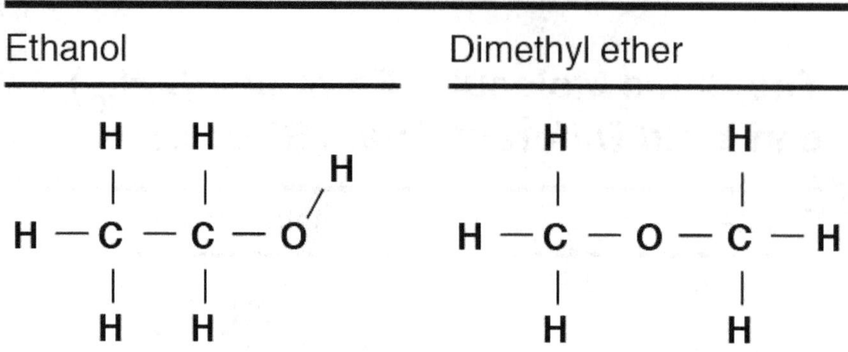

4. *Tautomerism* refers to a special type of structural isomerism resulting from spontaneous inter-conversion of functional groups to form two different compounds. This process primarily results in migration of a proton and switching between single and double bonds. Tautomerization is a chemical reaction that reaches equilibrium between the two tautomers (isomers). One example of tautomerism is "keto-enol tautomerism." It causes conversion of keto (-C=O) group to from a double bond ("ene" from alk<u>ene</u>) and an alcohol group (-OH) ("ol" from alcoho<u>l</u>). Therefore, it is called keto-enol tautomerism. See the example below in which a ketone, acetone (propanone), undergoes tautomerization to form an alcohol, 2-propenol:

The Tautomerization of a Ketone to an Alcohol

Acetone	2 - Propenol
Propanone	
$CH_3-C(=O)-CH_2-H$	$CH_3-C(OH)=CH_2$

Stereoisomerism is the type of isomerism in which molecules have similar molecular and structural formula, but they differ in their three-dimensional configurations and orientation of atoms in space. There are two types of stereoisomers: diastereomers and enantiomers.

1. Also called configurational or cis-trans isomers, the *diastereomers* have different orientations of atoms/groups along the C-C bond axis. Diastereomers generally contain a double bond or cyclic structure that has restricted bond rotation. The different isomers are designated "cis" and "trans." "Cis" isomers have similar atoms or groups on *the same side* of the C-C bond axis. "Trans" isomers have similar atoms or groups positioning on *the other side or across* the C-C bond axis. Examples of cis and trans isomers in double bond and cyclic structures are presented below:

Examples of cis and trans isomers in double bond and cyclic structures are presented below

Cis - 1, 2 - dichloro ethene	Cis - butene - 2	Cis - 1, 2 - dimethylcyclopropane
H, Cl > C = C < H, Cl	H, CH_3 > C = C < H, CH_3	CH_2 ring; H, CH_3 > C – C < H, CH_3
Trans - 1, 2 - dichloro ethene	**Trans - butene - 2**	**Trans - 1, 2 - dimethylcyclopropane**
Cl, H > C = C < H, Cl	CH_3, H > C = C < H, CH_3	CH_2 ring; CH_3, H > C – C < H, CH_3

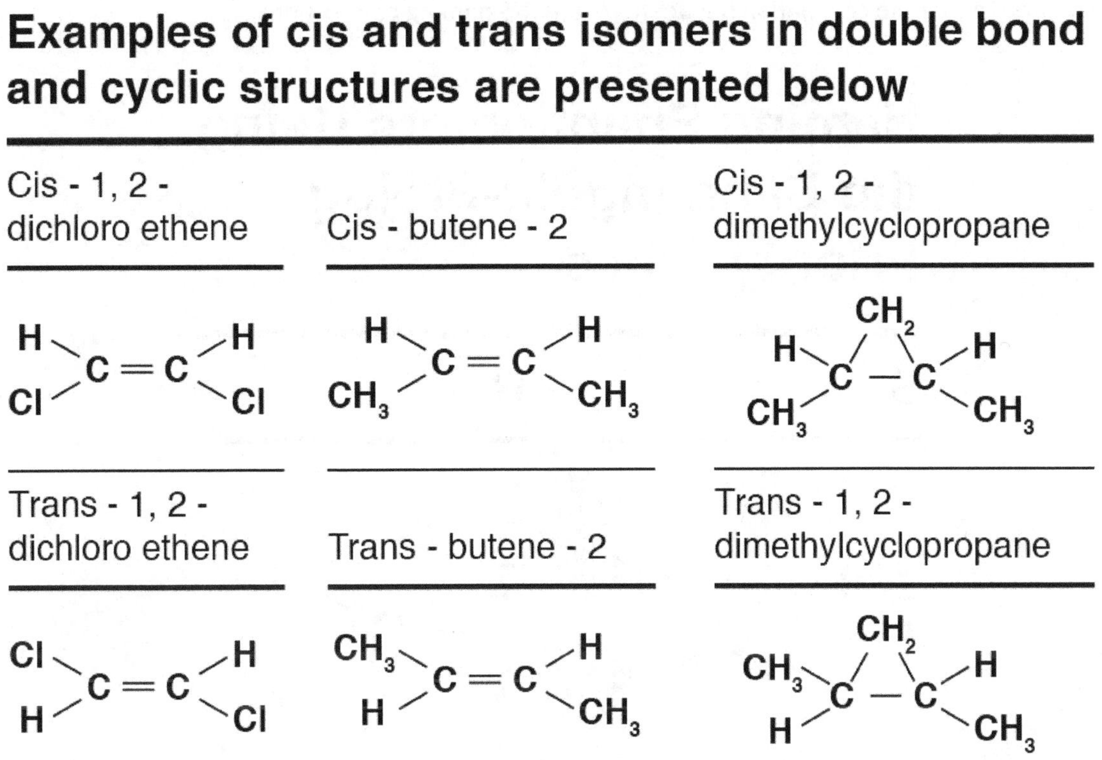

2. *Enantiomers* are stereoisomers that have a different arrangement around a chiral (asymmetric) center (usually a C atom). Enantiomers are mirror images of each other that cannot be superimposed on top of each other. A non-chemistry example this concept is your hands. If you hold them facing each other, you can see they are mirror images of each other. However, it is impossible to superimpose your left hand on top of your right hand.

When these isomers are in a symmetric environment, they have the same physical and chemical properties, but they behave differently in symmetric environments. Also, enantiomers can rotate plane-polarized light.

Most enantiomers are formed from a *chiral carbon*, which is a C atom that has four different atoms or functional groups attached to it. They are also called an asymmetric carbon. The four different atoms/groups can be arranged in two different ways around the chiral carbon, creating left-handed and right-handed configurations. These configurations are mirror images and do not superimpose. The number of optical isomers that can be formed from an organic compound is 2^n, where n equals the number of chiral C atoms in the molecule.

There are two naming conventions for enantiomers. One stems from their ability to rotate plane-polarized light. The enantiomer that rotates the light to the right is called the *dextrorotatory* or (+) or *d*-isomer. The enantiomer that rotates plane-polarized light left is called the *levorotatory* or (-) or *l*-isomer. The other naming method uses the Cahn-Ingold-Prelog priority rules, which ranks the functional groups based on their atomic number (a higher number has a higher priority). If the molecule is rotated so that the lowest priority group (4) faces you, the remaining three groups will either increase priority in a clockwise direction (the R enantiomer), or will increase priority in a counterclockwise direction (the S enantiomer). There is no correlation between d/l and R/S naming conventions.

Naming Enantiomers Using the Cahn-Ingold-Prelog Priority Rules

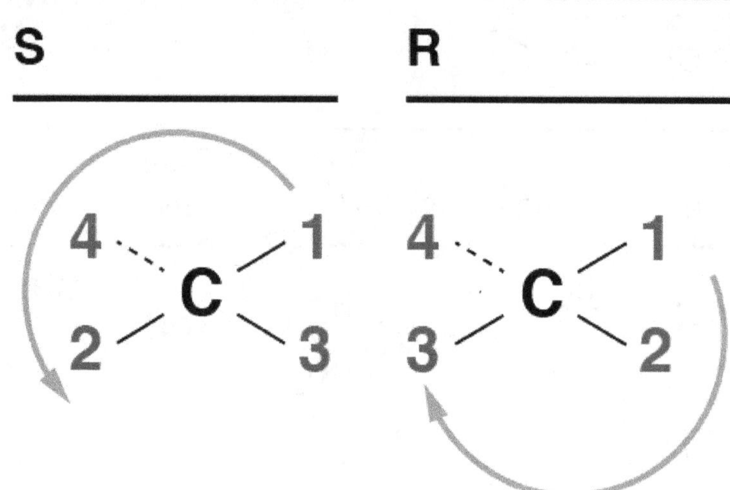

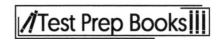

The example below shows a chiral carbon-containing compound, lactic acid [CH_3-CH(OH)-COOH]:

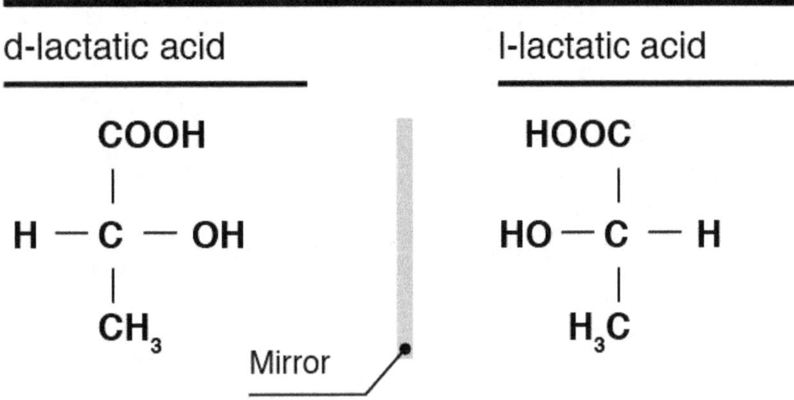

Normal visible light is a mixture of electromagnetic waves. The waves oscillate (up and down motion of the light wave) perpendicular to the direction the wave moves. In normal visible light, this oscillation can occur in all planes (directions) around the wave. *Plane polarized light* is light that is monochromatic (has only one wavelength), and all of the waves oscillate on the same plane. Plane polarized light is created by using a lamp that only produces light with one wavelength and then passing that light through an optical filter called a polarizer.

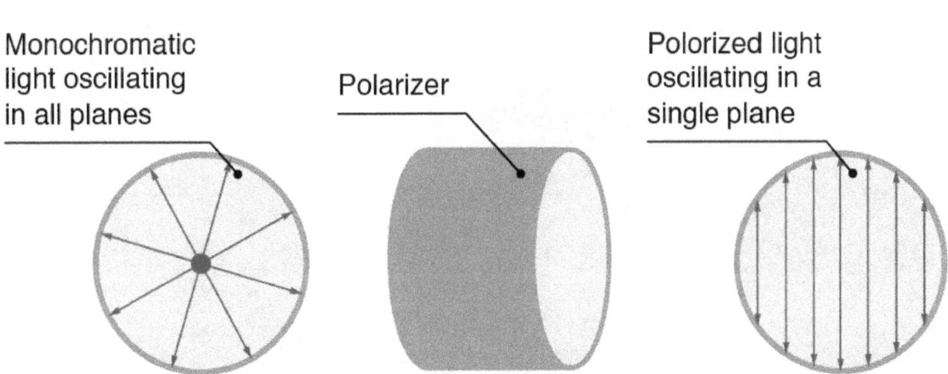

Optically-active compounds have the ability to rotate the plane polarized light. The instrument used to measure the angle of rotation of plane polarized light, while passing through an optically-active compound, is called *polarimeter*. The overall process of studying the properties of optically-active compounds is presented in the figure below:

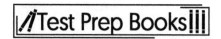

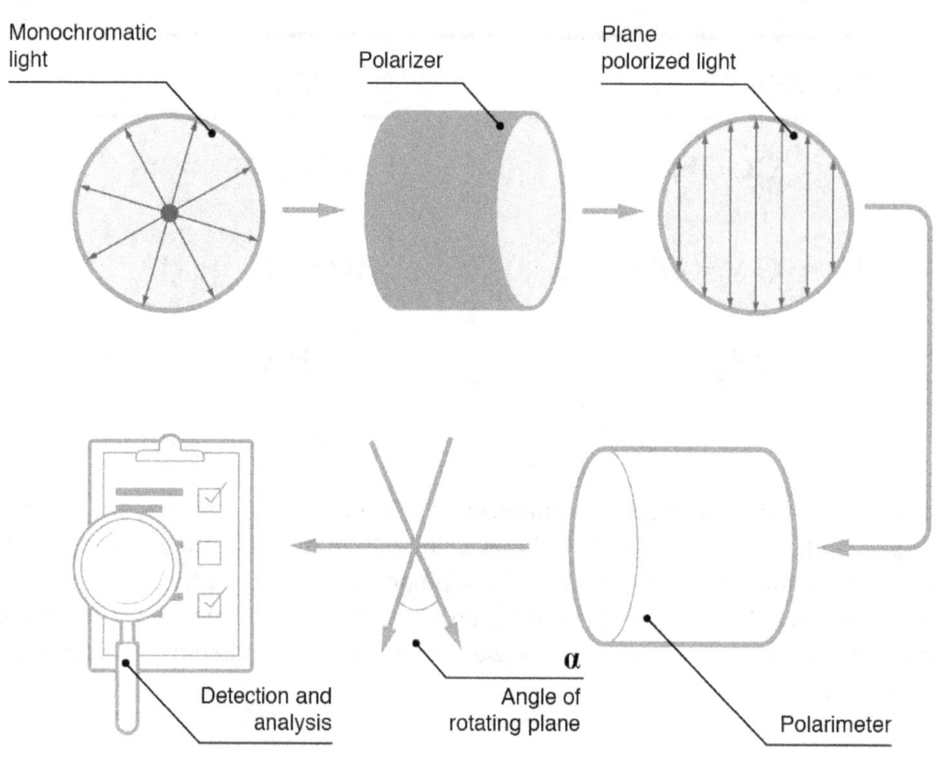

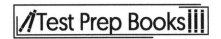

A *racemic mixture* contains an equal amount of *d*-(also called *R)* and *l*-(also called *S)* isomers, which do not rotate plane polarized light. For example, the mixture of equal ratio (1:1) of *d*-lactic acid and *l*-lactic acid is a racemic mixture. A racemic mixture is presented by *dl* or ± or *RS*. If the mixture is not a 1:1 ratio, a slash is used instead (i.e. *d/l* or *(+)/(-)* or *R/S)*.

The Classification of Isomers

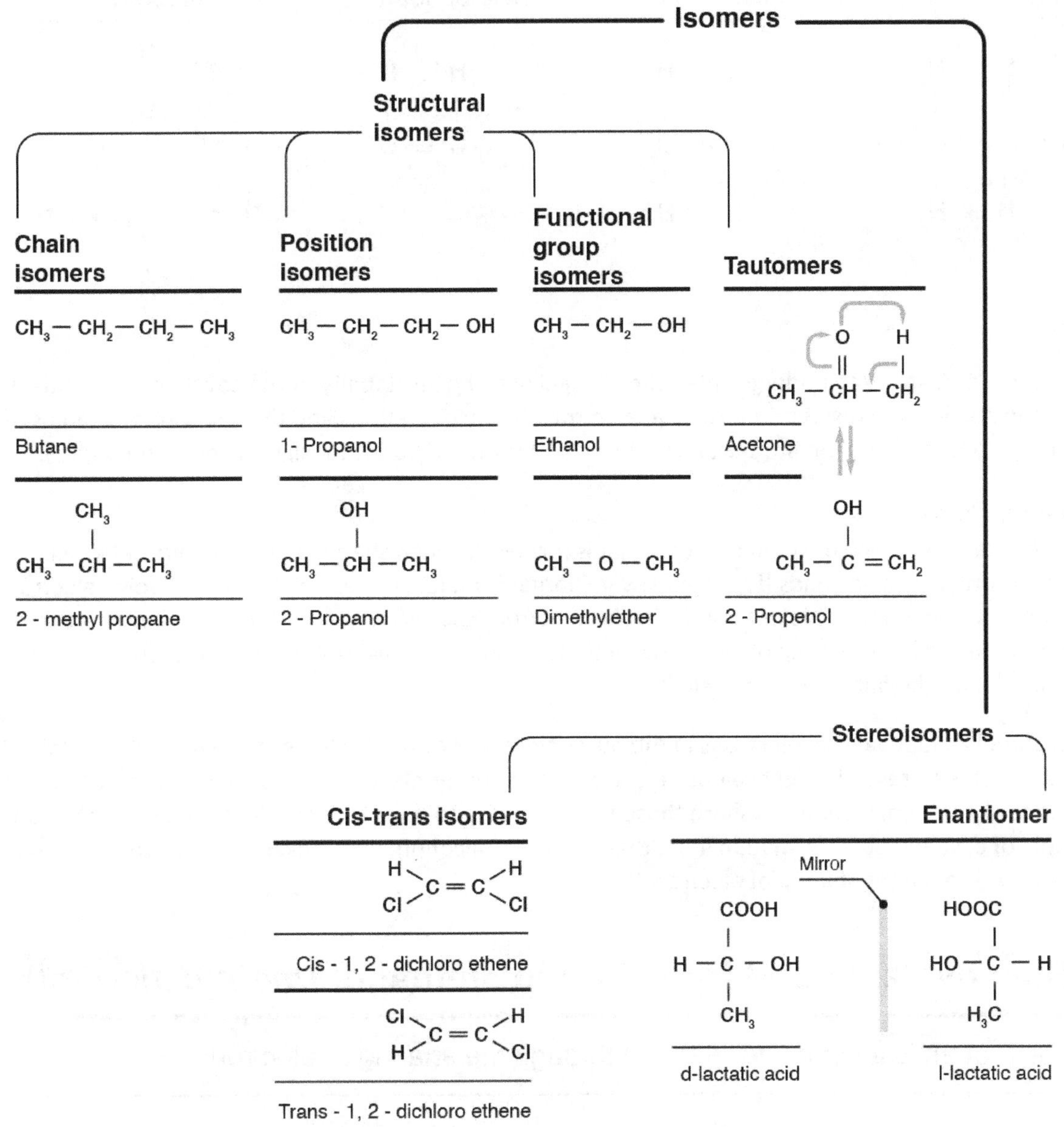

Isomers

Structural isomers

Chain isomers	**Position isomers**	**Functional group isomers**	**Tautomers**
$CH_3-CH_2-CH_2-CH_3$	$CH_3-CH_2-CH_2-OH$	CH_3-CH_2-OH	$CH_3-C(=O)-CH_3$
Butane	1- Propanol	Ethanol	Acetone
$CH_3-CH(CH_3)-CH_3$	$CH_3-CH(OH)-CH_3$	CH_3-O-CH_3	$CH_3-C(OH)=CH_2$
2 - methyl propane	2 - Propanol	Dimethylether	2 - Propenol

Stereoisomers

Cis-trans isomers	
H(Cl)C=C(Cl)H	Cis - 1, 2 - dichloro ethene
Cl(H)C=C(Cl)H	Trans - 1, 2 - dichloro ethene

Enantiomer		
COOH, H — C — OH, CH_3	Mirror	HOOC, HO — C — H, H_3C
d-lactatic acid		l-lactatic acid

Catenation

Carbon atoms can undergo a unique process called catenation, which make them able to form a vast number of organic compounds found in nature. *Catenation* refers to the linkage of the same kind of atom to form longer chains and structures. Carbon catenation helps build numerous types of structures, containing open chain, branch chain, or cyclic configurations in organic compounds. C atoms can form single bonds (a, in the figure below), double bonds (b), or triple bonds (c). C atoms can also form ring structures (d).

The Catenation of Carbon

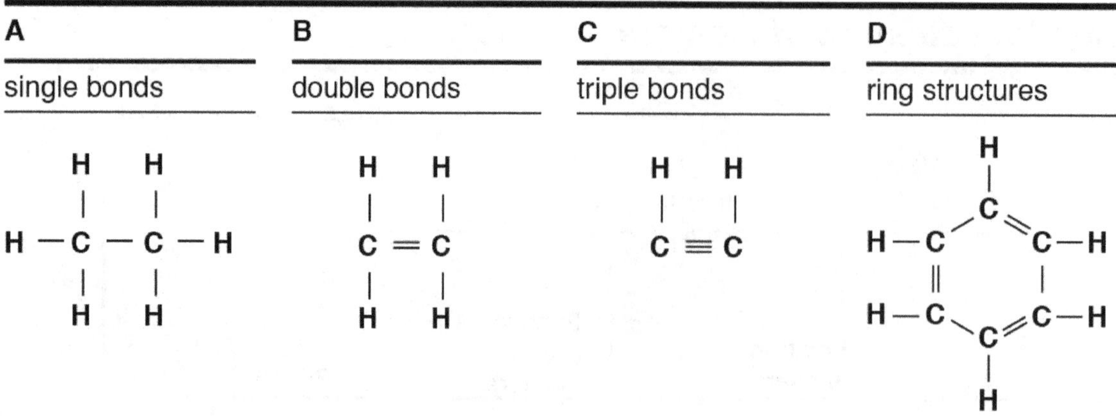

The success of C atoms to undergo catenation is because of high stability of the covalent C-C bonds. This high bond stability is a result of the relative electron affinity of C atoms and the small atomic radius of the atoms to face across the intra-atomic orbitals and form C-C bonds (σ (sigma) and π (pi) bonds).

Covalent Bonds

A *covalent bond* is a type of chemical bond that is formed through sharing electron pairs between atoms. Contrary to ionic bonds (found mostly in inorganic molecules, e.g. Na^+Cl^-) that involve electron *transfer* between atoms, covalent bonds involve electrons *shared* between atoms. A covalent bond formation, through the sharing of electrons, helps the corresponding atoms attain a stable electronic configuration at the outer valence shell.

The C atom has four valence electrons in the outer electron orbital. The octet rule states that most atoms combine to result in eight valence electrons in the outer electron orbital. In order to get a stable atomic configuration, carbon can share those four electrons to form four covalent bonds. Below is an example of covalent bond formation in methanol (methyl alcohol). In this example, a C atom is attached to H and O through the sharing of electrons.

The covalent bond formation in methanol *(methyl alcohol)*

The C atom is attached to H and O through the sharing of electrons

CH_3- OH → C + 4 H + O → H C O H

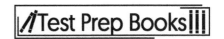

Atomic orbitals are the space, relative to the atom's nucleus, where one or more electrons persist. Covalent bonds are formed through an overlapping of the atomic orbitals. There are two types of covalent bonds: *sigma* (σ) and *pi* (π). Typically, a single bond is a σ-bond, and a multiple bond has both σ-bonds and π-bonds. For example, a double bond has one σ-bond and one π-bond, while a triple bond has one σ-bond and two π-bonds.

Sigma (σ) Bonds

A *sigma (σ) bond* is the strongest type of covalent bond. It forms from the direct and linear overlapping of atomic orbitals.

1. Formation of σ-bond by overlapping s-orbitals:

Sigma (*σ*) Bonds

1. Formation of σ-bond by overlapping s-orbitals

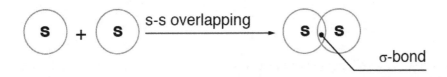

2. Formation of σ-bond by overlapping s-orbitals and p-orbitals

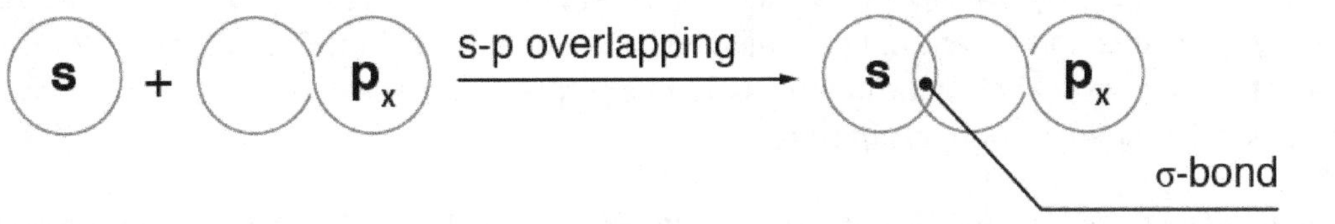

3. Formation of σ-bond by overlapping two p-orbitals

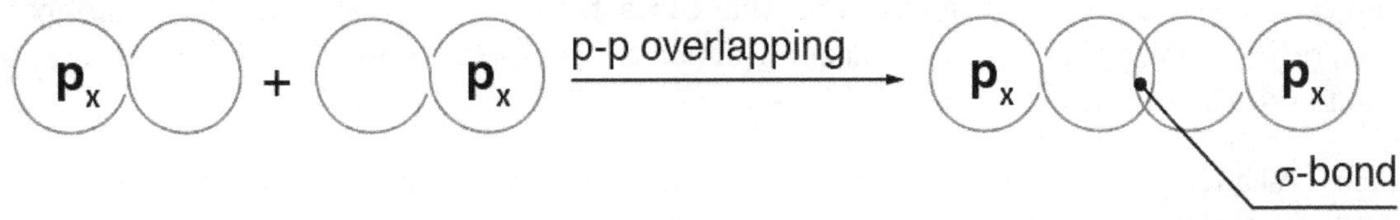

The nature of a σ-bond allows for rotation around the bond.

Pi (π) Bonds

Pi (π) bonds are formed as a result of parallel overlapping between two p-orbitals, which is a weaker and more diffuse bond than the linear σ-bond. π-bonds are weaker than σ-bonds and more susceptible to fission in chemical reactions. The parallel nature of a π-bond prevents rotation around the bond. Any rotation would cause the π-bond to break.

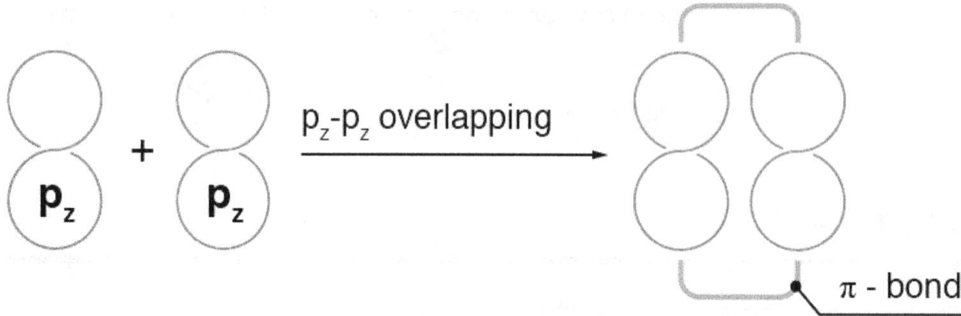

Properties of Organic Compounds

Alkanes

Alkanes are saturated hydrocarbons with a general molecular formula of C_nH_{2n+2}. Some examples of alkanes are methane (CH_4), ethane (C_2H_6), propane (C_3H_8), and butane (C_4H_8).

The physical properties of alkanes are as follows:

1. *Physical State:* Lower molecular weight alkanes (C_1 to C_4) are odorless gases at room temperature (i.e., methane, ethane, propane, and butane). Higher alkanes with C numbers from C_5 to C_{17} are colorless liquids with a petroleum odor. The alkanes with a C number equal or greater than C_{18} are colorless, odorless, and a wax-like solid at room temperature.

2. *Melting and Boiling Points:* The melting and boiling temperatures of straight chain alkanes increase as the number of C atoms increases. Branched chain alkanes have lower melting and boiling points than the straight chain alkanes with the same number of carbons. For example, pentane, iso-pentane, and neo-pentane have the boiling points of 36°C, 28°C, and 10°C, respectively. This happens because the branched chain alkanes have a less surface area that contacts each other (the molecules cannot pack in as tightly), resulting in weaker intra-molecular attraction (van der Waals force). Therefore, this causes lower melting/boiling points.

3. *Solubility:* Alkanes are insoluble in water and other polar liquids. Instead, they are soluble in organic liquids. Alkanes are non-polar, so they are soluble in other non-polar liquids (e.g. benzene, ethanol, ether etc.).

4. *Relative Density:* The relative density, or specific gravity, of alkanes is less than 1. Therefore, alkanes are not as dense as water. With the increase in the chain length of alkanes, the relative density is gradually increased, but always remains less than 1.

5. *Combustion:* Alkanes are flammable, catch fire easily, and burn with a blue flame. The complete combustion of an alkane leads to the formation of carbon dioxide and water. During combustion, the

supply of oxygen has to be sufficient. Insufficient oxygen leads to the production of carbon monoxide, and the heat generated is less if sufficient oxygen is unavailable.

Alkanes only have sigma (σ) bonds, which are relatively stable in chemical reactions. Therefore, alkanes generally do not react with acids, alkalis, and oxidizing/reducing agents. However, in the presence of high temperature and pressure, σ-bonds undergo fission to produce free radicals. Free radicals are highly reactive, since they carry unpaired valence electrons. Once alkyl-free radicals are formed, they interact with the attacking reagents to form new compounds. The chemical reactions of alkanes are categorized three ways: substitution reactions, thermal decomposition reactions or pyrolysis, and isomerizations.

Alkenes

Alkenes are unsaturated hydrocarbons with one or more double bonds. Alkenes are represented by the general formula C_nH_{2n}. Examples of alkenes are ethene ($CH_2=CH_2$) and propene ($CH_3—CH=CH_2$).

The physical properties of alkenes are as follows:

1. *Physical State:* Lower molecular weight alkenes (C_2 to C_4) are gases at room temperature (i.e., ethene, propene and butene). Higher alkenes with the carbon number of C_5 to C_{15} are liquids. C_{16} and higher alkenes are solid. Ethene has a sweet odor, but other alkenes are colorless and odorless.

2. *Melting and Boiling Points:* The melting and boiling points of alkenes increase with the molecular weight. However, branched chain alkenes have lower melting and boiling points than those of the corresponding straight chain alkenes.

3. *Solubility:* Alkenes are insoluble in water, but soluble in organic solvents like benzene, ethanol, ether, etc.

4. *Relative Density:* The relative density of alkenes is less than 1. Therefore, they are less dense than water. With the increase in the chain length of alkanes, the relative density increases, but always remains less than 1.

5. *Combustion:* Alkenes are flammable, and they burn with a yellow flame. Complete combustion of an alkene in the presence of adequate oxygen produces carbon dioxide and water. When enough oxygen is not available, partial combustion of alkenes primarily produces carbon monoxide.

Alkenes are unsaturated hydrocarbons, which have double bonds. The double bond consists of one sigma (σ) bond and one pi (π) bond. The π-bond is prone to electrophilic addition reactions. Alkenes undergo three types of reactions: addition reactions, oxidation reactions, and polymerizations.

Alkynes

Alkynes are unsaturated hydrocarbons with one or more triple bonds. They are represented by the general formula C_nH2_{n-2}, where *n* equals 1, 2, 3 . . .n. Examples of alkynes are ethyne and 2-butyne.

The physical properties of alkynes are as follows:

1. *Physical State:* Lower molecular weight alkynes (C_2 to C_4) are gases at room temperature (i.e., ethyne, propyne and butyne). Alkynes with the carbon number of C_5 to C_{12} are liquids. Higher alkynes are colorless and odorless solids.

2. *Melting and Boiling Points:* The melting and boiling points of alkynes are higher than that of alkanes and alkenes of similar C-chain length. With the increase in molecular weight of the alkynes, the melting and boiling points increase accordingly.

3. *Solubility:* Alkynes are insoluble in water, but soluble in organic solvents.

4. *Relative Density:* The relative density of alkynes is higher than that of alkanes and alkenes, but still less than water.

5. *Combustion:* Alkynes are flammable, and they burn with a yellow flame. Like alkanes and alkenes, complete combustion of an alkyne in the presence of adequate oxygen produces carbon dioxide and water. When oxygen is inadequate, combustion of alkynes produces carbon monoxide.

A triple bond in an alkyne contains one σ-bond and two π-bonds. The presence of π-electrons in alkynes makes them suitable to interact with electrophiles. Alkynes undergo the following types of chemical reactions: addition reactions, oxidation reactions, and polymerizations.

Aromatic Compounds

Aromatic compounds are also called arenes. The term "aromatic" is a historical term related to the belief that aromatic compounds have a pleasant aroma. We now know this is not true. These molecules all contain a planar ring structure with conjugated, delocalized π-electrons. This configuration renders the aromatic structure unusually stable. Therefore, they are relatively more resistant to chemical fission or participation in chemical reactions. Aromatic compounds include benzene, benzene derivatives, and compounds that behave like benzene.

Aromatic Compounds are Stable Because of Their Structure

Benzenoid structure with delocalized π-electrons in the planar molecular orbital

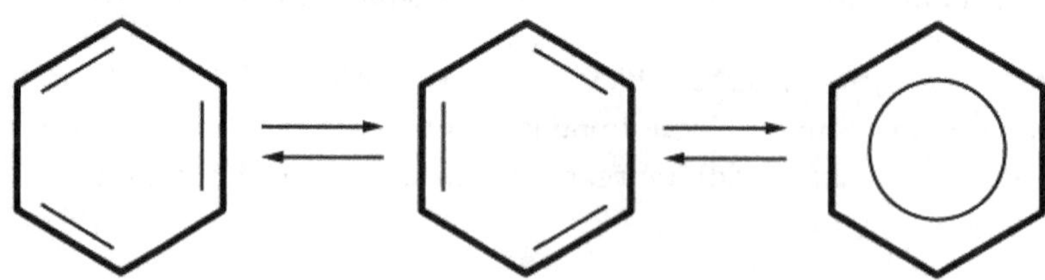

Aromatic compounds are classified into three major groups:

1. Benzene and substituted benzene compounds
2. Polycyclic or fused aromatic compounds
3. Heterocyclic aromatic compounds

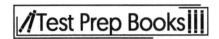

Benzene and substituted benzene compounds contain a benzene ring with/without substituted groups or atoms in the ring. Examples are benzene, toluene (methyl benzene), ethyl benzene, and phenol.

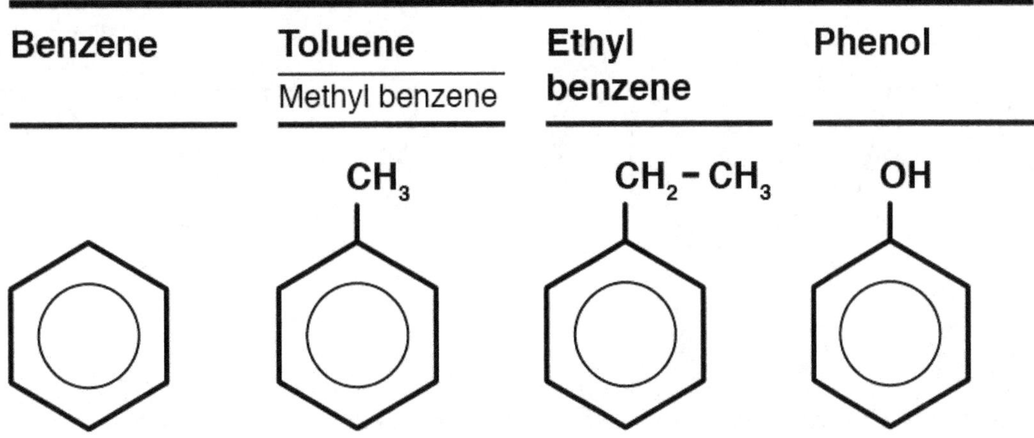

Polycyclic aromatic compounds contain two or more benzene rings fused together while sharing two adjacent C atoms. Examples of this type of compounds are naphthalene, anthracene, and phenanthrene.

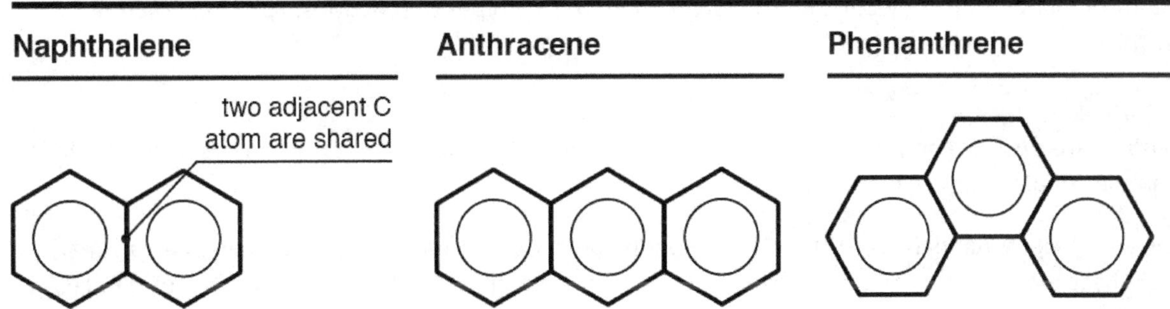

Heterocyclic aromatic compounds contain one or more heteroatoms (other than C atoms), like O, N, S, as a part of the aromatic ring. This causes a decrease in the ring's aromaticity and stability, and therefore increases its reactivity. Some examples of heteroaromatic compounds are furan, pyridine, imidazole, oxazole, and thiophene (or thiofuran).

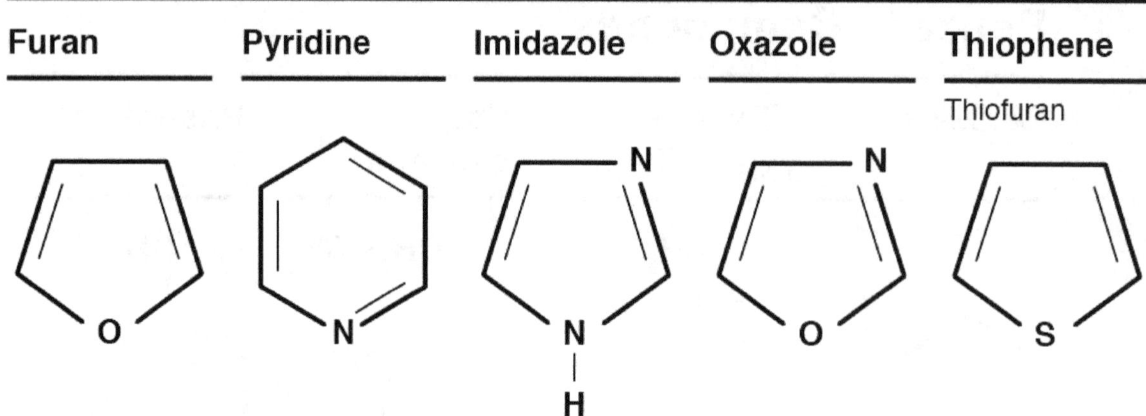

Benzene is a colorless liquid with a sweet smell. Benzene's melting and boiling points are 5.5°C and 80.1°C, respectively. Its specific gravity is less than water, and therefore it is less dense than water. It is a constituent of crude oil and it is flammable. It burns with a black flame. Because of its high stability, it is a good solvent for organic compounds.

Benzene has a hexagonal planar structure. Six H atoms remain attached to C atoms by σ-bonds. The functional group of an aromatic hydrocarbon formed by removing one H atom is called aryl functional group. For example, the function groups of benzene (C_6H_6) is called phenyl group (C_6H_5-).

The high stability of the benzene ring makes the molecule resistant to any reaction that would destroy the aromaticity of the molecule. Benzene can undergo two types of reactions: addition reactions and substitution reactions.

Alcohols

Alcohols are organic compounds that contain one or more hydroxyl (-OH) group in the aliphatic chain. Examples of alcohols are methanol

(CH_3—OH) and ethanol (CH_3—CH_2—OH). Alcohols can exist on an aliphatic side-chain of an aromatic ring. These alcohols are called aromatic alcohols or aryl alcohols. Examples are phenyl methanol (C_6H_5—CH_2—OH) and phenyl ethanol (C_6H_5—C_2H_4—OH).

Most alcohols contain one hydroxyl group. For example, methyl alcohol is CH_3-OH, ethyl alcohol is CH_3—CH_2—OH, and propyl alcohol is CH_3—CH_2—CH_2—OH.

Depending on the position of –OH on the C chain, monohydric alcohols are further classified as:

1. Primary or 1° alcohols have an –OH group attached to a C atom bound to two or three H atoms. See the classification examples below:

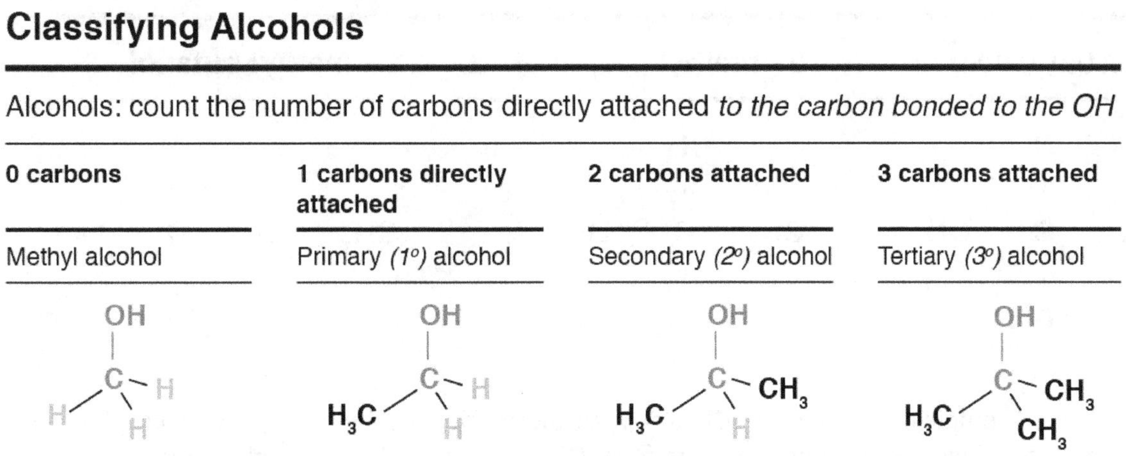

Classifying Alcohols

Alcohols: count the number of carbons directly attached *to the carbon bonded to the OH*

0 carbons	**1 carbons directly attached**	**2 carbons attached**	**3 carbons attached**
Methyl alcohol	Primary *(1°)* alcohol	Secondary *(2°)* alcohol	Tertiary *(3°)* alcohol
OH | H–C–H H	OH | H_3C–C–H H	OH | H_3C–C–CH_3 H	OH | H_3C–C–CH_3 CH_3

2. Secondary or 2° alcohols have an –OH group attached to a C atom bound to only one H atom. See the examples below:

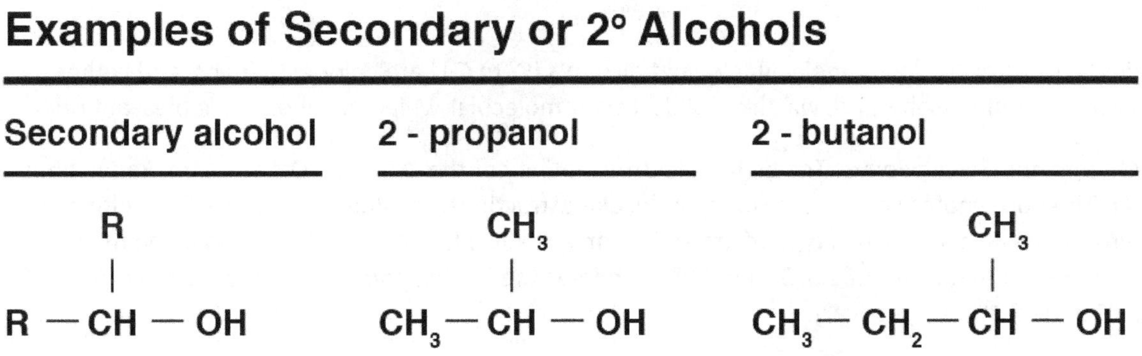

Examples of Secondary or 2° Alcohols

Secondary alcohol	**2 - propanol**	**2 - butanol**
R | R — CH — OH	CH_3 | CH_3— CH — OH	CH_3 | CH_3— CH_2— CH — OH

3. Tertiary or 3° alcohols have an –OH group attached to a C atom not bound to any H atoms. All of the side chains have been substituted. Examples are illustrated below:

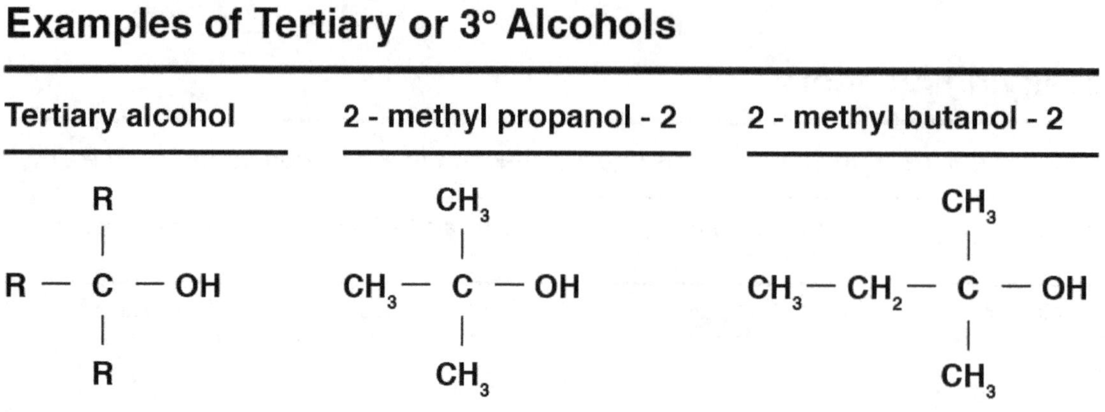

Examples of Tertiary or 3° Alcohols

Tertiary alcohol	2 - methyl propanol - 2	2 - methyl butanol - 2
$R-\underset{R}{\overset{R}{\mid}}{C}-OH$	$CH_3-\underset{CH_3}{\overset{CH_3}{C}}-OH$	$CH_3-CH_2-\underset{CH_3}{\overset{CH_3}{C}}-OH$

Some alcohols contain more than one -OH group. Alcohols with two –OH groups are called "diols," three –OH groups are called "triols" and those with four –OH groups are called "tetraols." Examples of alcohols with more than one –OH group are shown below.

$OH-CH_2-CH_2-OH$	$OH-CH_2-CH_2-CH_2-OH$	$OH-CH_2-CH(OH)-CH_2-OH$
Ethane-1,2-diol	Propane-1,3-diol	Propane-1,2,3-triol (glycerol)

The physical properties of alcohols are as follows:

1. *Physical State:* The lower molecular weight alcohols (C_1 to C_{12}) are colorless liquids, and higher molecular weight alcohols are wax-like solids. Lower molecular weight alcohols have pleasant odors.

2. *Melting and Boiling Points:* The higher electronegativity of the O in the –OH group makes alcohols polar. The polar molecules produce intra-molecular attractions, resulting in increases in melting and boiling points. In alkanes, this type of attractive force is absent. For example, the boing points of methane and ethane are -161.5°C, and -89°C, whereas the boiling points of methanol and ethanol are 64.7°C and 78.4°C, respectively.

3. *Solubility:* The –OH group makes alcohols polar. Methanol, ethanol and propanol are readily-soluble in water. However, as the size of the C chain increases, the solubility in water decreases because the C chain is non-polar.

4. *Relative Density:* The relative densities of alcohols are less than water.

5. *Combustion:* Alcohols are flammable, and they burn in the presence of oxygen to produce carbon dioxide and water.

Alcohols can act as a weak acid by donating a proton (H atom) in aqueous solutions.

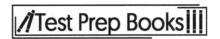

An Alcohol Can Act as a Weak Acid

$$R-OH + H_2O \longrightarrow R-O + H_3O^+$$

Alcohol — Hydronium ion

Therefore, alcohols can interact with different chemical species including alkali metals, carboxylic acids, acyl halides, and oxidizing agents.

In reactions with alkali metals, the –OH group releases its proton to alkali metals to form alkoxide and hydrogen.

The Reaction between Alcohols and Alkali Metals

$$2R-O-H + 2Na \longrightarrow 2R-ONa + H_2$$

Alcohol — Sodium alkoxide

$$2CH_3-O-H + 2Na \longrightarrow 2CH_3-ONa + H_2$$

Methanol — Sodium methoxide

Alkoxides can react with water to reproduce an alcohol.

The Reaction between Alkoxides and Water can Produce an Alcohol

$$R-O-Na + H_2O \longrightarrow 2R-OH + NaOH$$

Alkoxide — Alcohol

Alcohols can react with organic acids (carboxylic acids) to produce esters and water. For example, the reaction between ethanol and acetic acid produces an ester, ethyl acetate.

An Example of an Alcohol Reacting with an Organic Acid to Produce an Ester and Water

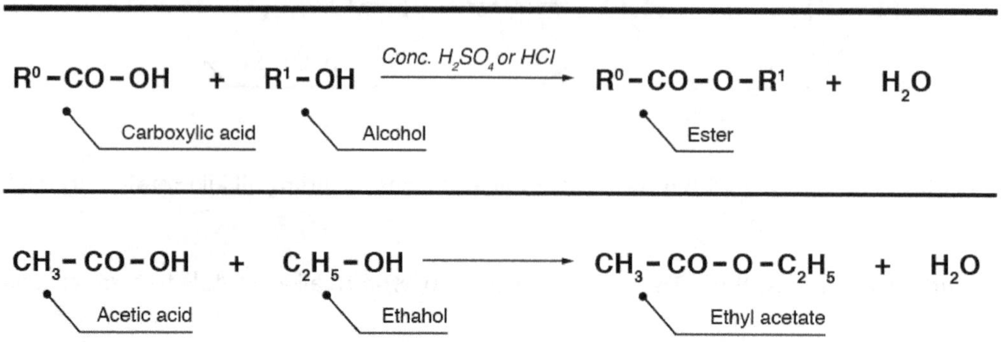

$$R^0\text{-}CO\text{-}OH + R^1\text{-}OH \xrightarrow{\text{Conc. } H_2SO_4 \text{ or } HCl} R^0\text{-}CO\text{-}O\text{-}R^1 + H_2O$$

Carboxylic acid; Alcohol; Ester

$$CH_3\text{-}CO\text{-}OH + C_2H_5\text{-}OH \longrightarrow CH_3\text{-}CO\text{-}O\text{-}C_2H_5 + H_2O$$

Acetic acid; Ethahol; Ethyl acetate

Alcohols react with acyl halide to form esters. For example, the reaction between ethanol and acetyl chloride forms ethyl acetate ester.

An Example of an Alcohol Reacting with an Acyl Halide

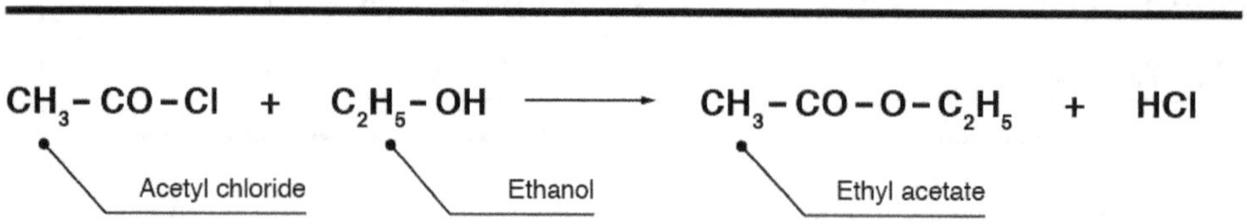

$$CH_3\text{-}CO\text{-}Cl + C_2H_5\text{-}OH \longrightarrow CH_3\text{-}CO\text{-}O\text{-}C_2H_5 + HCl$$

Acetyl chloride; Ethanol; Ethyl acetate

Phenols

Aromatic hydrocarbons that have one or more H atoms replaced by hydroxyl (-OH) groups are collectively called *phenols*. When a single H atom is replaced by an –OH group, it is called a carbolic acid (generally termed as phenol). Phenols are generally slightly acidic in nature. See examples below of certain phenolic compounds with different substituents in the ring:

Examples of Phenols

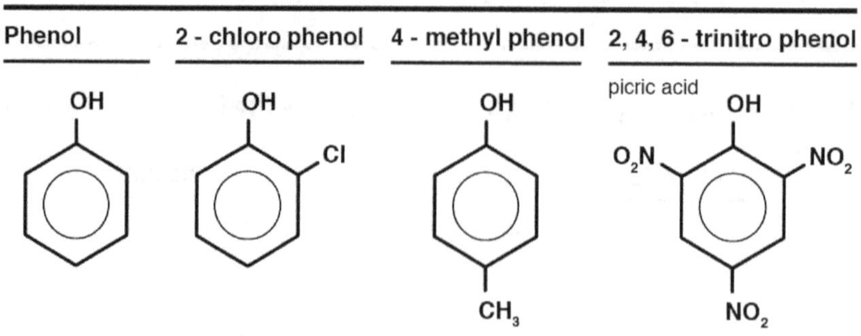

Phenol; 2 - chloro phenol; 4 - methyl phenol; 2, 4, 6 - trinitro phenol (picric acid)

OH; OH, Cl; OH, CH_3; OH, O_2N, NO_2, NO_2

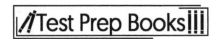

Phenol, carbolic acid, specifically, is colorless crystalline solid. The –OH group in phenol is polar and forms intra-molecular hydrogen bonds. Therefore, phenol's molecular weight (94.1 g/mol), melting point (40.5°C), and boiling (181.7°C) points are higher than that of other organic compounds, such as toluene, with a similar molecular weight (92.1 g/mol), melting point, (-95°C), and boiling point (111°C).

As a class of organic compounds, phenols do not dissolve in water at room temperature. At higher temperatures hydrogen bonds break down, and phenols dissolve in water. Similarly, phenols are insoluble in other polar solvents, like alcohol and ether, at room temperature but dissolve at higher temperatures.

The chemical properties of phenols are as follows:

Phenols are more reactive than benzene due to the presence of the –OH group attached to the ring. However, the –OH group of a phenol is less reactive than that of an alcohol. This is because the delocalized π-electrons stabilize the O atom and the –OH group remains strongly attached to the benzene ring. Therefore, unlike alcohols, phenols do not react with the Lucas reagent. The bond between the –OH molecules in phenols is more polarized than that in alcohols and thus, they can readily donate a proton. Because of this, phenols are more acidic than alcohols.

Phenols Can Act as Acids

$$C_6H_5OH + H_2O \longrightarrow C_6H_5O^- + H_3O^+$$

Benzene — Phenoxide ion — Hydronium ion

Phenols react with different chemicals. The major reactions of phenols are discussed below.

1. *Reduction of Phenol by Zinc:* When a phenol is passed through zinc crystals at high temperatures, it is reduced to form benzene, with the formation of zinc oxide.

Reduction of Phenol by Zinc

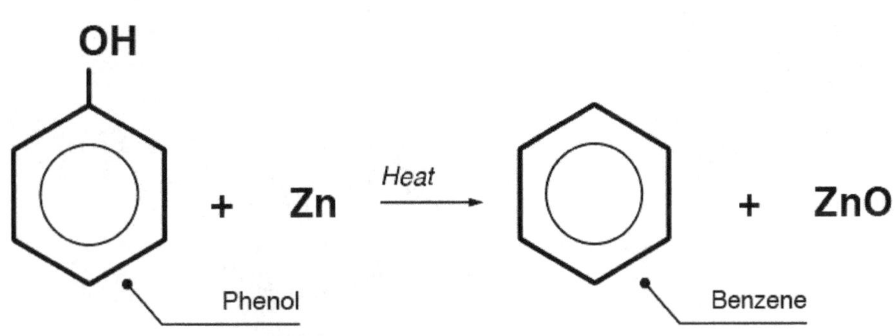

2. *Reduction of Phenol by Hydrogen:* When a phenol is treated with H_2 at 150°–175°C in the presence of a nickel catalyst, three molecules of H_2 are attached to form cyclohexanol.

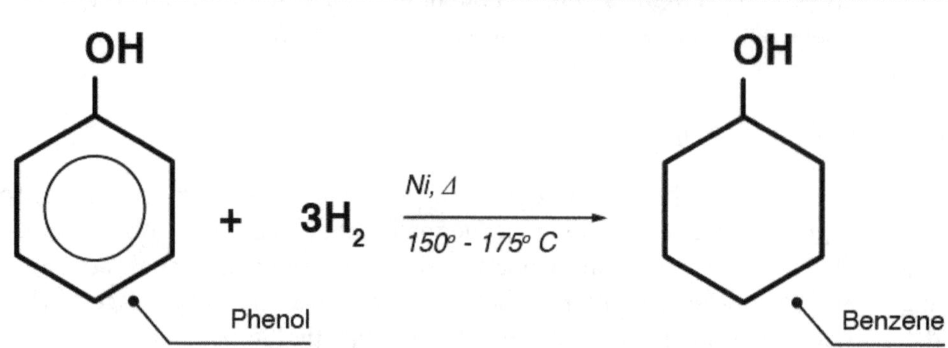

3. *Reaction with Ammonia*: At a high temperature and pressure, phenol reacts with ammonia to produce aniline (also called phenylamine or aminobenzene). The reaction uses zinc chloride as the reaction catalyst.

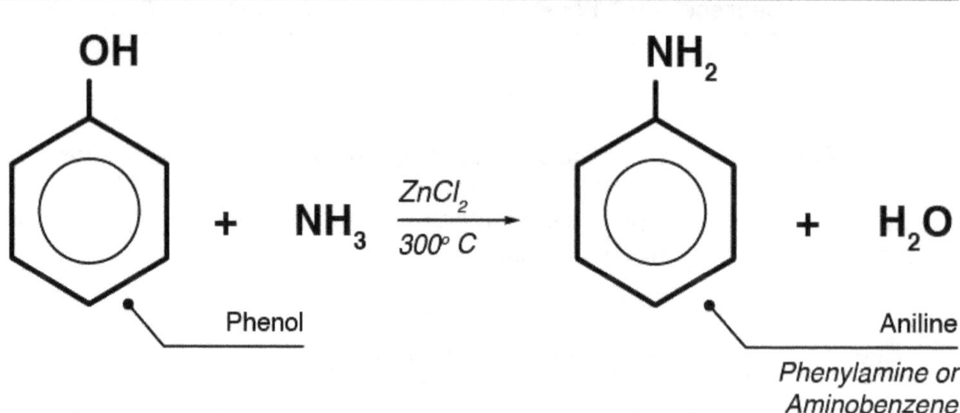

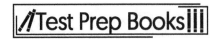

4. *Formation of Esters*: Like alcohols, phenols can also form esters. However, the reaction progresses slowly. Therefore, a phenol is first converted to a phenoxide, which further reacts with acyl halide or acid anhydride to form an ester. For example, sodium phenoxide reacts with acetyl chloride (CH_3COCl) or acetic anhydride (ethanoic anhydride) [$(CH_3CO)_2O$] to form phenyl acetate ester.

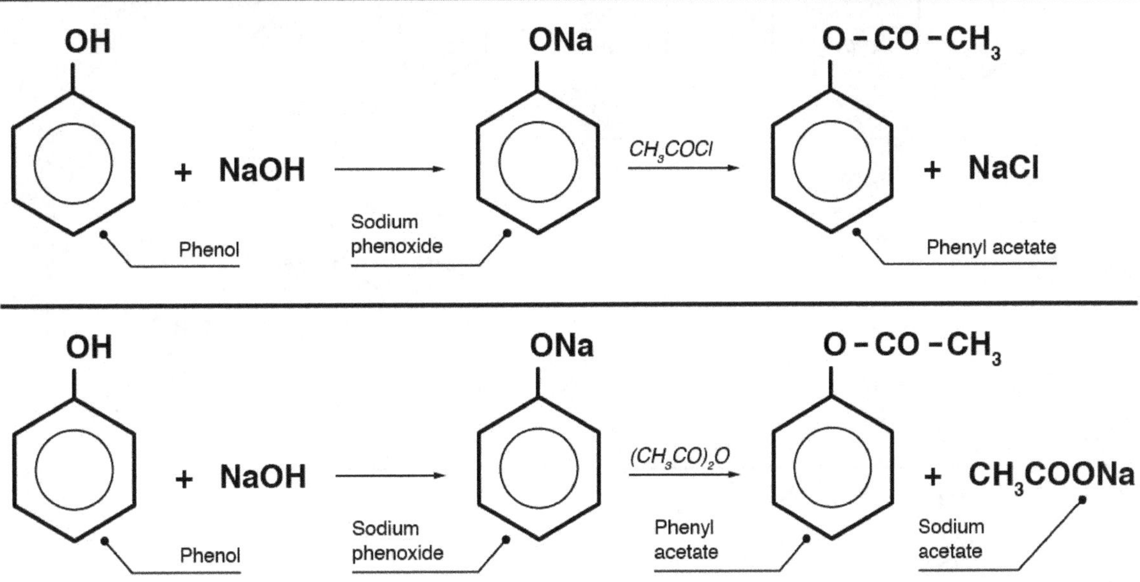

The above reactions can be used to commercially-synthesize aspirin (acetylsalicylic acid, ASA) and acetaminophen, which are widely used to treat fevers and pain.

The syntheses of aspirin and acetaminophen are shown below:

The syntheses of Aspirin and Acetaminophen

ONa

Pressure

CO_2

125° C+

Sodium phenoxide

OH

COONa

H_2O

HCl

Sodium salicylate

OH

COOH

+ NaCl

Salicylic acid

$(CH_3CO)_2O$

$OCOCH_3$

COOH

+ CH_3COOH

Acetylsalicylic acid

Asprin

Acetic acid

OH

NH_2

4-aminophenol

+ $(CH_3CO)_2O$

Acetic anhydride

OH

$NHCOCH_3$

Acetaminophen

+ CH_3COOH

Acetic acid

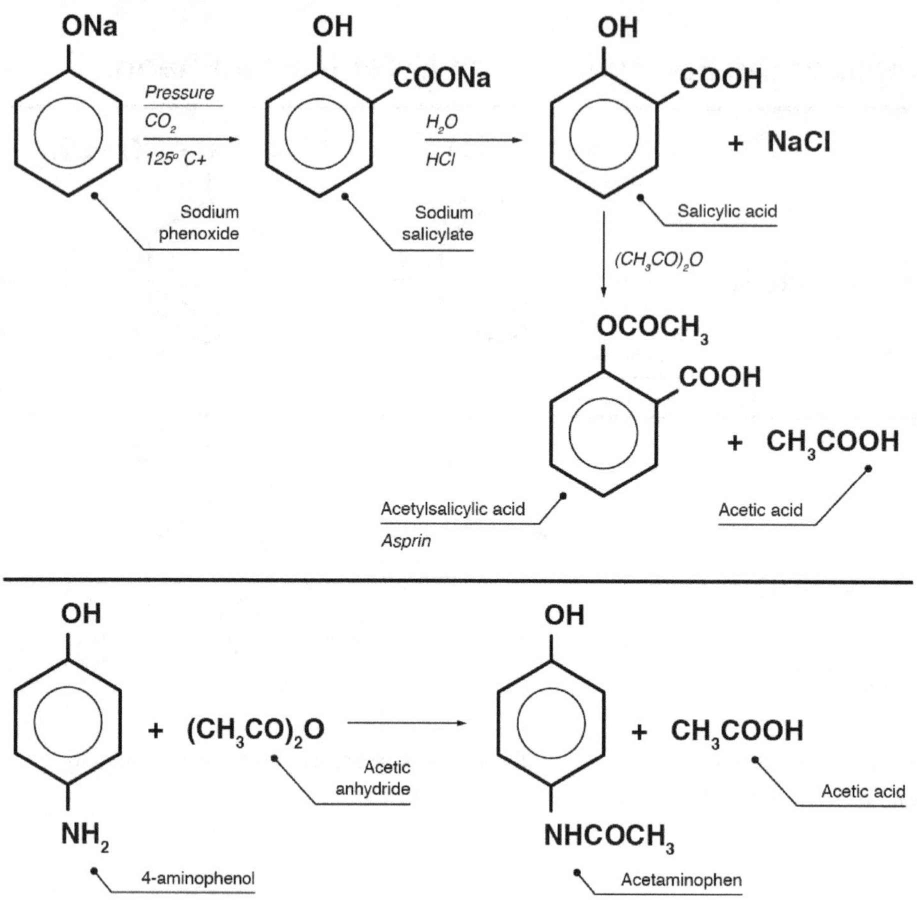

5. *Williamson Ether Synthesis:* This refers to the formation of an ether from an organohalide and an alcohol. For example, phenol reacts with sodium hydroxide to form sodium phenoxide, which further reacts with methyl bromide to form an ether, methoxybenzene.

Williamson Ether Synthesis

OH

Phenol

+ NaOH

ONa

Sodium phenoxide

CH_3Br

$O-CH_3$

Methoxybenzene

+ NaBr

Sodium bromide

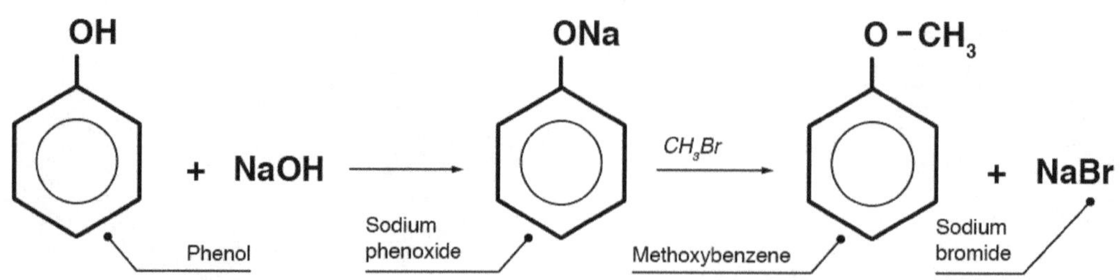

6. *Friedel-Crafts Alkylation:* In the presence of anhydrous aluminum chloride, phenols react with alkyl halides to form ortho- and para-alkyl phenol. For example, phenol reacts with methyl chloride to form ortho-methyl phenol and para-methyl phenol.

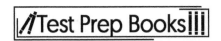

An Example of Friedel-Crafts Alkylation

$$2\,C_6H_5OH + 2CH_3Cl \xrightarrow[AlCl_3]{Anhydrous} o\text{-}CH_3C_6H_4OH + p\text{-}CH_3C_6H_4OH + 2HCl$$

Phenol, Methychloride, o-methyl phenol, p-methyl phenol

7. *Friedel-Crafts Acylation:* In the presence of anhydrous aluminum chloride, phenol reacts with acetyl chloride to form ortho- and para-acetyl phenol.

An Example of Friedel-Crafts Acylation

$$2\,C_6H_5OH + 2CH_3COCl \xrightarrow[AlCl_3]{Anhydrous} o\text{-}CH_3COC_6H_4OH + p\text{-}CH_3COC_6H_4OH + 2HCl$$

Phenol, Acetylchloride, o-acetyl phenol, p-acetyl phenol

8. *Reimer-Tiemann Reaction:* When phenol is mixed with chloroform and sodium hydroxide and heated to around 60°C, then phenol is converted into salicylaldehyde or 2-hydroxybenzaldehyde.

An Example of a Reimer-Tiemann Reaction

$$C_6H_5OH + CHCl_3 + 3NaOH \xrightarrow{60^\circ} o\text{-}OHC\text{-}C_6H_4OH + 3NaCl + 2H_2O$$

Phenol, Chloroform, Sodium hydroxide, Salicylaldehyde

Ethers

Ethers are organic compounds with two alkyl or aryl groups connected by an oxygen atom. They can be represented by R—O—R[1], where R and R[1] are alkyl or aryl groups.

Ethers can be classified into the following categories:

1. *Simple ethers* have the same alkyl group on each side of the O atom. Examples are dimethyl ether (CH_3—O—CH_3) and diethyl ether (C_2H_5—O—C_2H_5).

2. *Mixed ethers* have different alkyl groups on each side of the O atom. Examples are methyl ethyl ether (CH_3—O—C_2H_5) and methyl propyl ether (CH_3—O—C_3H_7).

3. *Cyclic ethers* form a ring structure. Three-membered ether rings (pictured below) are called epoxide compounds and are highly reactive (e.g. ethylene oxide).

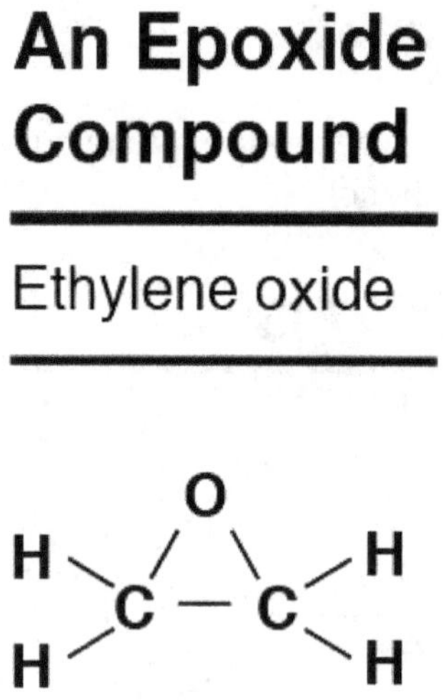

An Epoxide Compound

Ethylene oxide

```
      O
H    / \    H
 \  /   \  /
  C  —  C
 /       \
H         H
```

4. *Aromatic ethers* contain at least one aryl group connected to the O atom (the other group can be an aryl or an alkyl group). Examples are methyl phenyl ether or methoxy benzene (C_6H_5—O—CH_3) and diphenyl ether (C_6H_5—O—C_6H_5).

The physical properties of ethers are as follows:

Low molecular weight ethers are gases. However, higher molecular weight ethers are colorless liquids. Ethers have slight solubility in water because of the formation of H bonds between the H atom of water and O atom of the ether. The solubility decreases with the increase in molecular weight.

Ethers have lower melting and boiling points than alcohols of similar molecular weight. This is because, unlike alcohol, ether molecules do not readily form intra-molecular hydrogen bonds. For example, dimethyl ether (CH_3—O—CH_3) and ethanol (CH_3—CH_2—OH) have the same molecular formula, C_2H_6O, but the boiling points of ethanol and dimethyl ether are 78.4°C and –24°C, respectively. At room temperature, dimethyl ether is a gas, but ethanol is a liquid.

Ethers are less dense than water because they have a lower specific gravity. With an increase in molecular weight, their specific gravity increases. However, it remains less dense than water.

Ethers are one of the least reactive classes of organic compounds. They are less reactive than alcohols and phenols. When an ether is treated with a hydrogen halide, it undergoes fission to form alkyl halide and alcohol. In the case of a mixed ether, the halogen atom joins with the smaller alkyl group. For example, reaction between methyl ethyl ether and hydrogen iodide forms methyl iodide and ethanol.

An Example of a Reaction of an Ether with a Hydrogen Halide

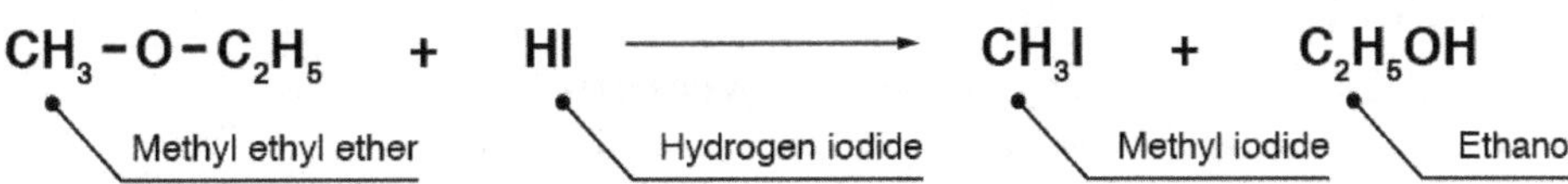

When treated with an excess of HI at a higher temperature, both alkyl groups are converted into alkyl halides.

An Example of a Reaction of an Ether with an Excess of a Hydrogen Halide at a High Temperature

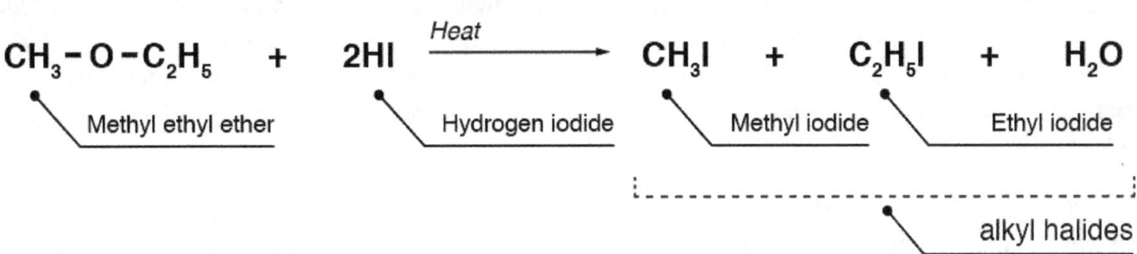

Carbonyl Compounds

Aldehydes and ketones are collectively termed *carbonyl compounds* because they contain the carbonyl (=C=O) functional group. The carbonyl group for aldehydes is on a terminal C atom. Some examples of aldehydes are formaldehyde or methanal (H—CHO), and acetaldehyde or ethanal (CH_3–CHO). The carbonyl group of ketones is on a central C atom. Examples of ketones are acetone or propanone (CH_3—CO—CH_3), and benzophenone or diphenylketone (C_6H_5—CO—C_6H_5).

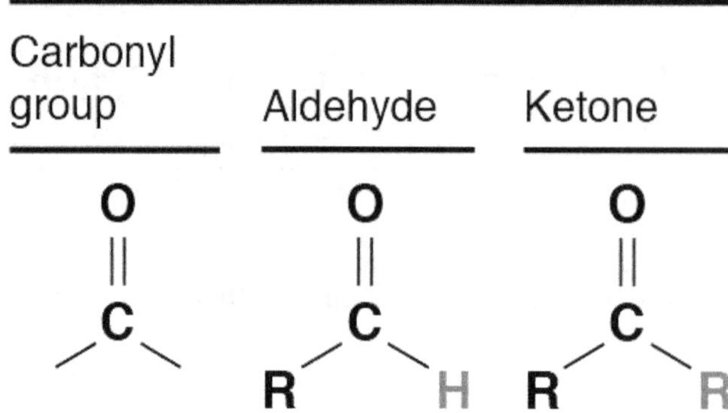

The physical properties of carbonyl compounds are as follows:

Formaldehyde (H—CHO) is a colorless gas, while acetaldehyde has a boiling point of 20.2°C. Aldehydes with C_3 to C_9 carbon numbers are colorless liquids, and higher carbon aldehydes are colorless solids. Ketones up to C_{11} are liquids, and C_{12} and higher ketones are solids. Lower C number aldehydes have an unpleasant odor, whereas higher C number aldehydes have a pleasant smell. Ketones have a pleasant smell as well.

Aldehydes and ketones with short C chains are fairly soluble in water through the formation of H bonds with water. Solubility decreases with the increase in molecular weight, and larger carbonyl compounds are insoluble in water. Carbonyl compounds are soluble in organic solvents.

Unlike alcohols, carbonyl compounds cannot readily form intra-molecular hydrogen bonds, resulting in relatively lower melting and boiling points.

The chemical properties of carbonyl compounds are as follows:

The bond between the C and O atoms in the carbonyl group is polarized ($–C^{\delta+}=O^{\delta-}$), making the carbonyl compounds highly reactive. The relatively positive-charged C atoms in carbonyl compounds are susceptible to nucleophile (electron-rich substrate) attack. Various chemical reactions of carbonyl compounds are summarized below.

1. *Grignard Reactions:* This reaction is used to produce a new C–C bond. The Grignard reagent reacts with the carbonyl group and is an organometallic compound with a general formula of R—MgX, in which R represents the alkyl or aryl groups, and X represents a halogen.

The Grignard reagent reacts with formaldehyde to form primary (1°) alcohols. For example, the reaction between formaldehyde and methyl magnesium bromide produces an unstable intermediate, which is further hydrolyzed to form ethanol.

A Grignard Reaction of a Carbonyl Compound

$$\underset{\text{Formaldehyde}}{H-\overset{\overset{\Large O}{\|}}{C}-H} + \underset{\text{Grignard reagent}}{CH_3-MgBr} \longrightarrow \underset{\text{Intermediate compound}}{H-\overset{\overset{OMgBr}{|}}{\underset{\underset{CH_3}{|}}{C}}-H} \xrightarrow{H^+/H_2O} \underset{\substack{\text{Ethanol} \\ 1^\circ \text{ alcohol}}}{CH_3-CH_2-OH} + BrMgOH$$

The Grignard reagent reacts with other aldehydes (except formaldehyde) to form secondary (2°) alcohols. For example, the reaction between acetaldehyde and methyl magnesium bromide forms a secondary alcohol, 2-propanol.

The Grignard Reagent Reacts with Aldehydes to Form Secondary *(2°)* Alcohols

$$\underset{\text{Acetaldehyde}}{CH_3-\overset{\overset{\Large O}{\|}}{C}-H} + \underset{\text{Grignard reagent}}{CH_3-MgBr} \longrightarrow \underset{\text{Intermediate compound}}{CH_3-\overset{\overset{OMgBr}{|}}{\underset{\underset{CH_3}{|}}{C}}-H} \xrightarrow{H^+/H_2O} \underset{\substack{\text{2 - propanol} \\ 2^\circ \text{ alcohol}}}{CH_3-\underset{\underset{CH_3}{|}}{CH}-OH} + BrMgOH$$

The Grignard reagent reacts with ketones to form tertiary (3°) alcohols. For example, the reaction between acetone and methyl magnesium bromide forms a tertiary alcohol, 2-methyl-2-propanol.

The Grignard Reagent Reacts with Ketones to Form Tertiary *(3°)* Alcohols

$$\underset{\text{Acetone}}{CH_3-\overset{\overset{\Large O}{\|}}{C}-CH_3} + \underset{\text{Grignard reagent}}{CH_3-MgBr} \longrightarrow \underset{\text{Intermediate compound}}{CH_3-\overset{\overset{OMgBr}{|}}{\underset{\underset{CH_3}{|}}{C}}-CH_3} \xrightarrow{H^+/H_2O} \underset{\substack{\text{2 - methyl - 2 -propanol} \\ 3^\circ \text{ alcohol}}}{CH_3-\overset{\overset{CH_3}{|}}{\underset{\underset{CH_3}{|}}{C}}-OH} + BrMgOH$$

2. *Oxidation Reactions:* Aliphatic aldehydes are readily oxidized by strong oxidizing agents, like potassium dichromate ($K_2Cr_2O_7$) and sulphuric acid (H_2SO_4), to form carboxylic acids. However, aromatic aldehydes are not easily oxidized.

An Oxidation Reaction of an Aliphatic Aldehyde Forms a Carboxylic Acids

$$\underset{\text{Aldehyde}}{R-\overset{\overset{\displaystyle O}{\|}}{C}-H} + [O] \xrightarrow[H_2SO_4]{K_2Cr_2O_7} \underset{\text{Carboxylic acid}}{R-\overset{\overset{\displaystyle O}{\|}}{C}-OH}$$

Ketones do not oxidize easily. When ketones are heated with strong oxidizing agents, a mixture of different organic acids is formed.

A Mixture of Organic Acids is Formed When Attempting to Oxidize Ketones

$$\underset{\text{Ketone}}{R^1-\overset{\overset{\displaystyle O}{\|}}{C}-R^2} + 3[O] \xrightarrow[H_2SO_4]{K_2Cr_2O_7} \underset{\text{Carboxylic acid -1}}{R^1-\overset{\overset{\displaystyle O}{\|}}{C}-OH} + \underset{\text{Carboxylic acid - 2}}{R^2-\overset{\overset{\displaystyle O}{\|}}{C}-OH}$$

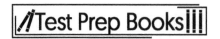

3. *Reduction Reactions:* Reduction of aldehydes by a mild reducing agent, like lithium aluminum hydride ($LiAlH_4$), sodium borohydride ($NaBH_4$), or sodium amalgam (NaHg), produces primary alcohols, whereas ketones are reduced to secondary alcohols.

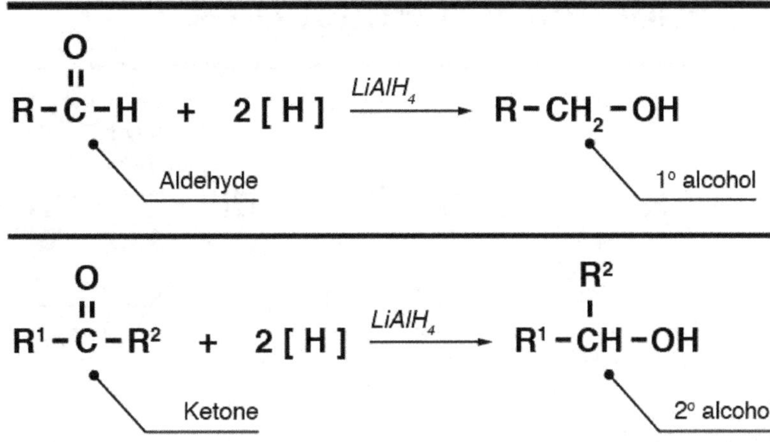

Reduction of carbonyl compounds with a strong reducing agent, like zinc amalgam and concentrated hydrochloric acid (ZnHg + HCl), causes conversion of the =C=O group into a $-CH_2-$ group, resulting in formation of saturated hydrocarbons. This reaction is termed a *Clemmensen reduction.*

A Clemmensen Reduction Produces a Saturated Hydrocarbon

$$R-\overset{O}{\overset{\|}{C}}-H + 4[H] \xrightarrow[HCl]{Zn/Hg} R-CH_2-H + H_2O$$

Aldehyde → Alkane

$$R^1-\overset{O}{\overset{\|}{C}}-R^2 + 4[H] \xrightarrow[HCl]{Zn/Hg} R^1-CH_2-R^2 + H_2O$$

Ketone → Alkane

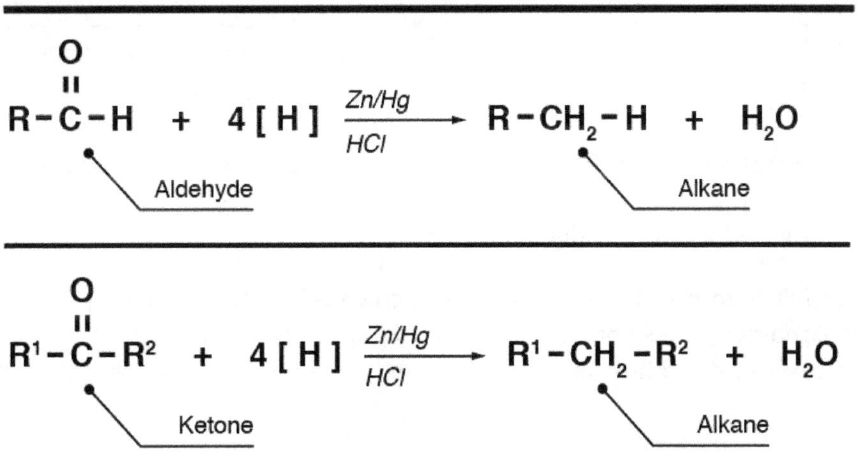

4. *Aldol Condensation Reaction:* In the presence of dilute acid or alkali, two molecules of an aldehyde or ketone containing α-hydrogen can undergo a condensation reaction to form a β-hydroxy aldehyde or β-hydroxy ketone. This reaction is termed "aldol condensation," as the product carries both the *ald*ehyde (–CHO) and alcoh*ol* (–OH) functional groups. Aldol condensation helps form a new C–C bond. For example, in the presence of dilute NaOH, two molecules of acetaldehyde condense to from an aldol, 3-hydroxybutanal (or β-hydroxybutanal).

An Aldol Condensation Reaction

$$CH_3-\overset{\overset{\displaystyle O}{\|}}{C}-H \;+\; H-\overset{\alpha}{CH_2}-CHO \xrightarrow{NaOH} \overset{4}{CH_3}-\overset{\overset{\displaystyle OH}{|}}{\underset{3}{CH}}-\overset{2}{CH_2}-\overset{1}{CHO}$$

Acetaldehyde
with α - hydrogen

Aldol
3 - hydroxybutanal

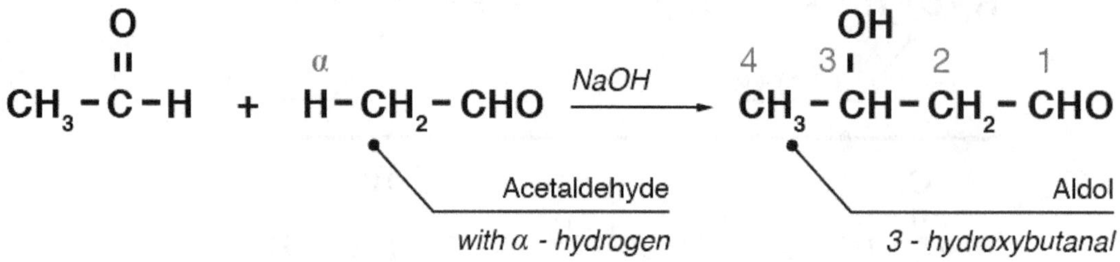

When aldol is heated in the presence of an acid (e.g. HCl), a water molecule is removed causing the formation of α-β unsaturated aldehyde or ketone.

Heating an Aldol in the Presence of an Acid

$$CH_3-\overset{\overset{\displaystyle OH}{|}}{\underset{\beta}{CH}}-\overset{\alpha}{CH_2}-CHO \xrightarrow{HCl} CH_3-\overset{\beta}{CH}=\overset{\alpha}{CH}-CHO \;+\; H_2O$$

Aldol
3 - hydroxybutanal

α - β unsaturated aldehyde
3 - hydroxybutanal

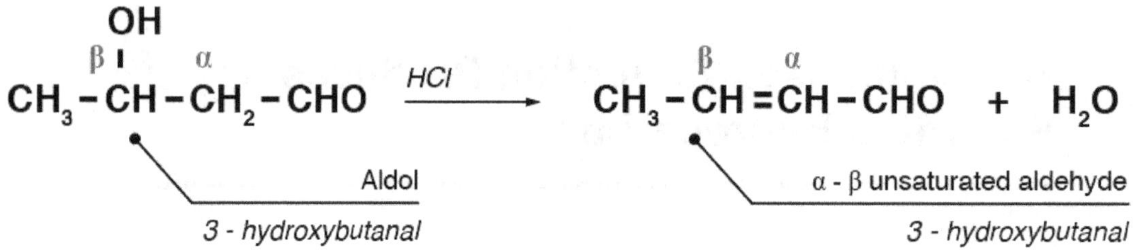

Carbonyl compounds that do not have α-hydrogen cannot participate in aldol condensation. For example, formaldehyde (H-CHO) and trimethyl-acetaldehyde [$(CH_3)_3C$–CHO] do not have an α-hydrogen, so they cannot undergo aldol condensation.

5. *Cannizzaro Reaction:* In the presence of a concentrated base (e.g. NaOH), aldehydes *lacking* an α-hydrogen undergo oxidation-reduction reaction. In such reactions, one aldehyde molecule is oxidized to form a salt of carboxylic acid and the other is reduced to form an alcohol. For example, when treated

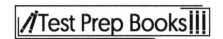

with NaOH, two molecules of formaldehyde undergo an oxidation-reduction reaction to form methanol and sodium formate.

An Example of an Aldehyde Undergoing the Cannizzaro Reaction

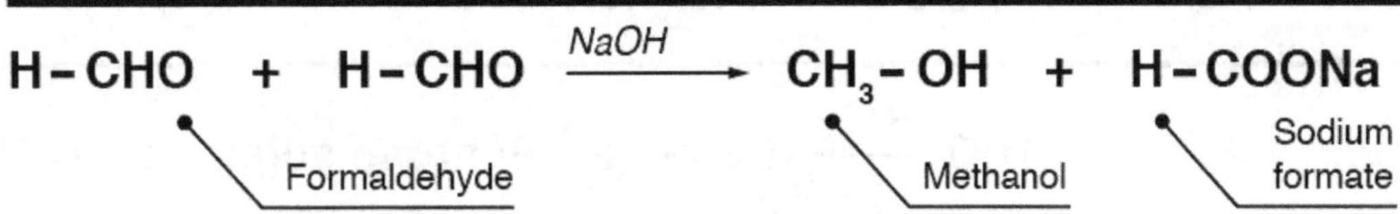

Biomolecules

Humans, animals, and plants are built with different biomolecules and vital life functions rely on them. *Biomolecules* are organic polymers that perform various functions in the human body. Among their many functions in the human body, biomolecules do the following: provide structure, provide nutrition and energy to cells, perform various enzymatic reactions, regulate the body's defense mechanism, and control genetic functions through heredity.

Classes of important biopolymers include:

1. Carbohydrates, such as starch (in animals) and cellulose (in plants).
2. Proteins, such as nucleoprotein, plasma protein, hormones, enzymes, and antibodies.
3. Nucleic acids, such as ribonucleic acid (RNA) and deoxyribonucleic acid (DNA).
4. Triglycerides, which are formed from fatty acids with a glycerol backbone.

All biomolecules are polymers, which are formed from repeated units of basic monomers. These polymers can be broken down (hydrolyzed) into their respective monomers.

Proteins can be hydrolyzed under acidic condition to form amino acids.

Hydrolyzing a Protein

Proteins can be hydrolyzed under acidic condition to form amino acids

$$\text{Protein} + nH_2O \xrightarrow{H^+} \text{Amino acids}$$

Nucleic acids are structurally associated with some proteins to form nucleoproteins. The hydrolysis of nucleic acids and nucleoproteins is illustrated below:

Nucleoprotein and Nucleic Acid Hydrolysis

$$\text{Nucleoprotein} + nH_2O \xrightarrow{H^+} \text{Nucleic acid} + \text{Protein}$$

$$\text{Nucleic acid} + nH_2O \xrightarrow{H^+} \underset{\substack{\textit{purine} \\ \textit{pyrimidine}}}{\text{Base}} + \text{Pentose sugar} + H_3PO_4$$

Carbohydrates are represented by a general formula,

$$(C_6H_{10}O_5)_n,$$

where $40 \leq n \leq 3000$. When hydrolyzed, starch produces the monosaccharide glucose ($C_6H_{12}O_6$).

Hydrolyzing a Starch

$$(C_6H_{10}O_5)_n + nH_2O \xrightarrow{H^+} C_6H_{12}O_6$$

However, glucose remains stored as glycogen in the liver and muscle. Glycogen stores energy in the body.

Storing Glucose as Glycogen in the body

$$n\, C_6H_{12}O_6 \xrightarrow{\textit{Glycogen Synthase}} (C_6H_{10}O_5)_n$$

Where n = approx. 6000 - 30000

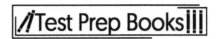

Carbohydrates are classified into three categories:

1. *Monosaccharides*: Monosaccharides are the monomers of carbohydrates. They are represented by a general formula $(CH_2O)_n$, where n = 3 – 6. Examples of monosaccharides are glucose (dextrose), fructose, and galactose.

They are named based on the number of C atoms in the molecule, such as triose (C3), tetrose (C4), pentose (C5) and hexose (C6). A monosaccharide with an aldehyde group is called an "aldose," and one with a ketone group is called a "ketose" (e.g. fructose).

Monosaccharides

D-ribose	D-Glucose	D-Fructose
	an aldohexose	a ketohexose
		H
H O	H O	
C	C	H — C — OH
H — C — OH	H — C — OH	C = O
H — C — OH	HO — C — H	HO — C — H
H — C — OH	H — C — OH	H — C — OH
CH_2OH	H — C — OH	H — C — OH
	CH_2OH	CH_2OH

2. *Disaccharides*: Disaccharides are two monosaccharides joined together. When hydrolyzed, disaccharides produce two monosaccharide molecules. See the examples below:

Hydrolysis of Disaccharides

$$C_{12}H_{22}O_{11} + H_2O \xrightarrow{H^+} C_6H_{12}O_6 + C_6H_{12}O_6$$

Sucrose → Glucose + Fructose

$$C_{12}H_{22}O_{11} + H_2O \xrightarrow{H^+} C_6H_{12}O_6 + C_6H_{12}O_6$$

Lactose → Glucose + Galactose

$$C_{12}H_{22}O_{11} + H_2O \xrightarrow{H^+} C_6H_{12}O_6 + C_6H_{12}O_6$$

Maltose → Glucose + Glucose

3. *Polysaccharides*: Polysaccharides are high molecular weight carbohydrates. When hydrolyzed, they produce many molecules of monosaccharides. Examples of polysaccharides are starch, glycogen, and cellulose.

Carbonyl compounds, aldehydes and ketones, can react with –OH group of an alcohol to form hemiacetal and acetal.

The Reaction of Carbonyl Compounds with Alcohols

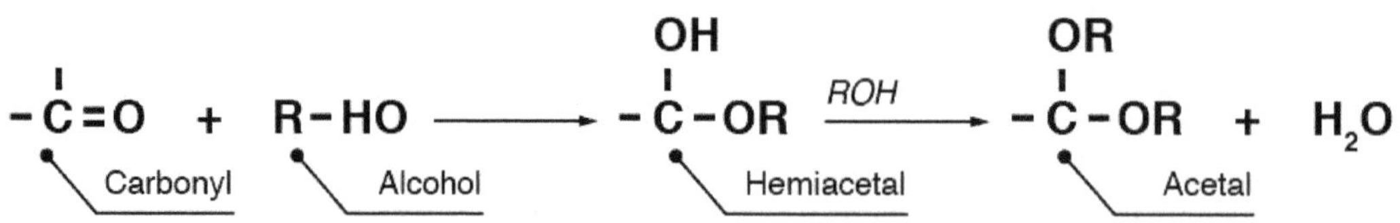

$$-\overset{|}{C}=O + R-HO \longrightarrow -\overset{OH}{\overset{|}{C}}-OR \xrightarrow{ROH} -\overset{OR}{\overset{|}{C}}-OR + H_2O$$

Carbonyl, Alcohol, Hemiacetal, Acetal

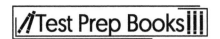

Glucose and fructose contain both carbonyl and hydroxyl groups, and therefore can form intramolecular hemiacetal to produce a cyclic structure. This hemiacetal formation takes place between C1 and C5 carbons to form a stable heterocyclic structure. The cyclic structure forms a pyranose ring, which is a six-membered ring consisting of five C atoms and one O atom. In a cyclic structure, C1 might have an –OH group at the right or left side, and therefore may be termed α-D-glucose and β-D-glucose, respectively. View the structures below as an example:

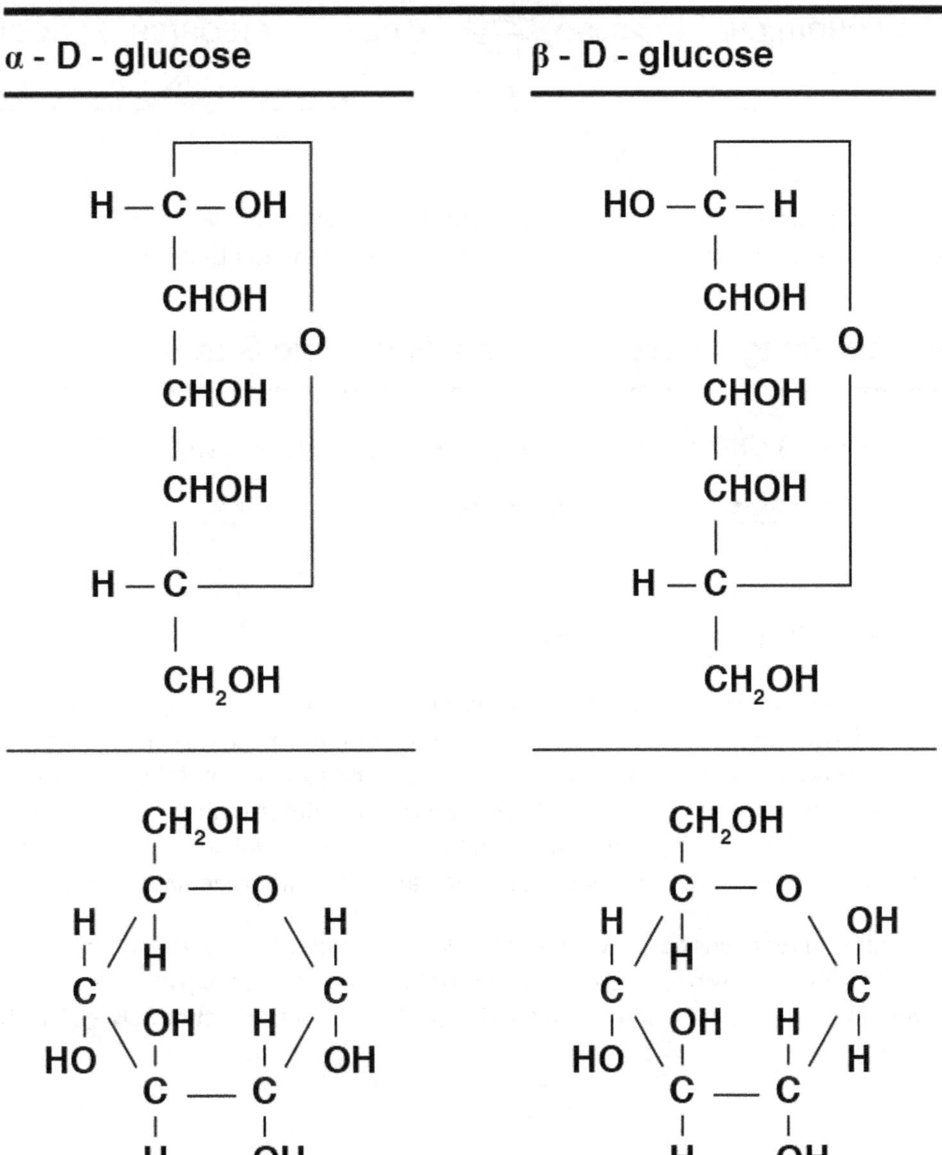

Reducing sugars are ones with a free aldehyde or ketone groups, and they can act as reducing agents. All monosaccharides, including glucose, fructose, and galactose, are reducing sugars. Many disaccharides, including lactose and maltose (except sucrose), are also reducing sugars. The reducing sugars are able to reduce Fehling's solution and Tollens' reagent.

When Fehling's solution is treated with a reducing sugar, the deep blue color of Fehling's solution fades and then forms a reddish precipitate. Fehling's solution is prepared by mixing a copper sulphate solution with potassium sodium tartrate in NaOH. See the reaction below as an example:

Fehling's Solution Treated with a Reducing Sugar

$$CH_2OH(CHOH)_4CHO + 2CuSO_4 \xrightarrow[Heat]{NaOH} Cu_2O + CH_2OH(CHOH)_4COONa + 3H_2O$$

Glucose; Deep blue; Reddish; Sodium gluconate

When a solution of reducing sugar is heated with Tollens' reagent, silver is precipitated and forms silver mirror on the inner surface of the reaction vessel. See the reaction that follows:

Tollens' Reagent Treated with a Reducing Sugar

$$CH_2OH(CHOH)_4CHO + 2Ag(NH_3)_2OH \longrightarrow 2Ag + CH_2OH(CHOH)_4COONH_4 + 3NH_3 + H_2O$$

Glucose; Tollens' reagent; Silver mirror

Reactions of Organic Compounds

In inorganic compounds, chemical reactions occur through the formation of electrically-charged ions and their polarization. However, organic compounds contain covalent bonds, and the chemical reactions of organic compounds involve simultaneous breakage and formation of these covalent bonds. The functional groups present in the molecule are important in determining the nature and rate of reactions. In addition to the functional groups, the reactions are also determined by the type of bonds present in the molecule (i.e. σ-bonds and π-bonds), and the nature of other reactants present.

Organic chemical reactions occur when an attacking reagent interacts with an organic molecule (substrate) to form a new organic compound (product). This can be explained with the reaction between chloromethane (CH_3—Cl) and sodium hydroxide (Na^+OH^-). In this reaction, CH_3—Cl is the organic substrate, OH^- is the attacking reagent, and CH_3-OH (methanol) is the product. There are three steps in this chemical reaction:

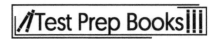

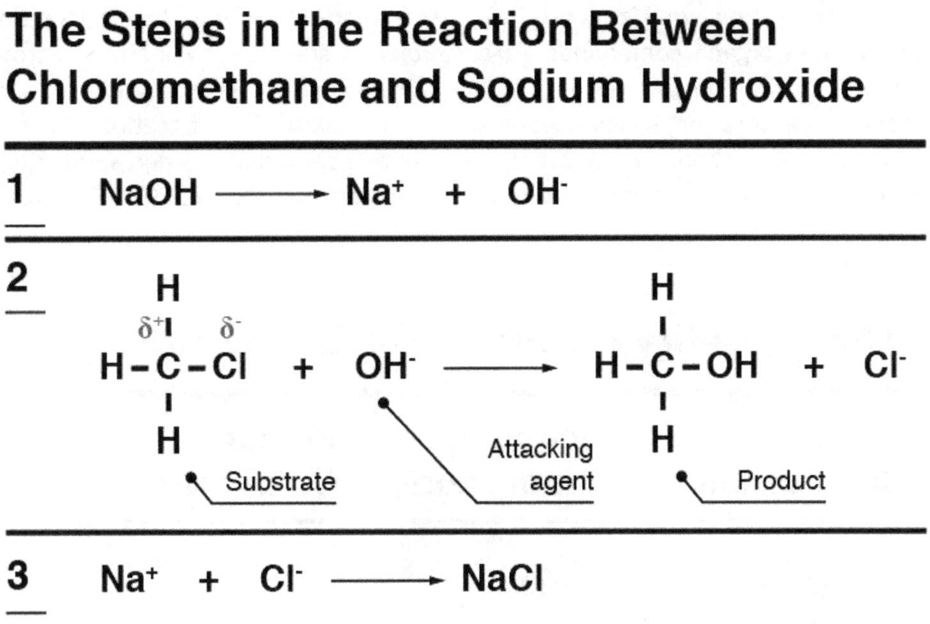

The Steps in the Reaction Between Chloromethane and Sodium Hydroxide

1 $NaOH \longrightarrow Na^+ + OH^-$

2

$$\underset{\text{Substrate}}{H{-}\overset{\overset{H}{|}}{\underset{\underset{H}{|}}{C}}{-}Cl} \quad (\delta^+ \text{ on C}, \ \delta^- \text{ on Cl}) \quad + \underset{\text{Attacking agent}}{OH^-} \longrightarrow \underset{\text{Product}}{H{-}\overset{\overset{H}{|}}{\underset{\underset{H}{|}}{C}}{-}OH} + Cl^-$$

3 $Na^+ + Cl^- \longrightarrow NaCl$

These chemical reactions take place through fission or breakdown of the C—C bonds and formation of carbon radical intermediates. There are two types of carbon radicals that are formed in chemical reactions: carbocation and carbanion.

A *carbocation* is a positively-changed carbon ion (i.e. cation). Examples are methyl carbocation ($^+CH_3$) and ethyl carbocation (CH_3—$^+CH_2$). Carbocation are formed due to an unequal distribution of the shared electrons from a bond cleavage. For example, in chloromethane (CH_3—Cl), the chlorine (Cl) atom is more electronegative than the C atom; therefore, electrons are drawn towards the Cl. Fission of the bond causes the Cl atom to take the shared electron of the C atom, which results in the formation of an electropositive carbocation.

The Formation of an Electropositive Carbocation

$$\underset{\text{Chloromethane}}{H{-}\overset{\overset{H}{|}}{\underset{\underset{H}{|}}{C}}{\cdot\cdot}Cl} \quad (\delta^+ \text{ on C}, \ \delta^- \text{ on Cl}) \longrightarrow \underset{\text{Carbocation}}{H{-}\overset{\overset{H}{|}}{\underset{\underset{H}{|}}{C^+}}} + \cdot\dot{Cl}^-$$

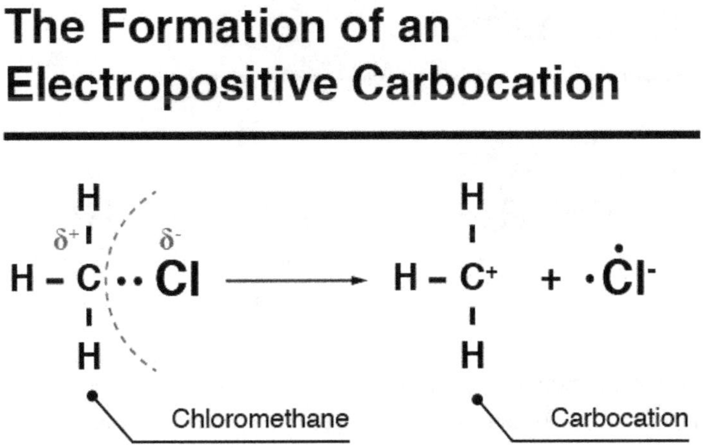

Carbocation groups are named after the parent alkyl group by "ium" (i.e. alkyl + ium = alkylium). For example, $^{+}CH_3$ is called methyl carbocation or "methylium." Similarly, $CH_3—^{+}CH_2$ is called ethyl carbocation ion or "ethylium."

The positively-charged carbocations are highly reactive and can readily bind with the electron-donating atoms or groups to form new organic compounds. Carbocations are stabilized by nearby electron donating groups, including alkyl groups. In terms of stability, the primary (1°) carbocation ion is less stable than secondary (2°) carbocation, which is less stable than tertiary (3°) carbocation. A 1° carbon is one that is bound to one other carbon, a 2° carbon is bound to two carbon atoms and a 3° carbon is bound to three carbon atoms. See the stability order below of carbocation where "R" refers to alkyl group(s).

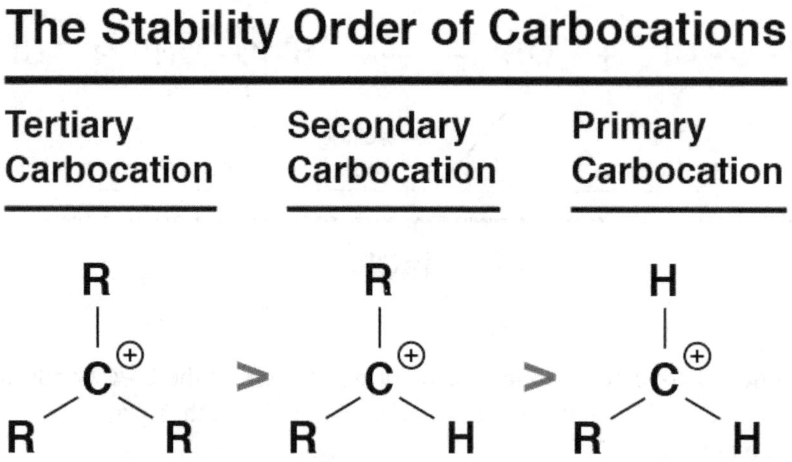

The Stability Order of Carbocations

A *carbanion* is a negatively-charged carbon atom that carries an unshared pair of electrons. Examples of carbanions are methyl carbanion ($^{-}CH_3$) and ethyl carbanion ($CH_3—^{-}CH_2$). A carbanion is formed through fission of an σ-bond and concentration of an unshared electron pair in a C atom. This type of fission takes place when the C atom carries relatively higher electronegativity compared to the attached atom or group.

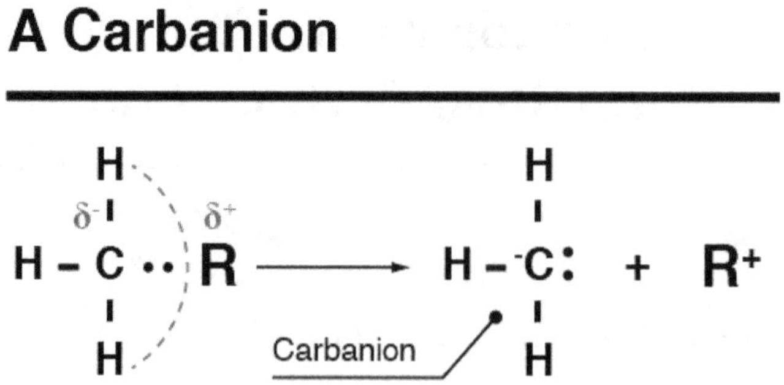

A Carbanion

The stability of a carbanion is increased in the presence of an electron-withdrawing (attracting) group that pulls the electron density toward itself and stabilizes the carbanion (e.g. $–NO_2$, –CO, –CN etc.). On

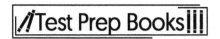

the other hand, the stability is decreased in the presence of the electron-donating (repelling) alkyl (R) groups, which push the electron cloud toward the carbanion

(e.g. $-CH_3$, $-C_2H_5$ etc.)

Therefore, the stability order is as follows:

The Stability Order of Carbanions

Tertiary Carbanion		Secondary Carbanion		Primary Carbanion
$\mathrm{R{-}\overset{\displaystyle R}{\underset{\displaystyle R}{C}}{:}^{-}}$	<	$\mathrm{R{-}\overset{\displaystyle R}{\underset{\displaystyle H}{C}}{:}^{-}}$	<	$\mathrm{H{-}\overset{\displaystyle R}{\underset{\displaystyle H}{C}}{:}^{-}}$

In chemical reactions, a carbocation or carbanion binds with the attacking reagent to form a new organic compound. The nature of the reaction depends significantly on the attacking reagent. The mechanism of interaction between the organic substrate and the attacking reagent can be illustrated in the steps below:

The Steps of the Interaction Between an Organic Substrate and an Attacking Reagent

$$\underset{\text{Attacking reagent}}{Z} + \underset{\text{Substrate}}{X{:}Y} \longrightarrow \left[\begin{array}{l} {:}X^- + Y^+ \xrightarrow{Z^+} XZ + Y^+ \\ X^+ + {:}Y^- \xrightarrow{Z^-} XZ + Y^- \end{array}\right.$$

Depending on the nature, attacking reagents (Z) can be categorized into an electrophile or electrophilic reagent and a nucleophile or nucleophilic reagent.

Electrophiles

Electrophiles are attacking species that have a strong attraction to electrons. Electrophiles are naturally electron-deficient, and therefore, they have electron-accepting characteristics. There are two types of electrophiles: positive (or charged) electrophiles and neutral electrophiles.

Positive electrophiles (E^+) are positively-charged, so they have a high affinity for electrons. Examples are proton (H^+), alkylium (R^+), nitronium (NO_2^+), nitrosonium (^+NO) etc., where R = alkyl groups.

Neutral electrophiles (E) do not have an electric charge but have a strong affinity for electrons to complete the octet in their valence shell. Examples of neutral electrophiles are aluminum chloride ($AlCl_3$), boron trifluoride (BF_3), and ferric chloride ($FeCl_3$).

Neutral Electrophiles *(E)*

Aluminum Chloride	Boron Trifluoride
Cl Cl : Al : Cl	F F : B : F

Nucleophiles

Nucleophiles are rich in electrons, so they act as electron donors. Nucleophiles are also categorized into negative (or charged) nucleophile and neutral nucleophile.

Negative nucleophiles (Nu^-) are negatively-charged attacking reagents. Examples include methyl carbanion ($^-CH_3$), chloride (Cl^-), bromide (Br^-), hydroxide ion (^-OH), and cyanide ion (^-CN).

Neutral nucleophiles (Nu) carry an unshared pair of electrons, but do not carry any negative charge. Examples are ammonia (NH_3), water (H_2O), and alcohol (R-OH).

Neutral Nucleophile *(Nu)*

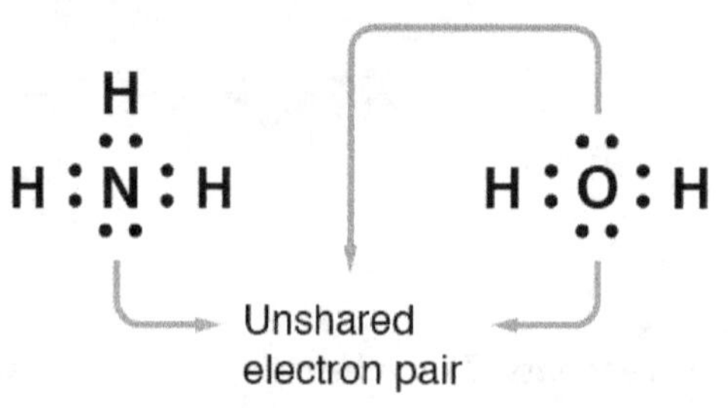

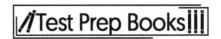

Based on the nature of the attacking agents, organic reactions can also be classified into following categories:

1. An *electrophilic addition* is an addition reaction in which an electrophile (electron-attracting species) is added to a molecule that is mostly carrying unsaturated bonds. For example, the electrophilic proton (H^+) attacks the double bond of ethene ($CH_2{=}CH_2$) to form ethane ($CH_3{-}CH_3$).

2. An *electrophilic substitution* is an elimination reaction in which an electrophile is eliminated from an organic molecule, e.g. elimination of protons from ethane (CH_3-CH_3) causes the formation of ethene ($CH_2{=}CH_2$).

3. A *nucleophilic addition* is an addition reaction in which an electron-rich reactant (i.e. nucleophile) attaches to an electrophile to form a new bond.

4. A *nucleophilic substitution* is an elimination reaction that causes the removal of a nucleophile from an organic molecule.

Oxidation and Reduction

Oxidation/reduction, or redox reactions, are reactions in which the oxidation state of an atom changes. This oxidation state change relates to the number of electrons lost or gained during the reaction. In the oxidation half of the reaction, an electron is lost. In the reduction half of the reaction, an electron is gained. These two parts are referred to as "half-reactions" because oxidation is always accompanied with reduction. Usually, the change in the oxidation state of the C atom determines if an organic redox reaction is termed an oxidation or a reduction reaction.

1. *Alkanes*: Alkanes are generally stable and unreactive. Therefore, alkanes rarely participate in chemical redox reactions. The most common redox reaction of alkanes is combustion, in which the burning of hydrocarbon chains in the presence of oxygen produces carbon dioxide, water, and energy. In the absence of adequate oxygen, oxidative combustion of hydrocarbons produces carbon monoxide, water, and energy. This is considered an oxidation reaction because the C atom loses electrons. In this equation, the O atoms are reduced. Linear and small chain alkanes are more readily oxidized than larger and branched chain alkanes. The figure below shows the oxidation of methane and is labeled with the oxidation numbers of each atom to illustrate the change in oxidation state. Here, carbon is oxidized and oxygen is reduced.

The Oxidation of Methane Showing the Oxidation Numbers

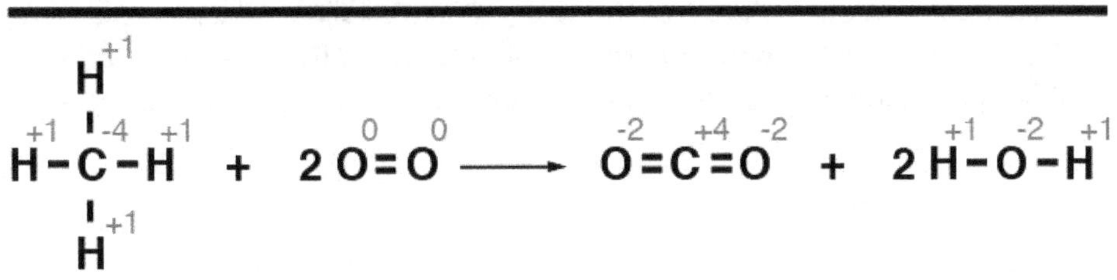

$$\overset{+1}{H}-\overset{-4}{C}(\overset{+1}{H})(\overset{+1}{H})-\overset{+1}{H} + 2\,\overset{0}{O}=\overset{0}{O} \longrightarrow \overset{-2}{O}=\overset{+4}{C}=\overset{-2}{O} + 2\,\overset{+1}{H}-\overset{-2}{O}-\overset{+1}{H}$$

2. *Alkenes:* In the presence of a weak oxidizing agent such as dilute potassium permanganate ($KMnO_4$) in alkaline (KOH) solution, alkenes undergo oxidation to produce glycols. This reaction is utilized to detect unsaturation (double and triple bonds) in organic compounds. While observing this test, called *Baeyer's Test,* the pink color of potassium permanganate gradually fades.

Oxidation of an Alkene and Using the Baeyer's Test

$$R^1-CH=CH-R^2 + H_2O + [O] \xrightarrow[KOH]{KMnO_4} R^1-HOCH-CHOH-R^2$$

Alkene — Glycol

However, in the presence of a strong oxidizing agent such as concentrated $KMnO_4$ in acidic (H_2SO_4) media, alkenes are oxidized to produce organic acids.

Oxidizing an Alkene to an Organic Acid

$$R-CH=CH_2 + 5[O] \xrightarrow[KOH]{KMnO_4} R-COOH + CO_2 + H_2O$$

Alkene — Carboxylic acid

In the presence of catalysts like platinum (Pt), palladium (Pd), or nickel (Ni), alkenes are reduced to alkanes.

Reducing an Alkene to an Alkane

$$R^1-CH=CH-R^2 + H_2 \xrightarrow{Pt\ or\ Pd} R^1-CH_2-CH_2-R^2$$

Alkene — Alkane

3. *Alkynes*: When alkynes are treated with an oxidizing agent like alkaline potassium permanganate ($KMnO_4$) in the presence of a high temperature, the π-bonds undergo fission and oxidation to form carboxylic acids. The type of carboxylic acids formed depends on the position of the triple bond in the C chain.

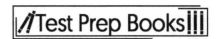

Alkynes can be reduced by H_2 at room temperature in the presence of Pt or Pd, or at a high temperature (150° – 180°C) in the presence of Ni.

Reduction of an Alkyne

$$R-C \equiv CH + H_2 \xrightarrow[180^\circ C]{Ni} R-CH = CH_2 \xrightarrow[180^\circ C]{H_2,\ Ni} R-CH_3-CH_3$$

Alkyne   Alkene   Alkane

4. *Aromatic Compounds:* The alkyl side chain on the benzene is susceptible to oxidation. For example, the $-CH_3$ group of toluene could be oxidized by $K_2Cr_2O_7/H_2SO_4$ or $KMnO_4$ or dilute heated HNO_3 to form benzoic acid.

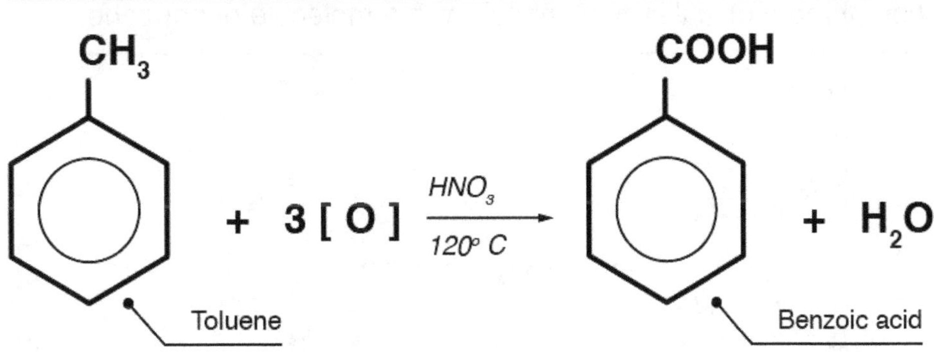

When treated with a weak oxidizing agent like chromyl chloride (CrO_2Cl_2), $-CH_3$ group of toluene is oxidized to form benzaldehyde. This is called the *Étard Reaction.*

The Étard Reaction

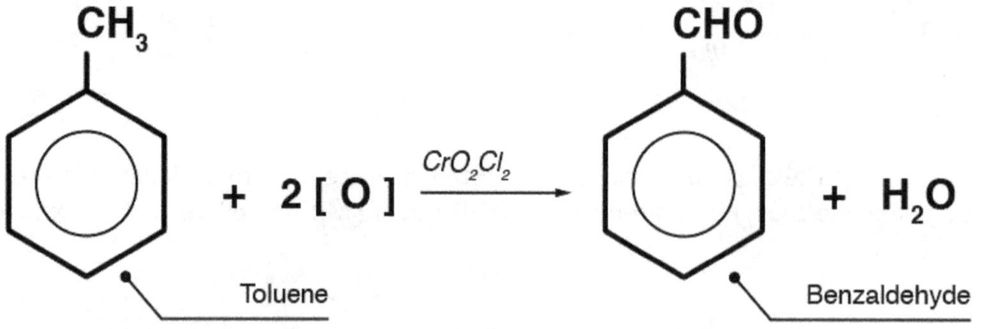

CH_3 / CHO

$$\text{Toluene} + 2[O] \xrightarrow{CrO_2Cl_2} \text{Benzaldehyde} + H_2O$$

Toluene

Benzaldehyde

In the presence of nickel (Ni) catalyst and at temperature 200°C, benzene (C_6H_6) is reduced by H_2 to form cyclohexane (C_6H_{12}). In this reaction, three molecules of H_2 attach with a molecule of benzene.

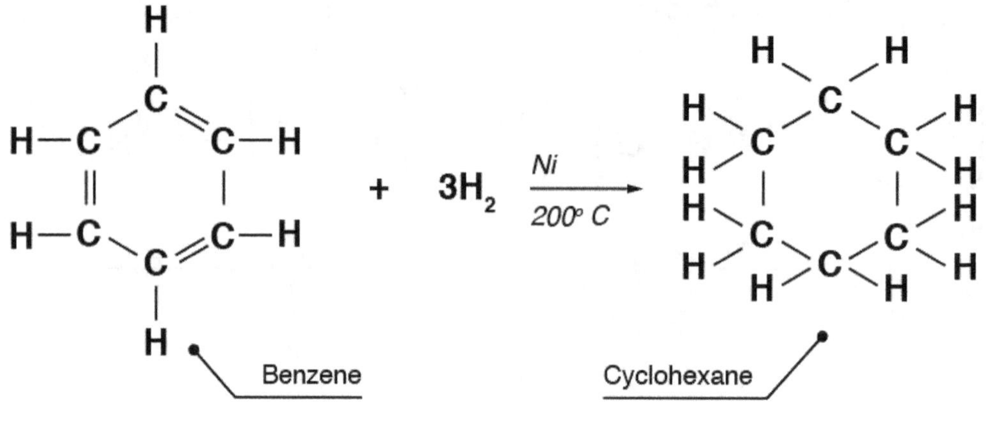

$$\text{Benzene} + 3H_2 \xrightarrow[200^\circ C]{Ni} \text{Cyclohexane}$$

Benzene

Cyclohexane

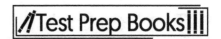

Under similar conditions, toluene is reduced to hexahydrotoluene.

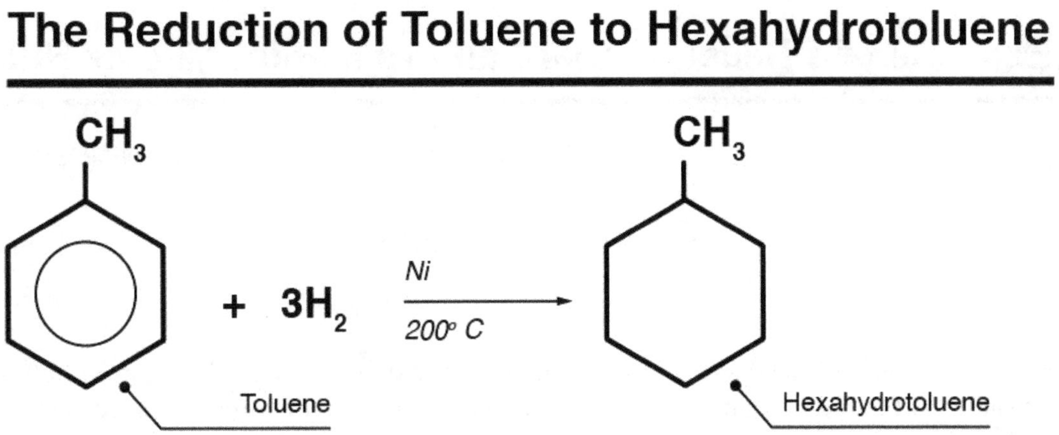

The Reduction of Toluene to Hexahydrotoluene

$$C_6H_5CH_3 + 3H_2 \xrightarrow[200^\circ C]{Ni} C_6H_{11}CH_3$$

Toluene → Hexahydrotoluene

5. *Alcohols:* Alcohols are oxidized to produce carbonyl compounds like aldehydes and ketones. The type of carbonyl compounds formed depends on the nature of alcohol (1°, 2°, or 3°) and oxidizing agent.

6. *Carbonyl Compounds:* Carbonyl compounds can be oxidized to organic acids, whereas reduction of carbonyl compounds produces alcohols.

Hydration and Dehydration

Hydration refers to the addition of water to a compound. Conversely, dehydration is the removal of water from a molecule.

1. Alkenes: Alkenes can be hydrated in the presence of concentrated sulphuric acid to form alcohol. In such reactions, an unstable intermediate, alkyl hydrogen sulphate, is formed. This is further degraded to yield an alcohol.

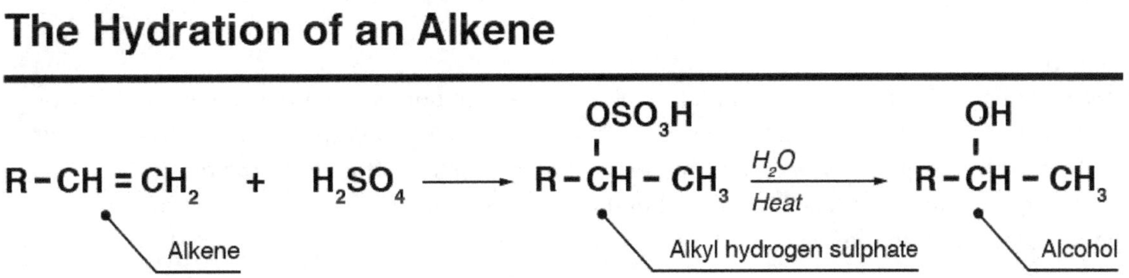

The Hydration of an Alkene

$$R-CH=CH_2 + H_2SO_4 \longrightarrow R-CH(OSO_3H)-CH_3 \xrightarrow[Heat]{H_2O} R-CH(OH)-CH_3$$

Alkene; Alkyl hydrogen sulphate; Alcohol

The above reaction follows *Markovnikov's Rule*. According to this rule, when an asymmetric alkene interacts with an asymmetric reagent, the H atom of the reagent attaches with the C atom that carries the greater number of H atoms. An example below shows how propene reacts with hydrogen bromide to yield 2-bromopropane as the principal yield in the reaction:

An Example of a Reaction that Follows Markovnikov's Rule

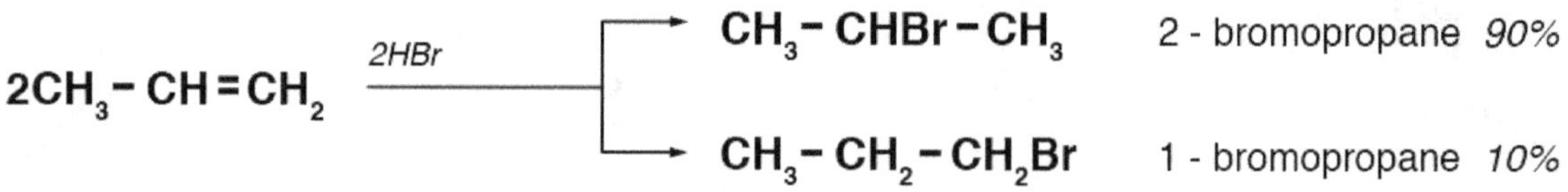

$$2CH_3-CH=CH_2 \xrightarrow{2HBr} \begin{cases} CH_3-CHBr-CH_3 & \text{2 - bromopropane } 90\% \\ CH_3-CH_2-CH_2Br & \text{1 - bromopropane } 10\% \end{cases}$$

2. *Alkynes*: When treated with sulphuric acid and in the presence of mercuric sulphate catalyst, alkynes are converted into carbonyl compounds. The reaction proceeds through the formation of an unstable intermediate that undergoes rearrangement to form the final carbonyl product.

The Conversion of Alkynes to Carbonyl Compounds

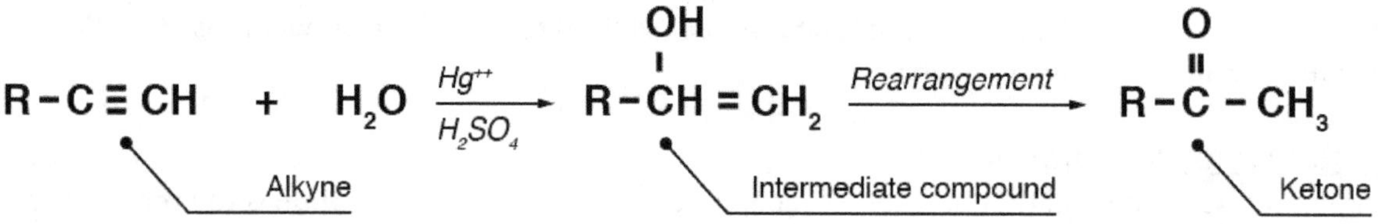

$$\underbrace{R-C\equiv CH}_{\text{Alkyne}} + H_2O \xrightarrow[H_2SO_4]{Hg^{++}} \underbrace{R-\overset{OH}{\overset{|}{C}}H=CH_2}_{\text{Intermediate compound}} \xrightarrow{\text{Rearrangement}} \underbrace{R-\overset{O}{\overset{\|}{C}}-CH_3}_{\text{Ketone}}$$

2. *Alcohols*: Alcohols undergo *dehydration* reactions in the presence of a *Lucas reagent*. This reaction causes the elimination of –OH group of alcohol, resulting in the formation of organic halide.

3. *Carbonyl Compounds*: Aldehydes and ketones can be hydrated to produce alcohols. Hydration of aldehydes produces 1° and 2° alcohols, whereas that of ketones produces 3° alcohols.

Hydrolysis

Hydrolysis refers to chemical reactions that involve cleavage of bonds in a molecule by the addition of water. In such reactions, a chemical bond in the organic molecule undergoes fission. The -OH group of water attaches to one part of the organic molecule, and proton (H) attaches to the other. The reactions are catalyzed by an acid or alkali. Hydrolytic bond cleavage is limited to certain classes of organic compounds, including amides, esters, ethers, and alkyl halides.

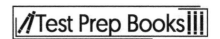

1. *Amides*: A primary amide is hydrolyzed to form a carboxylic acid and ammonia, whereas a secondary amide produces a carboxylic acid and primary amine.

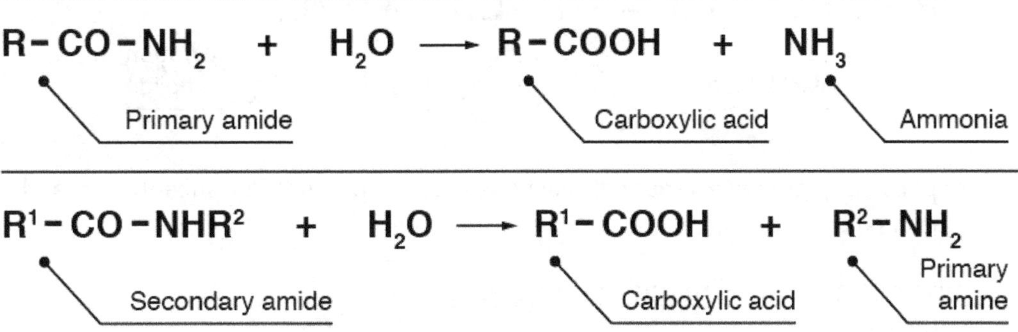

2. *Esters*: Hydrolysis of an ester produces a carboxylic acid and an alcohol.

Hydrolysis of Esters

$R^1-CO-OR^2 + H_2O \rightarrow R^1-COOH + R^2-OH$

Ester — Carboxylic acid — Alcohol

3. *Ethers*: Ethers are hydrolyzed to form alcohols.

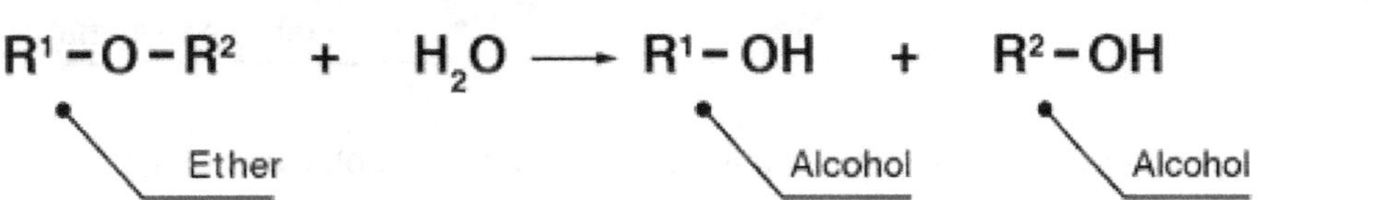

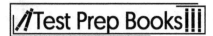

4. *Alkyl Halides*: Hydrolysis of alkyl halides produces alcohol.

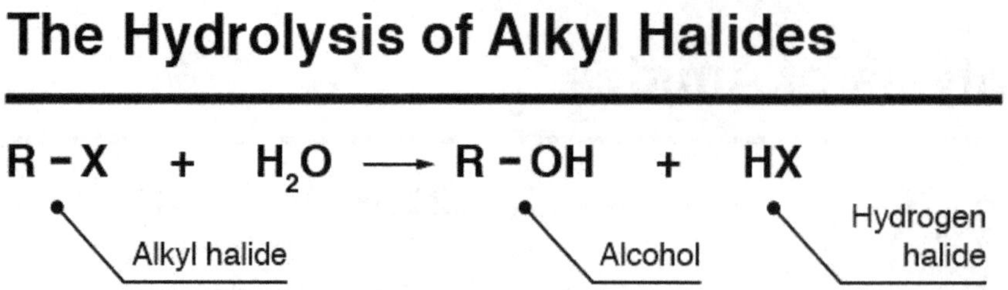

The Hydrolysis of Alkyl Halides

$$R-X + H_2O \longrightarrow R-OH + HX$$

Alkyl halide

Alcohol

Hydrogen halide

Organic compounds also undergo a variety of reactions that involve addition, substitution, and elimination of atom(s) or group(s).

Addition, Substitution, and Elimination Reactions

Addition Reactions

In *addition reactions*, two different molecules are combined to form a new organic compound. Generally, unsaturated compounds with π-bonds undergo addition reactions. These reactions involve breaking a π-bond to form more stable σ-bond. An example is the reaction between ethene and bromine, which causes the formation of 1,2-dibromo ethane.

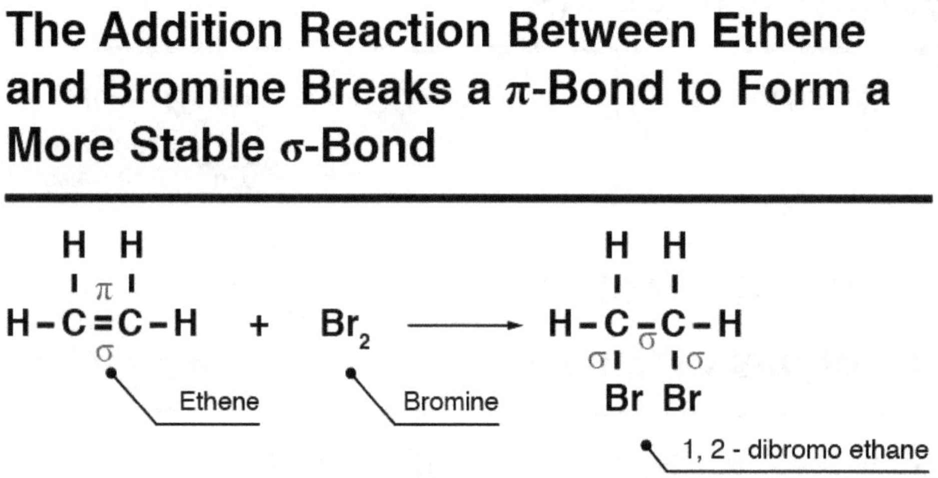

The Addition Reaction Between Ethene and Bromine Breaks a π-Bond to Form a More Stable σ-Bond

$$H_2C=CH_2 + Br_2 \longrightarrow BrH_2C-CH_2Br$$

Ethene

Bromine

1, 2 - dibromo ethane

Addition reactions are chemical reactions that involve the addition of a molecule to an organic compound that contains a double bond. Alkenes can undergo addition reactions with hydrogen (H_2), halogens (X_2), hydrogen halide (HX), hypohalous acid (HOX), and sulphuric acid (H_2SO_4). In such reactions, the above electrophilic reagents interact with π-electrons to form new compounds. Below are examples of addition reactions of alkenes with various reagents:

Addition Reactions of Alkenes

1. Reaction with H_2

$$CH_2=CH_2 + H_2 \longrightarrow CH_3-CH_3$$

Ethene → Ethane

2. Reaction with X_2

$$CH_2=CH_2 + Cl_2 \longrightarrow ClCH_2-CH_2Cl$$

Ethene → 1,2-dichloro ethane

3. Reaction with HX

$$CH_2=CH_2 + HCl \longrightarrow CH_3-CH_2Cl$$

Ethene → Ethyl chloride

4. Reaction with HOX

$$CH_2=CH_2 + HOCl \longrightarrow ClCH_2-CH_2OH$$

Ethene → 2 - chloroethanol

5. Reaction with H_2SO_4

$$CH_2=CH_2 + H_2SO_4 \longrightarrow CH_3-CH_2-OSO_3H + H_2O \longrightarrow CH_3-CH_2-OH + H_2SO_4$$

Ethene → Ethyl hydrogen sulphate → Ethanol

The π-bond in alkenes is readily oxidized by different oxidizing agents. In such reactions, the different compounds formed include glycols, ketones, carboxylic acid, and carbon dioxide. The reaction pattern, however, depends on the nature of the oxidizing agent. For example, in the presence of a weak oxidizing agent, such as dilute potassium permanganate (KMnO4), in alkaline (KOH) solution, ethene undergoes oxidation to produce an alcohol, ethylene glycol.

An Example of Oxidizing the π-Bond in in Alkene

$$CH_2=CH_2 + 2MnO_4^- + 2OH^- \longrightarrow \underset{OH}{CH_2}-\underset{OH}{CH_2} + 2MnO_4^-$$

dark green solution

However, in the presence of a strong oxidizing agent, such as concentrated $KMnO_4$, in acidic (H_2SO_4) conditions, propene undergoes oxidation to produce carboxylic acid, acetic acid.

$$CH_3—CH=CH_2 + 5[O] \rightarrow CH_3—COOH + CO_2 + H_2O$$

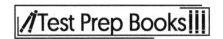

Like alkenes, alkynes can undergo addition reactions with hydrogen (H_2), halogens (X_2), hydrogen halide (HX), hypohalous acid (HOX), and sulphuric acid (H_2SO_4). In such reactions, these electrophilic reagents interact with π-electrons to form new compounds. Examples of addition reactions are illustrated below:

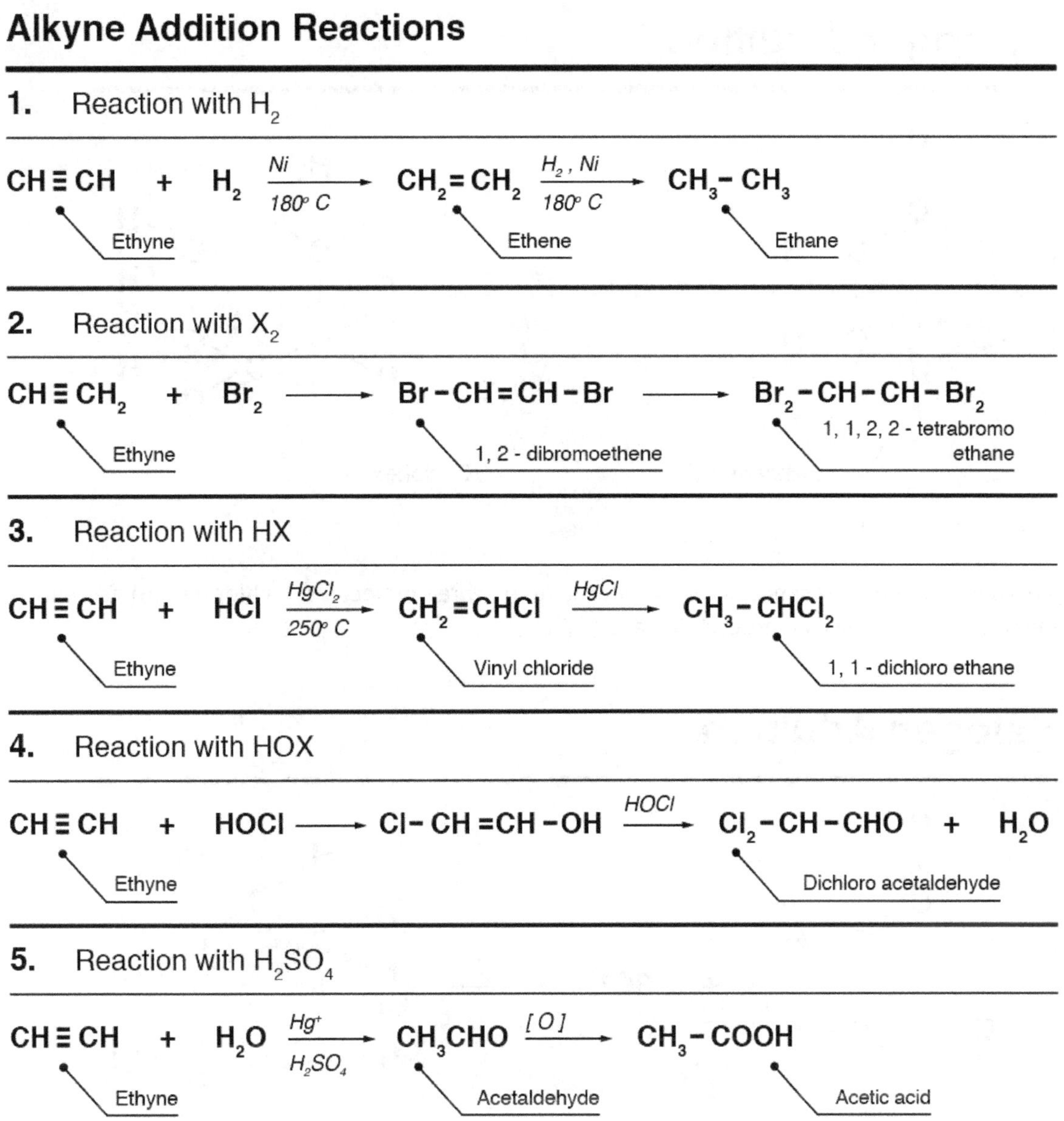

Alkyne Addition Reactions

1. Reaction with H_2

$$CH \equiv CH + H_2 \xrightarrow[180^\circ C]{Ni} CH_2 = CH_2 \xrightarrow[180^\circ C]{H_2,\, Ni} CH_3 - CH_3$$

Ethyne; Ethene; Ethane

2. Reaction with X_2

$$CH \equiv CH_2 + Br_2 \longrightarrow Br - CH = CH - Br \longrightarrow Br_2 - CH - CH - Br_2$$

Ethyne; 1, 2 - dibromoethene; 1, 1, 2, 2 - tetrabromo ethane

3. Reaction with HX

$$CH \equiv CH + HCl \xrightarrow[250^\circ C]{HgCl_2} CH_2 = CHCl \xrightarrow{HgCl} CH_3 - CHCl_2$$

Ethyne; Vinyl chloride; 1, 1 - dichloro ethane

4. Reaction with HOX

$$CH \equiv CH + HOCl \longrightarrow Cl - CH = CH - OH \xrightarrow{HOCl} Cl_2 - CH - CHO + H_2O$$

Ethyne; Dichloro acetaldehyde

5. Reaction with H_2SO_4

$$CH \equiv CH + H_2O \xrightarrow[H_2SO_4]{Hg^+} CH_3CHO \xrightarrow{[O]} CH_3 - COOH$$

Ethyne; Acetaldehyde; Acetic acid

Benzene also undergoes addition reactions including hydrogen addition and halogen addition.

Hydrogen Addition: In the presence of a nickel (Ni) catalyst and at temperature 200°C, hydrogen (H_2) undergoes an addition reaction with benzene (C_6H_6) to form cyclohexane (C_6H_{12}). In this reaction, three molecules of H_2 attach with a molecule of benzene.

Hydrogen Addition

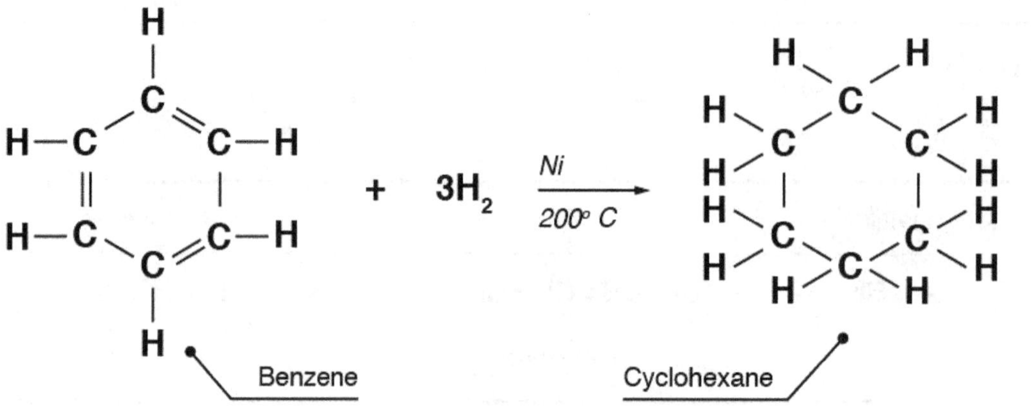

$$C_6H_6 + 3H_2 \xrightarrow[200^\circ C]{Ni} C_6H_{12}$$

Benzene

Cyclohexane

Halogen Addition: In the presence of ultraviolet radiation, three molecules of chlorine (Cl_2) add with benzene (C_6H_6) to form hexachlorocyclohexane ($C_6H_6Cl_6$).

Halogen Addition

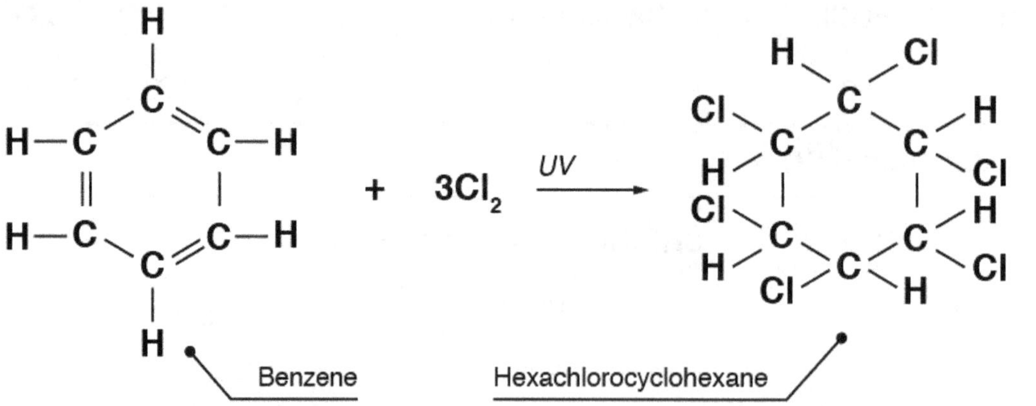

$$C_6H_6 + 3Cl_2 \xrightarrow{UV} C_6H_6Cl_6$$

Benzene

Hexachlorocyclohexane

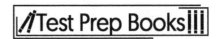

Substitution Reactions

A *substitution reaction* is when an atom or group is substituted by another atom or group to form a new compound. An example is a reaction between chloroethane and sodium hydroxide, where the chloride group of chloroethane is replaced by the hydroxyl group to form ethanol.

A Substitution Reaction

The chloride group of chloroethane is replaced by the hydroxyl group to form ethanol

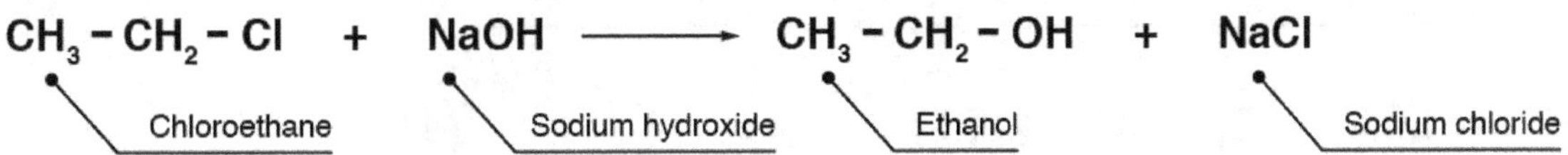

In substitution reactions, one functional group is replaced with another. For alkanes, H atoms (R-H) are replaced by attacking reagents such as halogens (X) or nitro (-NO_2) groups. Introduction of a halogen is called *halogenation*, and introduction of a nitro group is called *nitration*.

Halogenation of alkanes requires UV light and high temperatures (300°–400° C) because alkanes are very stable. Halogenation can occur at every available H atom. For example, halogenation of alkanes by chlorine (Cl_2) will produce methyl chloride (CH_3Cl), dichloromethane (CH_2Cl_2), trichloromethane or chloroform ($CHCl_3$), and carbon tetrachloride (CCl_4), respectively. The steps of reaction are illustrated below.

1. $CH_4 + Cl_2 \rightarrow CH_3Cl + HCl$
2. $CH_3Cl + Cl_2 \rightarrow CH_2Cl_2 + HCl$
3. $CH_2Cl_2 + Cl_2 \rightarrow CHCl_3 + HCl$
4. $CHCl_3 + Cl_2 \rightarrow CCl_4 + HCl$

The chlorination reaction takes place in three steps:

1. Chlorine free-radical is formed in the presence of high temperature and UV radiation.
2. A chlorine free-radical attacks a C—H bond of alkane to form an alkyl (R) free-radical and HCl.

3. The other chlorine free-radical binds with the alkyl free-radical to form chlorinated (halogenated) alkane (R—Cl).

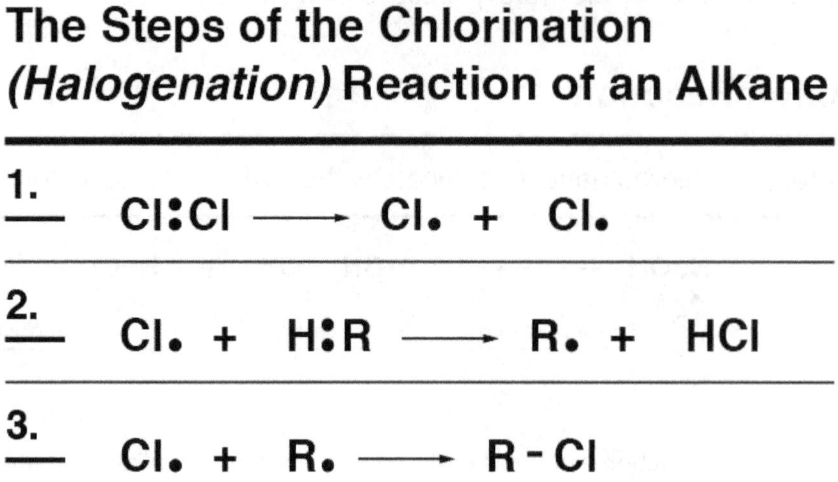

The Steps of the Chlorination *(Halogenation)* Reaction of an Alkane

1. Cl:Cl ⟶ Cl• + Cl•

2. Cl• + H:R ⟶ R• + HCl

3. Cl• + R• ⟶ R - Cl

Because a carbon free-radical is formed, the rate and extent of halogenation depends on the stability of the carbon free-radical. For example, a H atom attached to a 3° carbon is more reactive than that attached with 2° and 1° carbon, respectively. Therefore, in the following reaction, the yield of 2-chloro propane (55%) is more than that of propyl chloride (45%).

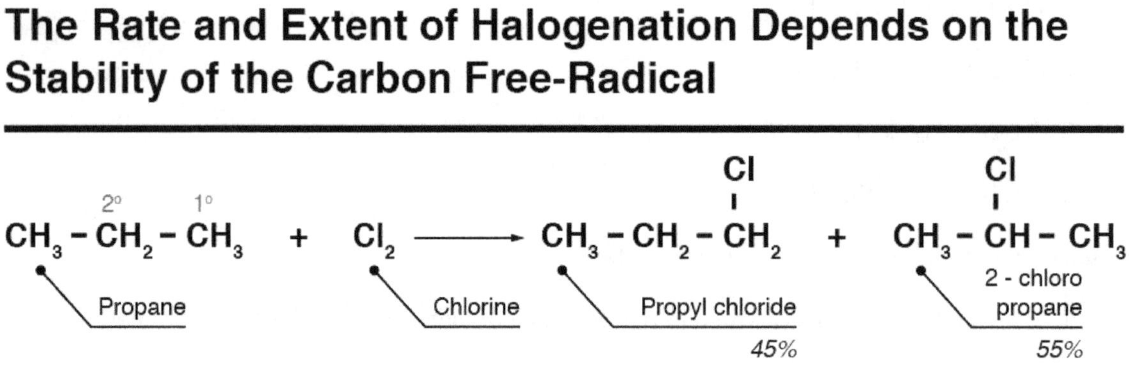

The Rate and Extent of Halogenation Depends on the Stability of the Carbon Free-Radical

$CH_3 - \overset{2°}{CH_2} - \overset{1°}{CH_3}$ (Propane) + Cl_2 (Chlorine) ⟶ $CH_3 - CH_2 - CH_2Cl$ (Propyl chloride, *45%*) + $CH_3 - CH(Cl) - CH_3$ (2 - chloro propane, *55%*)

Halogenation with any halogen occurs through the same general steps. However, the different halogens have different reactivities. The order of reactivity is as follows: $F_2 > Cl_2 > Br_2 > I_2$.

Benzene and aromatic compounds undergo substitution reactions. Since benzene is quite stable, each H atom is substituted sequentially. The substituent groups/atoms take specific positions on the benzene ring during those substitution reactions.

1. *Halogenation:* Halogen substitution is a catalyst-dependent reaction, commonly using ferric chloride ($FeCl_3$), ferric bromide ($FeBr_3$) and aluminum chloride ($AlCl_3$) as catalysts. Halogenation is an electrophilic

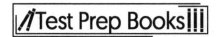

addition reaction. For example, in the presence of anhydrous $AlCl_3$, chlorine (Cl_2) substitutes an H atom to form chlorobenzene (see below).

Halogenation of Benzene is an Electrophilic Addition Reaction

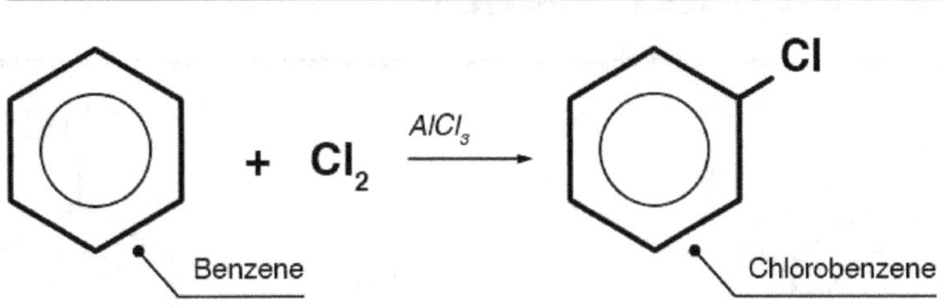

These substitutions can eventually replace all of the H atoms. In the example above, continued reaction would form dichlorobenzene, trichlorobenzene, tetrachlorobenzene, pentachlorobenzene and hexachlorobenzene, respectively.

Subsequent Halogen Substitutions

1. $C_6H_6 + Cl_2 \xrightarrow{AlCl_3} C_6H_5Cl + HCl$

   Benzene → Chlorobenzene

2. $C_6H_5Cl + Cl_2 \xrightarrow{AlCl_3} C_6H_4Cl_2 + HCl$

   Chlorobenzene → Dichlorobenzene

3. $C_6H_4Cl_2 + Cl_2 \xrightarrow{AlCl_3} C_6H_3Cl_3 + HCl$

   Dichlorobenzene → Trichlorobenzene

4. $C_6H_3Cl_3 + Cl_2 \xrightarrow{AlCl_3} C_6H_2Cl_4 + HCl$

   Trichlorobenzene → Tetrachlorobenzene

5. $C_6H_2Cl_4 + Cl_2 \xrightarrow{AlCl_3} C_6HCl_5 + HCl$

   Tetrachlorobenzene → Pentachlorobenzene

6. $C_6HCl_5 + Cl_2 \xrightarrow{AlCl_3} C_6Cl_6 + HCl$

   Pentachlorobenzene → Hexachlorobenzene

2. *Nitration:* This electrophilic substitution reaction replaces H atoms with a nitro ($-NO_2$) group. For example, when benzene is treated with concentrated sulphuric acid (H_2SO_4) and concentrated nitric acid (HNO_3) at around 50°C, one H atom is substituted by a $-NO_2$ group to produce nitrobenzene and water.

Nitration of Benzene is an Electrophilic Substitution Reaction

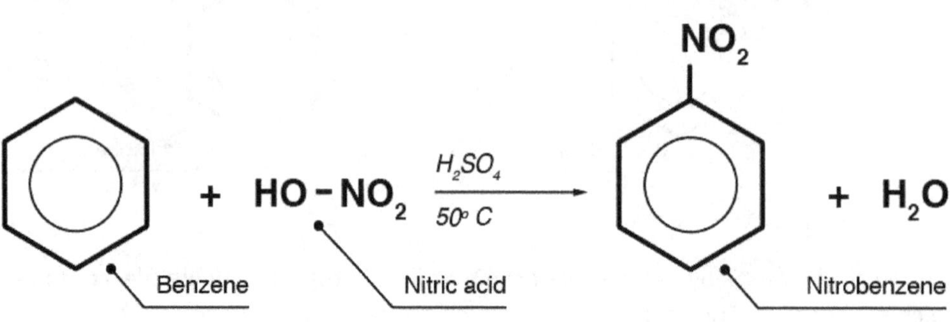

When the reaction is carried out at 100°C in the presence of concentrated H_2SO_4 and HNO_3, 1,3-dinitrobenzene (meta-dinitrobenzene) is formed.

Nitration of Benzene at 100°C in the Presence of Concentrated H_2SO_4 and HNO_3

$$C_6H_5NO_2 + HO-NO_2 \xrightarrow[100^\circ C]{H_2SO_4} C_6H_4(NO_2)_2 + H_2O$$

Nitrobenzene

Nitric acid

1, 3 - dinitrobenzene

Meta-dinitrobenzene

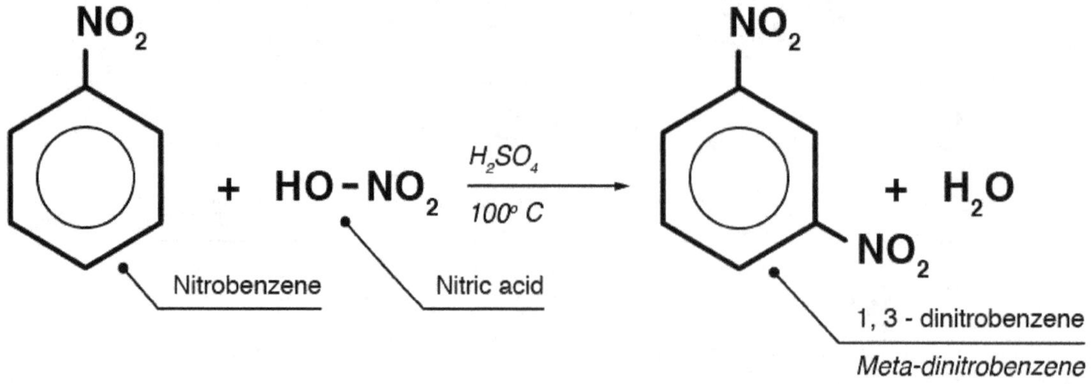

3. *Friedel-Crafts Alkylation:* When benzene is treated with an alkyl halide (R—X) in the presence of a Lewis acid catalyst (e.g. anhydrous $AlCl_3$ or $FeCl_3$), one H atom of the ring is substituted by the alkyl group to form alkyl benzene. This is called Friedel-Crafts alkylation. For example, in a reaction between benzene and methyl chloride, methyl benzene (toluene) is formed.

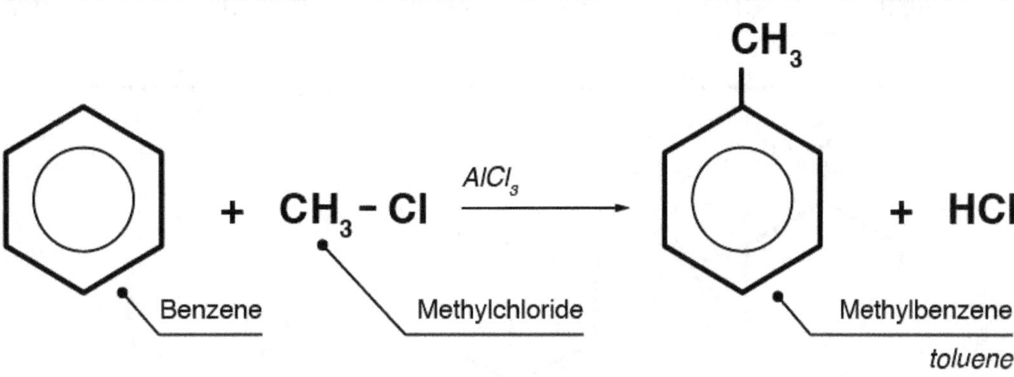

4. *Friedel-Crafts Acylation:* When benzene reacts with an acyl halide (RCO—X) in the presence of a Lewis acid, like $AlCl_3$ or $FeCl_3$, an acyl group (RCO-) is introduced in the benzene ring to form an aromatic ketone. For example, the reaction between benzene and acetyl chloride produces acetophenone (methyl phenyl ketone).

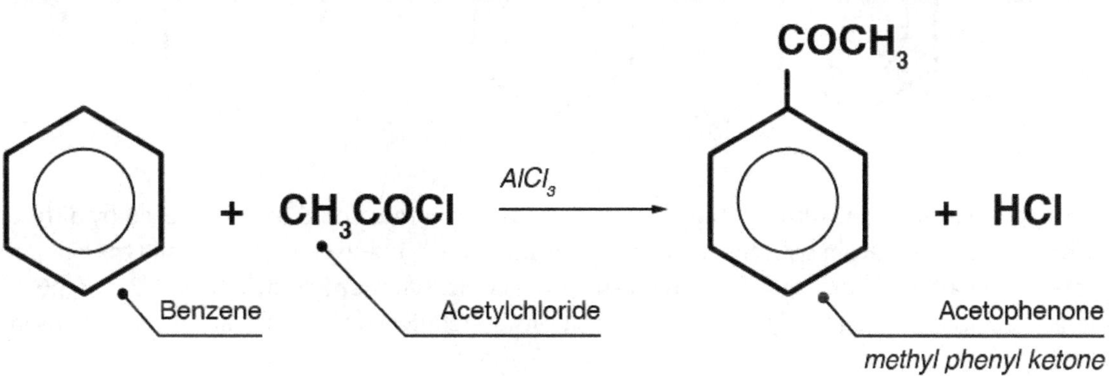

When a single H atom is substituted from the benzene ring, it makes mono-substituted benzene derivatives. Examples are methylbenzene (toluene), chlorobenzene, phenol, phenyl amine (aniline), benzaldehyde, and benzoic acid.

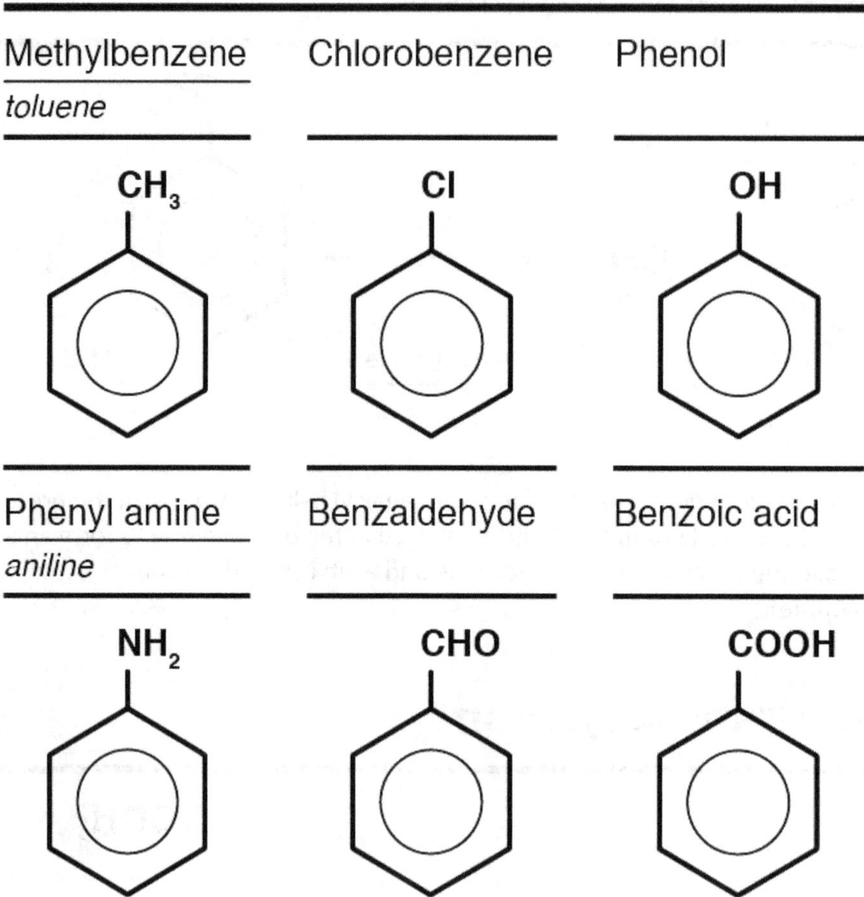

When a single H atom is substituted, there are still five H atoms that could be substituted by different atoms or groups. The C atom with first substitution is numbered 1, and other C atoms in the ring are numbered and named accordingly. Since benzene has a cyclic, symmetrical structure, 1:2 and 1:6 positions are equivalent. Similarly, 1:3 and 1:5 positions are equivalent. The 1:2 and 1:6 positions are nearest, and called "ortho" or "*o*." The 1:3 and 1:5 positions are termed "meta" or "*m*", and the 1:4 position is the farthest, and termed "para" or "*p*."

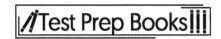

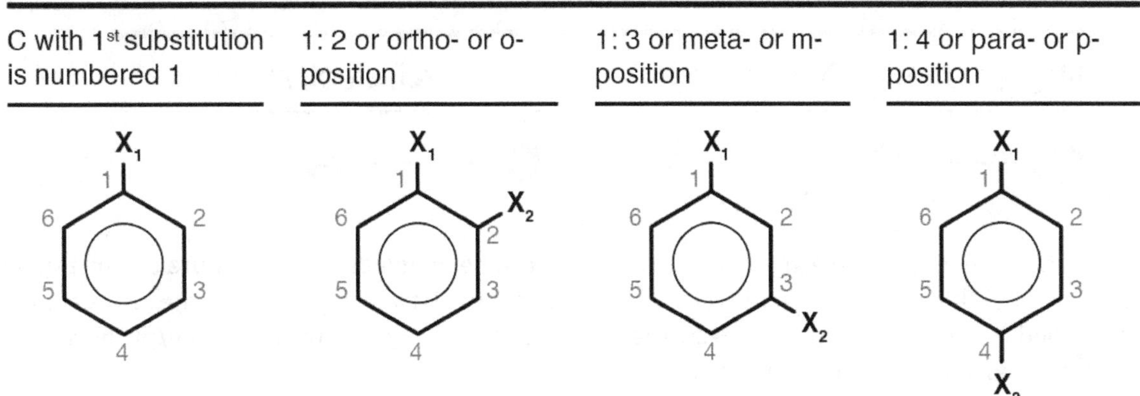

The following example shows three possible isomers of dichlorobenzene based on the relative positions of the substituent atoms.

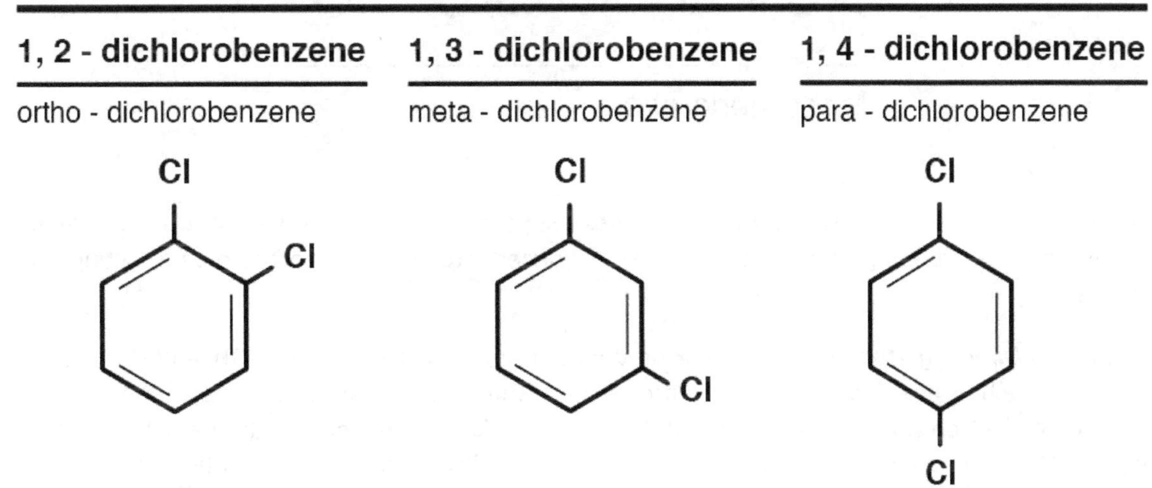

The substituents on benzene ring could have two types of effects: an inductive effect or a mesomeric effect.

1. *Inductive Effect (I):* The electronegativity of substituent atoms or groups can cause polarization of the bond between the C atom in benzene ring and the substituent group. When the electronegativity of the substituent (e.g. halogens, X: F, Cl, B, I) is higher than carbon, it pulls the σ-electrons and causes polarization of the bond. This is called a negative (–) inductive effect. In contrast, if the electronegativity

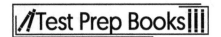

of substituent atoms or groups (e.g. alkyl groups, R: $-CH_3$, $-C_2H_5$) is lower than the ring C atom, it pushes the σ-electrons toward C atom, and is called a positive (+) inductive effect.

The Inductive Effect *(I)* Involves σ-Electrons

Negative inductive effect	Positive inductive effect
C ⟶ X	C ⟵ R

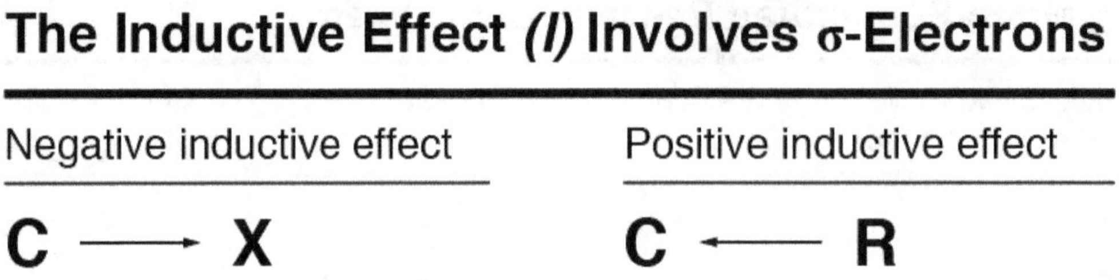

2. *Mesomeric Effect (M):* The electron cloud in a π-bond can be influenced by the nature of substituent atoms or groups. The delocalization of π-electrons toward the relatively higher electronegative atom or group is called a negative mesomeric effect. The opposite effect by an electron repelling/pushing atom or group is called a positive mesomeric effect.

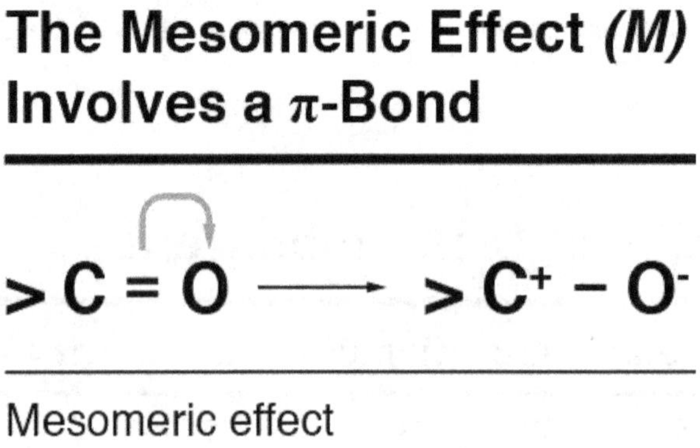

The Mesomeric Effect *(M)* Involves a π-Bond

$$>C=O \longrightarrow >C^{+}-O^{-}$$

Mesomeric effect

The nature of substituent group or atom determines the position of further substitutions in the ring. Therefore, the substituent groups/atoms can be categorized into two types: ortho-para directing and meta directing.

1. *Ortho-Para Directing Atoms/Groups:* Electron-donating substituents like $-CH_3$, -OH, and $-NH_2$ donate electrons to the benzene ring and make it more reactive. Due to the positive mesomeric effect, they push into the electron cloud and the electron density gets relatively higher at ortho-para positions. Therefore, the ortho-para position becomes more reactive, allowing further substitutions on those positions. In the case of halogens, the effect is relatively complicated. X atoms have a negative inductive effect, but they provide a positive mesomeric effect by pushing unpaired electrons to the benzene ring. Therefore, halogens are ortho-para directing substituents.

2. *Meta Directing Atoms/Groups:* Certain atoms/groups, due to their negative mesomeric effects, pull the electron cloud from the benzene ring. These atoms and groups make benzene ring less reactive. Examples are $-NO_2$, -CHO, -COOH, and $-SO_3H$. By withdrawing the electron cloud, these groups decrease the electron density significantly at the ortho-para positions. However, meta position is less affected, and thus, the second electrophile attacks the meta position. These groups are called meta-directing substituents.

Elimination Reactions

In *elimination reactions*, atoms or groups are eliminated from two adjacent C atoms to form π-bonds. This is opposite to addition reactions. As an example, in the presence of concentrated sulphuric acid, a water molecule is removed from ethanol to form a C-C π-bond, i.e. ethene.

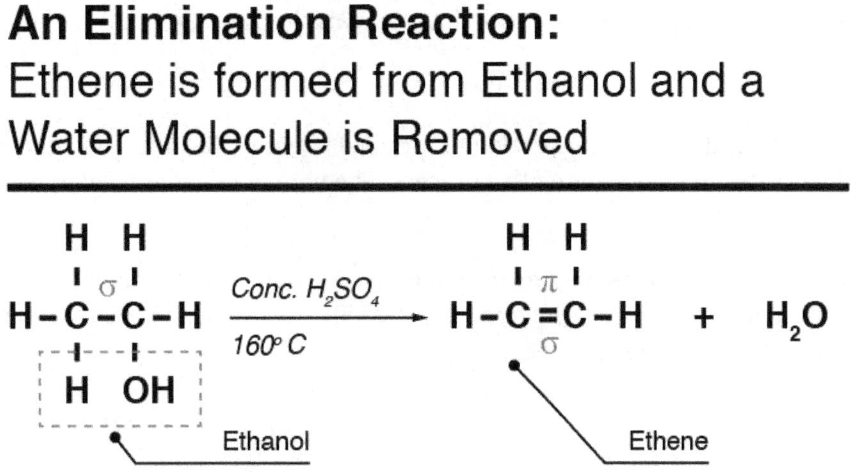

An Elimination Reaction:
Ethene is formed from Ethanol and a Water Molecule is Removed

$$H_3C{-}CH_2OH \xrightarrow[160^\circ C]{Conc.\ H_2SO_4} H_2C{=}CH_2 + H_2O$$

Ethanol   Ethene

Isomerization

Isomerization refers to a rearrangement of atoms or groups in an organic molecule to form an isomer. The newly formed compound has a similar molecular formula, but has a different structural arrangement than the parent compound. As an example, in the presence of aluminum chloride and hydrochloric acid, butane undergoes atomic rearrangement to form 2-methyl propane.

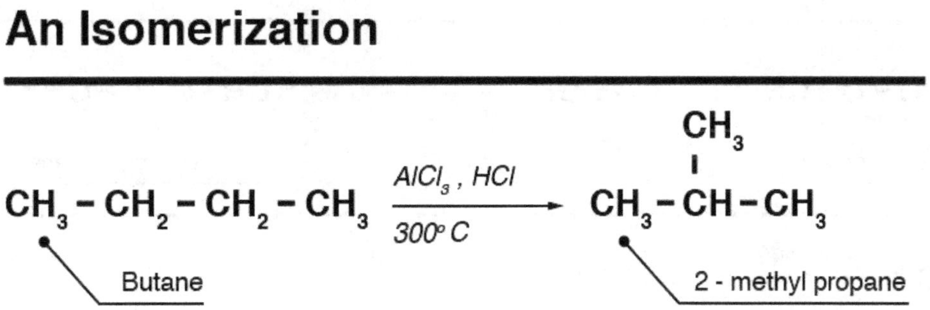

An Isomerization

$$CH_3-CH_2-CH_2-CH_3 \xrightarrow[300^\circ C]{AlCl_3,\ HCl} CH_3-CH(CH_3)-CH_3$$

Butane   2 - methyl propane

Alkanes can undergo *isomerization* to produce isomers. In such reactions, straight chain alkanes can be converted into corresponding branched-chain isomers. For example, in the presence of aluminum chloride ($AlCl_3$) and hydrochloric acid (HCl) and at 250°–300°C, butane is converted into iso-butane (2-methyl propane).

$$CH_3\text{-}CH_2\text{-}CH_2\text{-}CH_3 \rightarrow CH_3\text{-}CH(CH_3)\text{-}CH_3$$

Butane   Isobutane

Polymerization

In the presence of a high temperature, pressure, and a catalyst, molecules of a same alkene can join together to form a large molecule. This process is called *polymerization* and it results in the formation a polymer from a monomer (single unit). Polymerization is used widely in industries to synthesize compounds with modified physical properties and shear withstanding capacities. For example, polymerization of ethene (ethylene) causes the formation of polyethylene, which is widely used as a plastic material in manufacturing industries. Note that *n* equals the number of monomers.

$$nCH_2{=}CH_2 \rightarrow (-CH_2-CH_2-)n$$

Like alkenes, alkynes also undergo polymerization to produce larger molecules. Alkynes can produce both aliphatic and aromatic polymers during this process. The type of polymer formed depends on the reaction conditions.

1. *Formation of Aliphatic Polymers:* In the presence of cuprous chloride (CuCl) and ammonium chloride (NH_4Cl), ethyne (or acetylene) undergoes polymerization to first form vinylacetylene, and the further addition of a molecule forms divinylacetylene.

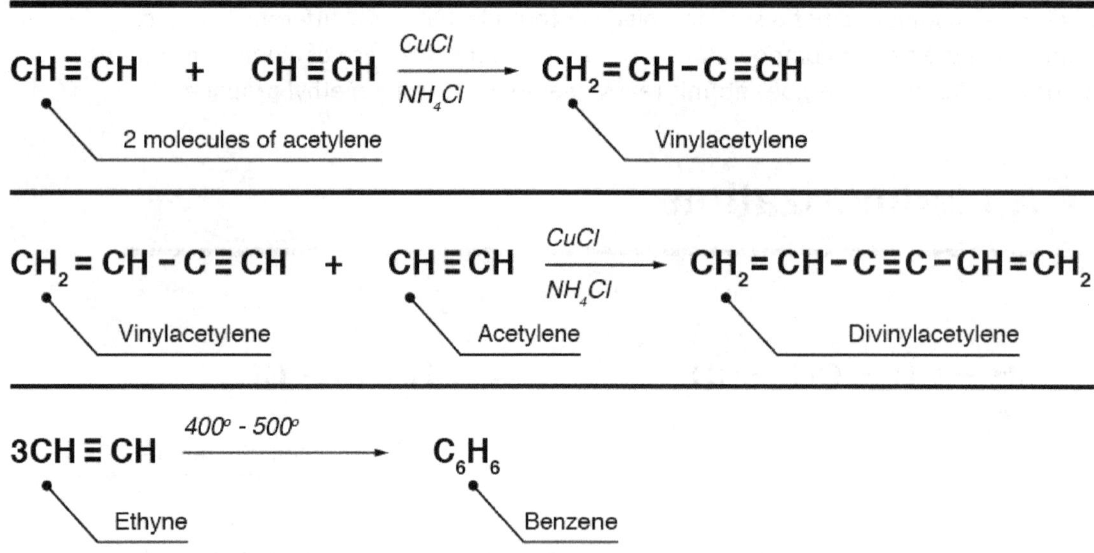

2. *Formation of Aromatic Polymers:* When ethyne (or acetylene) is passed through a heated iron pipe at a temperature of 400°–500°C, then three molecules join together to form aromatic compound benzene.

Basic Biochemistry Processes

Basic units of organic compounds are often called *monomers*. Repeating units of linked monomers are called *polymers*. The most important polymers found in all living things can be divided into just four categories: carbohydrates, lipids, proteins, and nucleic acids. This may be surprising since there is so much diversity in the outward appearances and functions of living things present on Earth. Carbon (C), hydrogen (H), oxygen (O), nitrogen (N), sulfur (S), and phosphorus (P) are the major elements of most biological molecules. Carbon is a common backbone of large molecules because of its ability to form four covalent bonds.

DNA and RNA

Nucleic acids have two important duties in the body. As monomers, they are crucial for energy transfer. As polymers, they are a fundamental component of genetic material. Nucleotides are the monomer units that assemble to form nucleic acids. Nucleotides have three components: a nitrogenous base and a phosphate functional group, both of which are attached to a five-carbon (pentose) sugar. There are two classes of nitrogenous bases, purines and pyrimidines. The two types of purines are guanine (G) and adenine (A), while the three types of pyrimidines are thymine (T), cytosine (C), and uracil (U). The two types of pentose sugars are deoxyribose and ribose. Nucleotides containing deoxyribose are termed deoxyribonucleic acid (DNA). DNA utilizes guanine, adenine, cytosine, and thymine as its nitrogenous bases. Nucleotides containing ribose are termed ribonucleic acid (RNA). RNA utilizes guanine, adenine, cytosine, and uracil as its nitrogenous bases.

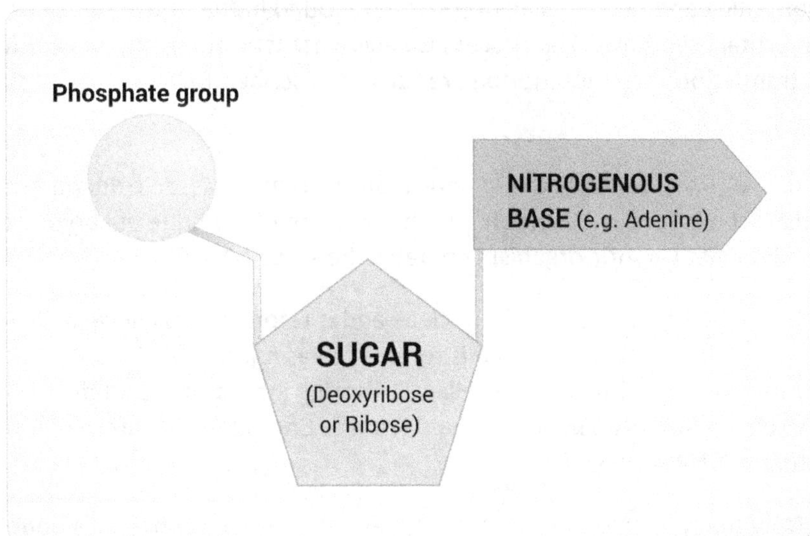

Chromosomes, Genes, Proteins, RNA, and DNA

Chromosomes are composed of hundreds to thousands of genes. Human cells contain 23 pairs of chromosomes for a total of 46 chromosomes. Genes are inherited in pairs, one from each parent.

Proteins are made of long chains of amino acids. In total, there are 20 amino acids, 11 of which humans can synthesize on their own and the remaining 9 of which are procured through diet. DNA contains the information for the synthesis of proteins, but that information on DNA has to undergo transcription and translation by RNA in order to produce proteins.

Codons

A *codon* represents a sequence of three nucleotides, which codes for either one specific amino acid or a stop signal during protein synthesis. Codons are found on messenger RNA (mRNA).

Twenty essential amino acids are utilized in the process of protein synthesis. The full set of codons encompasses 64 possible combinations and is termed the *genetic code*. In the genetic code, 61 codons represent amino acids and three codons are stop signals. The genetic code is redundant due to the fact that a single amino acid may be produced by multiple codons. For example, the codons AAA and AAG produce the amino acid lysine. The codons UAA, UAG, and UGA are stop signals. The codon AUG codes for both the amino acid methionine and the start signal. As a result, AUG when found in mRNA, marks the initiation point of protein translation.

RNA

Ribonucleic acid (RNA) plays crucial roles in protein synthesis and gene regulation. RNA is made of nucleotides consisting of ribose (a sugar), a phosphate group, and one of four possible nitrogen bases—adenine (A), cytosine (C), guanine (G), and uracil (U). RNA utilizes the nitrogenous base uracil in place of the base thymine found in DNA. Another difference between RNA and DNA is that RNA is typically found as a single-stranded structure, while DNA typically exists in a double-stranded structure.

RNA can be categorized into three major groups—messenger RNA (mRNA), ribosomal RNA (rRNA), and transfer RNA (tRNA). Messenger RNA (mRNA) transports instructions from DNA in the nucleus of a cell to the areas responsible for protein synthesis in the cytoplasm of a cell. This process is known as *transcription*. Transfer RNA (tRNA) deciphers the amino acid sequence for the construction of proteins found in mRNA. Both tRNA and ribosomal RNA (rRNA) are found in the ribosomes of cells. Ribosomes are responsible for protein synthesis. The process is known as *translation*, and both tRNA and rRNA play crucial roles. Both translation and transcription are further described below.

DNA

Deoxyribonucleic acid, or DNA, contains the genetic material that is passed from parent to offspring. It contains specific instructions for the development and function of a unique eukaryotic organism. The great majority of cells in a eukaryotic organism contains the same DNA.

The majority of DNA can be found in the cell's nucleus and is referred to as *nuclear DNA*. A small amount of DNA can be located in the mitochondria and is referred to as *mitochondrial DNA*. Mitochondria provide the energy for a properly functioning cell. All offspring inherit mitochondrial DNA from their mother. James Watson, an American geneticist, and Frances Crick, a British molecular biologist, first outlined the structure of DNA in 1953.

The structure of DNA visually approximates a twisting ladder and is described as a double helix. DNA is made of nucleotides consisting of deoxyribose (a sugar), a phosphate group, and one of four possible nitrogen bases—thymine (T), adenine (A), cytosine (C), and guanine (G). It is estimated that human DNA contains three billion bases. The sequence of these bases dictates the instructions contained in the DNA making each species singular. The bases in DNA pair in a particular manner—thymine (T) with adenine (A) and guanine (G) with cytosine (C). Weak hydrogen bonds between the nitrogenous bases ensure easy uncoiling of DNA's double helical structure in preparation for replication.

Transcription

Transcription refers to a portion of DNA being copied into RNA, specifically mRNA. It represents the first crucial step in gene expression. The process begins with the enzyme RNA polymerase binding to the promoter region of DNA, which initiates transcription of a specific gene. RNA polymerase then untwists the double helix of DNA by breaking weak hydrogen bonds between its nucleotides. Once DNA is untwisted, RNA polymerase travels down the strand reading the DNA sequence and adding complementary nitrogenous bases. With the assistance of RNA polymerase, the pentose sugar and phosphate functional group are added to the nitrogenous base to form a nucleotide. Lastly, the weak hydrogen bonds uniting the DNA-RNA complex are broken to free the newly formed mRNA. The mRNA travels from the nucleus of the cell out to the cytoplasm of the cell where translation occurs.

Translation

Translation refers to the process of ribosomes synthesizing proteins. It represents the second crucial step in gene expression. The instructions encoding specific proteins to be made are contained in codons on mRNA, which have previously been transcribed from DNA. Each codon represents a specific amino acid or stop signal in the genetic code.

Amino acids are the building blocks of proteins. Ribosomes contain transfer RNA (tRNA) and ribosomal RNA (rRNA). Translation occurs in ribosomes located in the cytoplasm of cells and consists of the following three phases:

1. Initiation: The ribosome gathers at a target point on the mRNA, and tRNA attaches at the start codon (AUG), which is also the codon for the amino acid methionine.

2. Elongation: A new tRNA reads the next codon on the mRNA and links the two amino acids together with a peptide bond. The process is repeated until a polypeptide, or long chain of amino acids, is formed.

3. Termination: The ribosome disengages from the mRNA when it encounters a stop codon (UAA, UAG, or UGA). The event releases the polypeptide molecule. Proteins are made of one or more polypeptide molecules.

Lipids

Lipids are a class of biological molecules that are hydrophobic, meaning they don't mix well with water. They are mostly made up of large chains of carbon and hydrogen atoms, termed hydrocarbon chains. When lipids mix with water, the water molecules bond to each other and exclude the lipids because they are unable to form bonds with the long hydrocarbon chains. The three most important types of lipids are fats, phospholipids, and steroids.

Fats are made up of two types of smaller molecules: glycerol and fatty acids. Glycerol is a chain of three carbon atoms, with a hydroxyl group attached to each carbon atom. A hydroxyl group is made up of an oxygen and hydrogen atom bonded together. Fatty acids are long hydrocarbon chains that have a backbone of sixteen or eighteen carbon atoms. The carbon atom on one end of the fatty acid is part of a carboxyl group. A *carboxyl group* is a carbon atom that uses two of its four bonds to bond to one oxygen atom (double bond) and uses another one of its bonds to link to a hydroxyl group. Fats are made by joining three fatty acid molecules and one glycerol molecule.

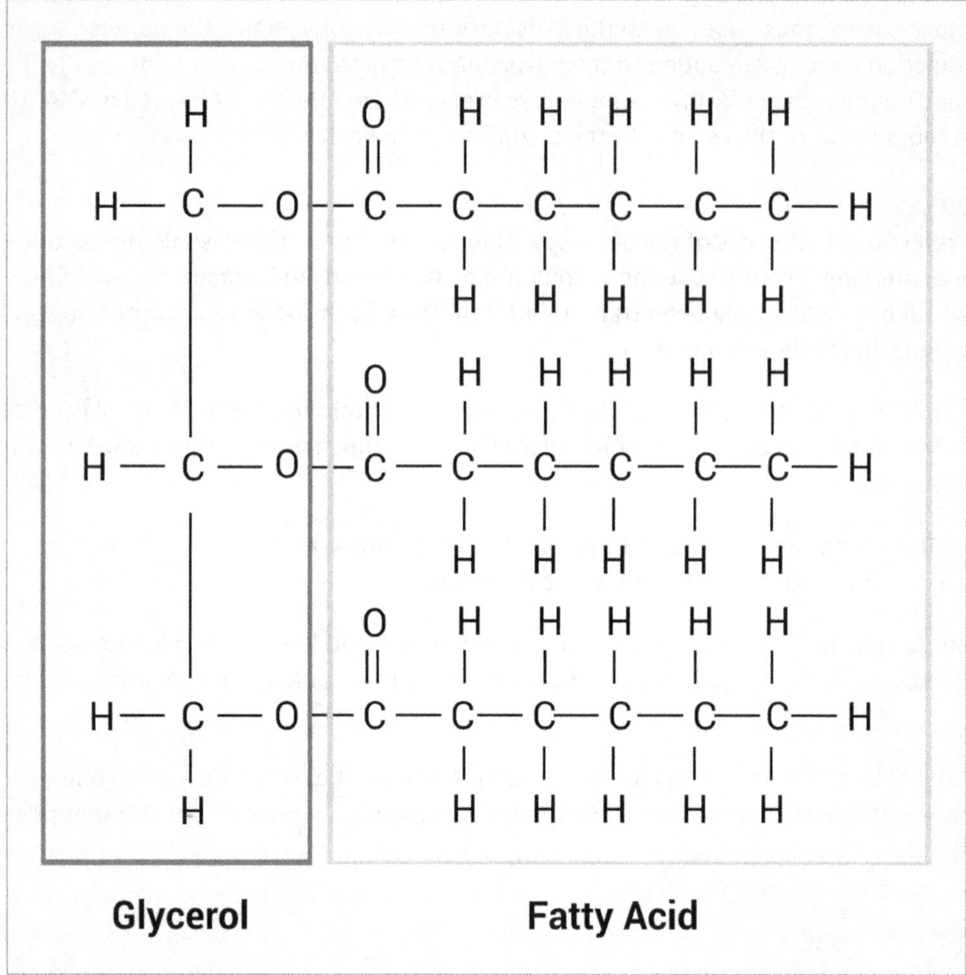

Phospholipids are made of two fatty acid molecules linked to one glycerol molecule. A phosphate group is attached to a third hydroxyl group of the glycerol molecule. A phosphate group has an overall negative charge and consists of a phosphate atom connected to four oxygen atoms.

Phospholipids have an interesting structure because their fatty acid tails are hydrophobic, but their phosphate group heads are hydrophilic. When phospholipids mix with water, they create double-layered structures, called bilayers, that shield their hydrophobic regions from water molecules. Cell membranes are made of phospholipid bilayers, which allow the cells to mix with aqueous solutions outside and inside, while forming a protective barrier and a semi-permeable membrane around the cell.

Steroids are lipids that consist of four fused carbon rings. The different chemical groups that attach to these rings are what make up the many types of steroids. Cholesterol is a common type of steroid found in animal cell membranes. Steroids are mixed in between the phospholipid bilayer and help maintain the structure of the membrane and aids in cell signaling.

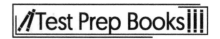

Proteins

Proteins are essential for most all functions in living beings. The name protein is derived from the Greek word *proteios*, meaning *first* or *primary*. All proteins are made from a set of twenty amino acids that are linked in unbranched polymers. The combinations are numerous, which accounts for the diversity of proteins. Amino acids are linked by peptide bonds, while polymers of amino acids are called *polypeptides*. These polypeptides, either individually or in linked combination with each other, fold up to form coils of biologically functional molecules, called proteins.

There are four levels of protein structure: primary, secondary, tertiary, and quaternary. The primary structure is the sequence of amino acids, similar to the letters in a long word. The secondary structure is beta sheets, or alpha helices, formed by hydrogen bonding between the polar regions of the polypeptide backbone. Tertiary structure is the overall shape of the molecule that results from the interactions between the side chains linked to the polypeptide backbone. Quaternary structure is the overall protein structure that occurs when a protein is made up of two or more polypeptide chains.

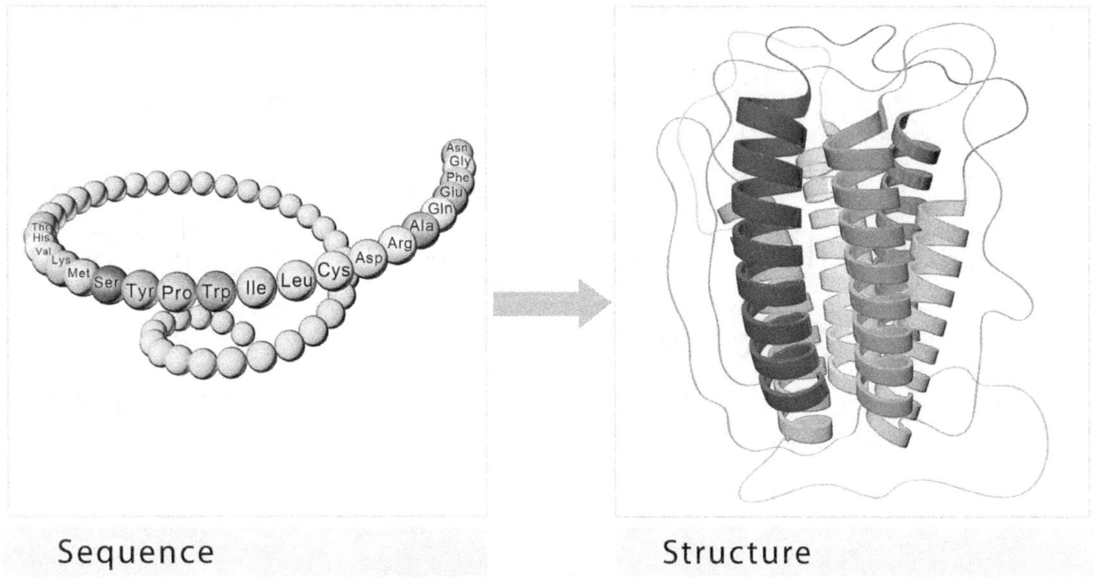

Carbohydrates

Carbohydrates consist of sugars and polymers of sugars. The simplest sugar type of sugar is a monosaccharide, which has the empirical formula of CH_2O. The formula for the monosaccharide glucose, for example, is $C_6H_{12}O_6$. Glucose is an important molecule for cellular respiration, the process of cells extracting energy by breaking bonds through a series of reactions. The individual atoms are then used to rebuild new small molecules. Polysaccharides are made up of a few hundred to a few thousand monosaccharides linked together. These larger molecules have two major functions. The first is that they can be stored as starches, such as glycogen, and then broken down later for energy. Secondly, they may be used to form strong materials, such as cellulose, which is the firm wall that encloses plant cells, and chitin, the carbohydrate insects use to build exoskeletons.

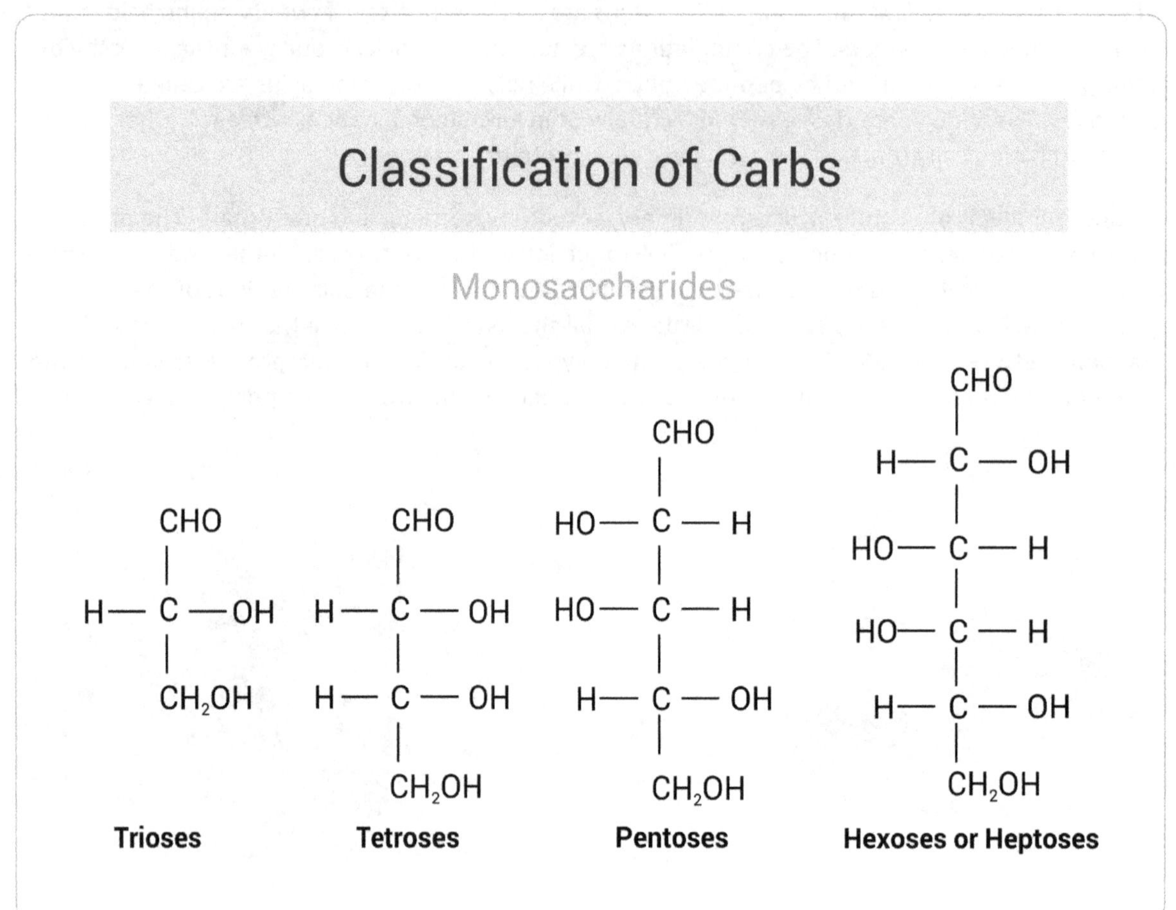

Practice Questions

1. Water has many properties due to its unique structure. Which of the following does NOT play a role in water's properties?
   a. Hydrogen bonding between molecules
   b. Polarity within one molecule
   c. Molecules held apart in solid state
   d. Equal sharing of electrons

2. Which is the metric prefix for 10^{-3}?
   a. Milli
   b. Centi
   c. Micro
   d. Deci

3. Which of the following must have an equal mass number?
   I. Isotopes
   II. Isotones
   III. Isobars
   a. I only
   b. I and II only
   c. II and III only
   d. III only

4. How are a sodium atom and a sodium isotope different?
   a. The isotope has a different number of protons.
   b. The isotope has a different number of neutrons.
   c. The isotope has a different number of electrons.
   d. The isotope has a different atomic number.

5. Which statement is true about nonmetals?
   a. They form cations.
   b. They form covalent bonds.
   c. They are mostly absent from organic compounds.
   d. They are all diatomic.

6. What is the basic unit of matter?
   a. Elementary particle
   b. Atom
   c. Molecule
   d. Element

7. Which particle is responsible for all chemical reactions?
   a. Electrons
   b. Neutrons
   c. Protons
   d. Orbitals

8. Which of these give atoms a negative charge?
   a. Electrons
   b. Neutrons
   c. Protons
   d. Orbital

9. How are similar chemical properties of elements grouped on the periodic table?
   a. In rows according to their total configuration of electrons
   b. In columns according to the electron configuration in their outer shells
   c. In rows according to the electron configuration in their outer shells
   d. In columns according to their total configurations of electrons

10. In a chemical equation, the reactants are on which side of the arrow?
   a. Right
   b. Left
   c. Neither right nor left
   d. Both right and left

11. What does the law of conservation of mass state?
   a. All matter is equally created.
   b. Matter changes, but is not created.
   c. Matter can be changed, and new matter can be created.
   d. Matter can be created, but not changed.

12. Which factor decreases the solubility of solids?
   a. Heating
   b. Agitation
   c Large surface area
   d. Decreasing solvent

13. What is the term for a homogeneous mixture that does not have the Tyndall effect?
   a. Solvent
   b. Suspension
   c. Solution
   d. Colloid

14. How does adding salt to water affect its boiling point?
   a. It increases it.
   b. It has no effect.
   c. It decreases it.
   d. It prevents it from boiling.

15. What is the effect of pressure on a liquid solution?
   a. It decreases solubility.
   b. It increases solubility.
   c. It has little effect on solubility.
   d. It has the same effect as with a gaseous solution.

16. Nonpolar molecules must have what kind of regions?
  a. Hydrophilic
  b. Hydrophobic
  c. Hydrolytic
  d. Hydrochloric

17. Which of these is a substance that increases the rate of a chemical reaction?
  a. Catalyst
  b. Helium
  c. Solvent
  d. Inhibitor

18. Based on collision theory, what is the effect of temperature on the rate of chemical reaction?
  a. Increasing the temperature slows the reaction.
  b. Decreasing the temperature speeds up the reaction.
  c. Increasing the temperature speeds up the reaction.
  d. Collision theory and temperature are unrelated.

19. What step happens first in protein synthesis?
  a. mRNA is pulled into the ribosome.
  b. Exons are spliced out of mRNA in processing.
  c. tRNA delivers amino acids.
  d. mRNA makes a complementary DNA copy.

20. Which type of bonding results from transferring electrons between atoms?
  a. Ionic bonding
  b. Covalent bonding
  c. Hydrogen bonding
  d. Dipole interactions

21. Which substance is oxidized in the following reaction?

$$4Fe + 3O_2 \rightarrow 2Fe_2O_3$$

  a. Fe
  b. O
  c. O_2
  d. Fe_2O_3

22. Which statements are true regarding nuclear fission?
  I. It involves the splitting of heavy nuclei
  II. It is utilized in power plants
  III. It occurs on the sun

  a. I only
  b. II and III only
  c. I and II only
  d. III only

23. Which type of nuclear decay is occurring in the equation below?

$$U_{92}^{236} \rightarrow He_2^4 + Th_{90}^{232}$$

a. Alpha
b. Beta
c. Gamma
d. Delta

24. Which statement is true about the pH of a solution?
a. A solution cannot have a pH less than 1.
b. The more hydroxide ions there are in the solution, the higher the pH will be.
c. If an acid has a pH of greater than -1, it is considered a weak acid.
d. A solution with a pH of 2 has ten times the amount of hydronium ions than a solution with a pH of

25. Which radioactive particle is the most penetrating and damaging and is used to treat cancer in radiation?
a. Alpha
b. Beta
c. Gamma
d. Delta

26. Which of the following choices contain the lowest coefficients that will balance the following combustion equation?

$$\_\_C_2H_{10} + \_\_O_2 \rightarrow \_\_H_2O + \_\_CO_2$$

a. 1:5:5:2
b. 4:10:20:8
c. 2:9:10:4
d. 2:5:10:4

27. What is the purpose of a catalyst?
a. To increase a reaction's rate by increasing the activation energy
b. To increase a reaction's rate by increasing the temperature
c. To increase a reaction's rate by decreasing the activation energy
d. To increase a reaction's rate by decreasing the temperature

28. Most catalysts found in biological systems are which of the following?
a. Special lipids called cofactors
b. Special proteins called enzymes
c. Special lipids called enzymes
d. Special proteins called cofactors

29. Which of the following is NOT a unique property of water?
a. High cohesion and adhesion
b. High surface tension
c. High density upon melting
d. High freezing point

30. Salts like sodium iodide (NaI) and potassium chloride (KCl) have what type of bond?
   a. Ionic bonds
   b. Disulfide bridges
   c. Covalent bonds
   d. London dispersion forces

31. Which of the following is unique to covalent bonds?
   a. Most covalent bonds are formed between the elements H, F, N, and O.
   b. Covalent bonds are dependent on forming dipoles.
   c. Bonding electrons are shared between two or more atoms.
   d. Molecules with covalent bonds tend to have a crystalline solid structure.

32. Which of the following describes a typical gas?
   a. Indefinite shape and indefinite volume
   b. Indefinite shape and definite volume
   c. Definite shape and definite volume
   d. Definite shape and indefinite volume

33. Which of the following is the type of the reaction between ethene and hydrogen bromide?
   a. Addition reaction
   b. Substitution reaction
   c. Elimination reaction
   d. Polymerization

34. Which of the following alcohols has a chiral carbon?
   a. 2-methyl-2-butanol
   b. 2-butanol
   c. 2-methyl-1-butanol
   d. 3-methyl-2-buten-1-ol

35. Which of the following aldehyde(s) can undergo a Cannizzaro reaction?
   a. Formaldehyde and benzaldehyde
   b. Benzaldehyde and trimethyl acetaldehyde
   c. Formaldehyde and trimethyl acetaldehyde
   d. All of the above

36. Which of the following does NOT involve Clemmensen reduction?
   a. Conversion of ethanal (acetaldehyde) to ethane
   b. Conversion of benzaldehyde to toluene (methylbenzene)
   c. Conversion of ethanoic acid (acetic acid) to ethanol
   d. Conversion of propanone (acetone) to propane

37. Which of the following is a nucleophilic reagent?
   a. Br^+
   b. NO_2^+
   c. $AlCl_3$
   d. NH_3

38. How many enantiomers are possible for a glucose molecule?
a. 4
b. 8
c. 16
d. 32

39. What is the IUPAC name of $CH_3CH_2CH_2C(CH_3)_2CH_2CH(CH_3)_2$?
a. 4,4,6,6-tetramethylhexane
b. 1,1,3,3-tetramethylhexane
c. 2,4,4-trimethylheptane
d. 4,4-dimethyloctane

40. Which product forms from a reaction between propene and bromine?
a. $CH_3–CHBr–CH_2Br$
b. $BrCH_2–CH_2–CH_2Br$
c. $CH_3–CH_2–CHBr_2$
d. None of the above

41. Aspirin is used as a non-steroidal anti-inflammatory drug (NSAID). It is available as an over-the-counter (OTC) medication for the treatment of pain, inflammation, and fever. A low dose of aspirin is also used for prevention of cardiovascular events including heart attack and stroke, which occurs secondary to blood clot formation. However, aspirin is a prodrug that needs to be bio-converted into an active drug, salicylic acid. Given that aspirin is chemically termed as acetyl salicylic acid, and salicylic acid is ortho-hydroxybenzoic acid, how would you best describe the bio-conversion reaction?
a. Oxidation
b. Ester hydrolysis
c. Hydrolysis
d. Reduction

42. Which of the following statements is true about an aldol condensation reaction?
I. Aldehydes with α-H can undergo the aldol condensation.
II. CH_3CHO can undergo aldol condensation.
III. Benzaldehyde can undergo aldol condensation.
a. I and II
b. I and III
c. II and III
d. I, II, and III

43. Which is NOT a disaccharide?
a. Sucrose
b. Lactose
c. Maltose
d. Mannose

44. Which is the most common reaction for alkenes and alkynes?
a. Nucleophilic addition
b. Electrophilic addition
c. Nucleophilic substitution
d. Electrophilic substitution

45. Which one of the following molecules has isomers that are optically active?

a. $CH_3—CH_2—COOH$

b. $C_5H_{10}O$

c. $CH_3—CH(NH_2)—COOH$

d. $CH_3—CH=CH—CH_3$

46. Which of the following compounds can be used to produce ethanol through an appropriate chemical reaction?

I. $CH_2=CH_2$

II. $C_2H_5—O—C_2H_5$

III. $CH_3—CHO$

a. I and II
b. I and III
c. II and III
d. I, II, and III

47. C_nH_{2n-2} is the general formula for which of the following?

a. Alkane
b. Alkene
c. Alkyne
d. Aromatic compound

48. Which of the following is NOT a function of lipids?

a. To provide cellular instructions
b. To provide chemical messages
c. To provide energy
d. To compose cell membranes

Answer Explanations

1. D: Equal sharing of electrons is correct. In water, the electronegative oxygen sucks in the electrons of the two hydrogen atoms, making the oxygen slightly negatively-charged and the hydrogen atoms slightly positively-charged. This unequal sharing is called "polarity." This polarity is responsible for the slightly-positive hydrogen atoms from one molecule being attracted to a slightly-negative oxygen in a different molecule, creating a weak intermolecular force called a hydrogen bond, so *A* and *B* are true. Choice *C* is also true, because this unique hydrogen bonding creates intermolecular forces that literally hold molecules with low enough kinetic energy (at low temperatures) to be held apart at "arm's length" (really, the length of the hydrogen bonds). This makes ice less dense than liquid, which explains why ice floats, a very unique property of water. Choice *D* is the only statement that is false, so it is the correct answer.

2. A: The metric prefix for 10^{-3} is "milli." 10^{-3} is $1/10^3$ or 1/1000 or 0.001. If this were grams, 10^{-3} would represent 1 milligram or 1/1000 of a gram. For multiples of 10, the prefixes are as follows: deca = 10^1, hecta = 10^2, kilo = 10^3, mega = 10^6, giga = 10^9, tera = 10^{12}, peta = 10^{15}, and so on. For sub-units of 10, the prefixes are as follows: deci=10^{-1}, centi=10^{-2}, milli=10^{-3}, micro=1^{-6}, nano=10^{-9}, pico=10^{-12}, femto=10^{-15}, and so on. Metric units are usually abbreviated by using the first letter of the prefix (except for micro, which is the Greek letter mu, or μ). Abbreviations for multiples greater than 10^3 are capitalized.

3. D: Isotones are atoms of different elements that have the same number of neutrons. Isotones will have different mass numbers, as will isotopes, which are atoms of the same element that have a different number of neutrons. Isobars are atoms that have the same number of nucleons (protons and neutrons), and therefore, they must have the same mass number.

4. B: Choices *A* and *D* both suggest a different number of protons, which would make a different element. It would no longer be a sodium atom if the proton number or atomic number were different, so those are both incorrect. An atom that has a different number of electrons is called an ion, so Choice *C* is incorrect as well.

5. B: They form covalent bonds. If nonmetals form ionic bonds, they will fill their electron orbital (and become an anion) rather than lose electrons (and become a cation), due to their smaller atomic radius and higher electronegativity than metals. Choice *A* is, therefore, incorrect. There are some nonmetals that are diatomic (hydrogen, oxygen, nitrogen, and halogens), but that is not true for all of them; thus, Choice *D* is incorrect. Organic compounds are carbon-based due to carbon's ability to form four covalent bonds. In addition to carbon, organic compounds are also rich in hydrogen, phosphorous, nitrogen, oxygen, and sulfur, so Choice *C* is incorrect as well.

6. B: The basic unit of matter is the atom. Each element is identified by a letter symbol for that element and an atomic number, which indicates the number of protons in that element. Atoms are the building block of each element and are comprised of a nucleus that contains protons (positive charge) and neutrons (no charge). Orbiting around the nucleus at varying distances are negatively-charged electrons. An electrically-neutral atom contains equal numbers of protons and electrons. Atomic mass is the combined mass of protons and neutrons in the nucleus. Electrons have such negligible mass that they are not considered in the atomic mass. Although the nucleus is compact, the electrons orbit in energy levels at great relative distances to it, making an atom mostly empty space.

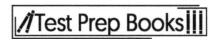

7. A: Nuclear reactions involve the nucleus, and chemical reactions involve electron behavior alone. If electrons are transferred between atoms, they form ionic bonds. If they are shared between atoms, they form covalent bonds. Unequal sharing within a covalent bond results in intermolecular attractions, including hydrogen bonding. Metallic bonding involves a "sea of electrons," where they float around non-specifically, resulting in metal ductility and malleability, due to their glue-like effect of sticking neighboring atoms together. Their metallic bonding also contributes to electrical conductivity and low specific heats, due to electrons' quick response to charge and heat, given to their mobility. Their floating also results in metals' property of luster as light reflects off the mobile electrons. Electron movement in any type of bond is enhanced by photon and heat energy investments, increasing their likelihood to jump energy levels. Valence electron status is the ultimate contributor to electron behavior as it determines their likelihood to be transferred or shared.

8. A: Electrons give atoms their negative charge. Electron behavior determines their bonding, and bonding can either be covalent (electrons are shared) or ionic (electrons are transferred). The charge of an atom is determined by the electrons in its orbitals. Electrons give atoms their chemical and electromagnetic properties. Unequal numbers of protons and electrons lend either a positive or negative charge to the atom. Ions are atoms with a charge, either positive or negative.

9. B: On the periodic table, the elements are grouped in columns according to the configuration of electrons in their outer orbitals. The groupings on the periodic table give a broad view of trends in chemical properties for the elements. The outer electron shell (or orbital) is most important in determining the chemical properties of the element. The electrons in this orbital determine charge and bonding compatibility. The number of electron shells increases by row from top to bottom. The periodic table is organized with elements that have similar chemical behavior in the columns (groups or families).

10. B: In chemical equations, the reactants are on the left side of the arrow. The direction of the reaction is in the direction of the arrow, although sometimes reactions will be shown with arrows in both directions, meaning the reaction is reversible. The reactants are on the left, and the products of the reaction are on the right side of the arrow. Chemical equations indicate atomic and molecular bond formations, rearrangements, and dissolutions. The numbers in front of the elements are called coefficients, and they designate the number of moles of that element accounted for in the reaction. The subscript numbers tell how many atoms of that element are in the molecule, with the number "1" being understood. In H_2O, for example, there are two atoms of hydrogen bound to one atom of oxygen. The ionic charge of the element is shown in superscripts and can be either positive or negative.

11. B: The law of conservation of mass states that matter cannot be created or destroyed, but that it can change forms. This is important in balancing chemical equations on both sides of the arrow. Unbalanced equations will have an unequal number of atoms of each element on either side of the equation and violate the law.

12. D: Solids all increase solubility with Choices *A, B,* and *C*. Powdered hot chocolate is an example to consider. Heating (*A*) and stirring (*B*) make it dissolve faster. Regarding Choice *C*, powder is in chunks that collectively result in a very large surface area, as opposed to a chocolate bar that has a very small relative surface area. The small surface area to volume area ratio dramatically increases solubility. Decreasing the solvent (most of the time, water) will decrease solubility.

13. C: A solution is the term for a homogeneous mixture. A solution contains a solute (particle) dissolved in a solvent (usually a liquid, such as water). Solutions have the smallest solutes of the mixtures, dissolving very easily, and the solute is spread out evenly, or homogeneous. A colloid has medium-sized particles that are somewhat evenly spread out, but their major difference from solutions is that they have the Tyndall effect. Because their particles are larger, they will reflect light that will appear as a beam (Tyndall). The sun's rays are an example of Tyndall; the light is reflecting off of the large gas particles in the atmosphere. A suspension has very large particles that actually settle, creating a heterogeneous mixture.

14. A: When salt is added to water, it increases its boiling point. This is an example of a colligative property, which is any property that changes the physical property of a substance. This particular colligative property of boiling point elevation occurs because the extra solute dissolved in water reduces the surface area of the water, impeding it from vaporizing. If heat is applied, though, it gives water particles enough kinetic energy to vaporize. This additional heat results in an increased boiling point. Other colligative properties of solutions include the following: their melting points decrease with the addition of solute, and their osmotic pressure increases (because it creates a concentration gradient that was otherwise not there).

15. C: Pressure has little effect on the solubility of a liquid solution because liquid is not easily compressible; therefore, increased pressure won't result in increased kinetic energy. Pressure increases solubility in gaseous solutions, since it causes them to move faster.

16. B: Nonpolar molecules have hydrophobic regions that do not dissolve in water. Oils are nonpolar molecules that repel water. Polar molecules combine readily with water, which is, itself, a polar solvent. Polar molecules are hydrophilic or "water-loving" because their polar regions have intermolecular bonding with water via hydrogen bonds. Some structures and molecules are both polar and nonpolar, like the phospholipid bilayer. The phospholipid bilayer has polar heads that are the external "water-loving portions" and hydrophobic tails that are immiscible in water. Polar solvents dissolve polar solutes, and nonpolar solvents dissolve nonpolar solutes. One way to remember these is "Like dissolves like."

17. A: A catalyst increases the rate of a chemical reaction by lowering the activation energy. Enzymes are biological protein catalysts that are utilized by organisms to facilitate anabolic and catabolic reactions. They speed up the rate of reaction by making the reaction easier (perhaps by orienting a molecule more favorably upon induced fit, for example). Catalysts are not used up by the reaction and can be used over and over again.

18. C: Increasing temperature increases the rate of reactions due to increases in the kinetic energy of atoms and molecules. This increased movement results in more collisions between reactants (with each other as well as with enzymes), which is the cause of the rate increase.

19. D: All statements are true, but nothing can happen without the message being available; thus, Choice *D* must occur first. After the copy is made in transcription (D), Choice *B* occurs because mRNA has to be processed before being exported into the cytoplasm. Once it has reached the cytoplasm, Choice *A* occurs as mRNA is pulled into the ribosome. Finally, Choice *C* occurs, and tRNA delivers amino acids one at a time until the full polypeptide has been created. At that point, the new protein (polypeptide) will be processed and folded in the ER and Golgi apparatus.

20. A: Ionic bonding is the result of electrons that have been transferred between atoms. When an atom loses one or more electrons, a cation, or positively-charged ion, is formed. An anion, or negatively-charged ion, is formed when an atom gains one or more electrons. Ionic bonds are formed from the attraction between a positively-charged cation and a negatively-charged anion. The bond between sodium and chloride in table salt or sodium chloride, Na^+Cl^-, is an example of an ionic bond.

21. A: Oxidation is when a substance loses electrons in a chemical reaction, and reduction is when a substance gains electrons. Any element by itself has a charge of 0, as iron and oxygen do on the reactant's side. In the ionic compound formed, iron has a +3 charge, and oxygen has a -2 charge. Because iron had a zero charge that then changed to +3, it means that it lost three electrons and was oxidized. Oxygen, which gained two electrons, was reduced.

22. C: Fission occurs when heavy nuclei are split and is currently the energy source that fuels power plants. Fusion, on the other hand, is the combining of small nuclei and produces far more energy, and it is the nuclear reaction that powers stars like the sun. Harnessing the extreme energy released by fusion has proven impossible so far, which is unfortunate since its waste products are not radioactive, while waste produced by fission typically is.

23. A: Alpha decay involves a helium particle emission (with two neutrons). Beta decay involves emission of an electron or positron, and gamma is just high-energy light emissions.

24. B: Choice *A* is false because it is possible to have a very strong acid with a pH between 0 and 1. Choice *C* is false because the pH scale is from 0 to 14, and while -1 is outside the usual scale, it would indicate a very strong acid (10M hydronium ions in solution), not a weak one. Choice *D* is false because a solution with a pH of 2 has ten times fewer hydronium ions than a solution with pH of 1.

25. C: Gamma is the lightest radioactive decay with the most energy, and this high energy is toxic to cells. Due to its weightlessness, gamma rays are extremely penetrating. Alpha particles are heavy and can be easily shielded by skin. Beta particles are electrons and can penetrate more than an alpha particle because they are lighter. Beta particles can be shielded by plastic.

26. C: 2:9:10:4. These are the coefficients that follow the law of conservation of matter. The coefficient times the subscript of each element should be the same on both sides of the equation.

27. C: A catalyst functions to increase reaction rates by decreasing the activation energy required for a reaction to take place. Inhibitors would increase the activation energy or otherwise stop the reactants from reacting. Although increasing the temperature usually increases a reaction's rate, this is not true in all cases, and most catalysts do not function in this manner.

28. B: Biological catalysts are termed *enzymes*, which are proteins with conformations that specifically manipulate reactants into positions which decrease the reaction's activation energy. Lipids do not usually affect reactions, and while cofactors can aid or be necessary to the proper functioning of enzymes, they do not make up the majority of biological catalysts.

29. D: Water's unique properties are due to intermolecular hydrogen bonding. These forces make water molecules "stick" to one another, which explains why water has unusually high cohesion and adhesion (sticking to each other and sticking to other surfaces). Cohesion can be seen in beads of dew. Adhesion can be seen when water sticks to the sides of a graduated cylinder to form a meniscus. The stickiness to neighboring molecules also increases surface tension, providing a very thin film that light things cannot penetrate, which is observed when leaves float in swimming pools. Water has a low freezing point, not a high freezing point, due to the fact that molecules have to have a very low kinetic energy to arrange themselves in the lattice-like structure found in ice, its solid form.

30. A: Salts are formed from compounds that use ionic bonds. Disulfide bridges are special bonds in protein synthesis that hold the protein in their secondary and tertiary structures. Covalent bonds are strong bonds formed through the sharing of electrons between atoms and are typically found in organic molecules like carbohydrates and lipids. London dispersion forces are fleeting, momentary bonds that occur between atoms that have instantaneous dipoles but quickly disintegrate.

31. C: As in the last question, covalent bonds are special because they share electrons between multiple atoms. Most covalent bonds are formed between the elements H, F, N, O, S, and C, while hydrogen bonds are formed nearly exclusively between H and either O, N, or F of other molecules. Covalent bonds may inadvertently form dipoles, but this does not necessarily happen. With similarly electronegative atoms like carbon and hydrogen, dipoles do not form, for instance. Crystal solids are typically formed by substances with ionic bonds like the salts sodium iodide and potassium chloride.

32. A: Gases like air will move and expand to fill their container, so they are considered to have an indefinite shape and indefinite volume. Liquids like water will move and flow freely, so their shapes change constantly, but do not change volume or density on their own. Solids change neither shape nor volume without external forces acting on them, so they have definite shapes and volumes.

33. A: The product of the addition reaction is ethyl bromide. Choice *B* is incorrect because no atom or group from ethene is substituted by the attacking atoms (i.e. hydrogen or bromide). Choice *C* is incorrect because no atom or group is eliminated from ethene in the reaction. Choice *D* is incorrect because polymerization involves bonding of similar molecules to form a larger molecule.

34. C: The correct answer is 2-methyl-1-butanol, which has a chiral C atom with 4 different groups/atoms. See the structures below:

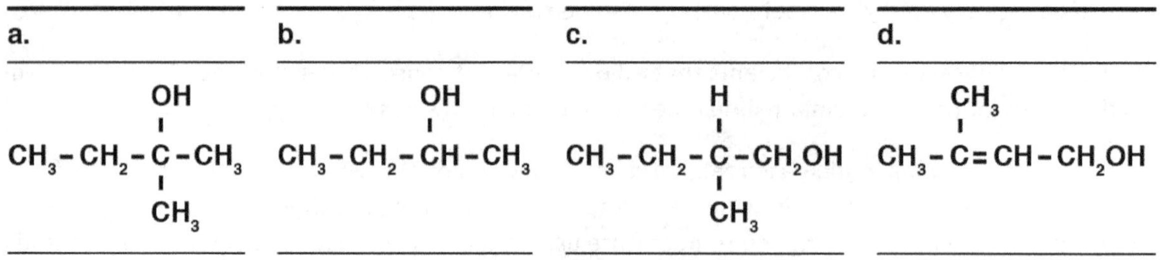

a.	b.	c.	d.
$CH_3-CH_2-C(OH)(CH_3)-CH_3$	$CH_3-CH_2-CH(OH)-CH_3$	$CH_3-CH_2-C(H)(CH_3)-CH_2OH$	$CH_3-C(CH_3)=CH-CH_2OH$

35. D: All the compounds in the list, including formaldehyde (H—CHO), trimethyl acetaldehyde [$(CH_3)_3C$—CHO], and benzaldehyde (C_6H_5—CHO), lack an α-hydrogen, and therefore can undergo a Cannizzaro reaction.

36. C: Clemmensen reduction converts carbonyl group (C=O) into -CH_2 groups, causing the formation of a saturated hydrocarbon. In Choices *A*, *B*, and *D*, carbonyl compounds are converted to hydrocarbons, and thus followed a Clemmensen reduction. According to Clemmensen reaction, acetic acid is reduced to form ethane, but not ethanol.

37. D: Choices *A* and *B* are positive electrophiles, while Choice *C* is a neutral electrophile. Choice *D* is a neutral nucleophile.

38. C: The number of enantiomers of an organic compound is 2^n, where "n" refers to the number of chiral C atoms in the molecule. Glucose has four chiral C atoms, and therefore the number of possible optical isomers would be $2^4 = 16$.

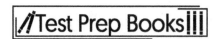

39. C: See the numbering of C-chain below and review IUPAC numbering section. The longest C-chain should be selected for numbering and naming as follows:

$$\overset{7}{CH_3}-\overset{6}{CH_2}-\overset{5}{CH_2}-\overset{4}{C}(CH_3)_2-\overset{3}{CH_2}-\overset{2}{CH}(CH_3)-\overset{1}{CH_3}$$

40. A: This is an addition reaction:

$$CH_3-CH=CH_2 + Br_2 \longrightarrow CH_3-CHBr-CH_2Br$$

Propene → 1, 2 - dibromopropane

41. B: Aspirin is an acetylated *ester* of salicylic acid. Therefore, the conversion of aspirin to salicylic acid is *best* described as an ester hydrolysis. See the reaction below.

The conversion of aspirin to salicylic acid via ester hydrolysis

$$C_6H_4(OCOCH_3)(COOH) + H_2O \xrightarrow{\text{Ester hydrolysis}} C_6H_4(OH)(COOH) + CH_3COOH$$

Acetylsalicylic acid (*Asprin*) → Salicylic acid + Acetic acid

42. A: For further review, see the aldol condensation section.

43. D: Sucrose, lactose, and maltose are disaccharides. Mannose is a monosaccharide.

44. B: Electrophilic addition refers to an addition reaction in which an electrophile (electron attracting species) is added to a molecule, mostly carrying unsaturated bonds.

45. C: This molecule has an asymmetric C atom attached with 4 different atoms/groups. Therefore, it would constitute isomers that are optically active.

46. D: Ethene, diethyl ether, and acetaldehyde could be converted to ethanol by appropriate chemical reactions that follow:

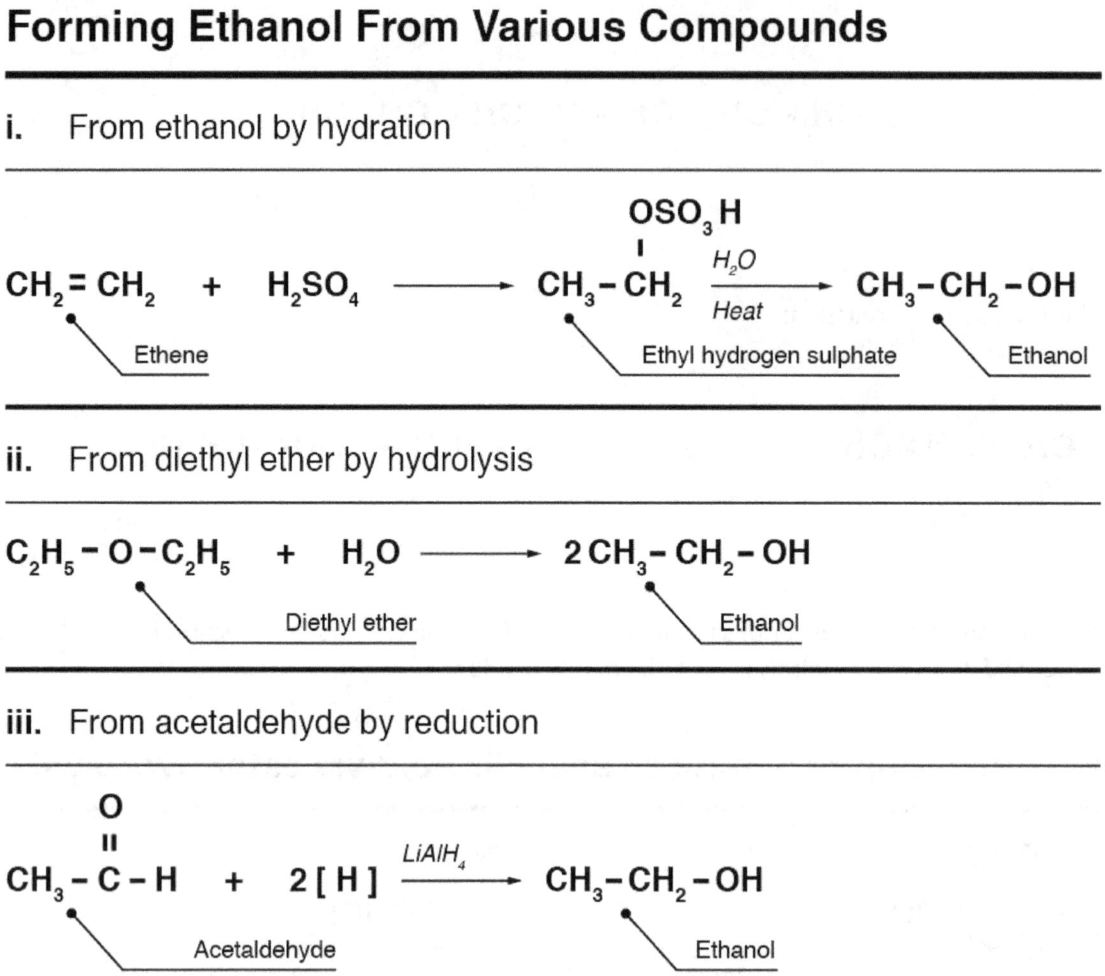

Forming Ethanol From Various Compounds

i. From ethanol by hydration

$$CH_2=CH_2 + H_2SO_4 \longrightarrow CH_3-CH_2(OSO_3H) \xrightarrow[Heat]{H_2O} CH_3-CH_2-OH$$

Ethene — Ethyl hydrogen sulphate — Ethanol

ii. From diethyl ether by hydrolysis

$$C_2H_5-O-C_2H_5 + H_2O \longrightarrow 2\,CH_3-CH_2-OH$$

Diethyl ether — Ethanol

iii. From acetaldehyde by reduction

$$CH_3-\overset{O}{\overset{\|}{C}}-H + 2[H] \xrightarrow{LiAlH_4} CH_3-CH_2-OH$$

Acetaldehyde — Ethanol

47. C: The general formula for an alkane, alkene, and alkyne are C_nH_{2n+2}, C_nH_{2n}, and C_nH_{2n-2}, respectively.

48. A: All the other answer choices are functions of lipids. Choice *B* is true because steroid hormones are lipid-based. Long-term energy is one of the most important functions of lipids, so Choice *C* is true. Choice *D* is also true because the cell membrane is not only composed of a lipid bilayer, but it also has cholesterol (another lipid) embedded within it to regulate membrane fluidity.

Critical Reading

Comprehension

Words in Context

Context Clues

Familiarity with common prefixes, suffixes, and root words assists tremendously in unraveling the meaning of an unfamiliar word and making an educated guess as to its meaning. However, some words do not contain many easily-identifiable clues that point to their meaning. In this case, rather than looking at the elements within the word, it is useful to consider elements around the word—i.e., its context. *Context* refers to the other words and information within the sentence or surrounding sentences that indicate the unknown word's probable meaning. The following sentences provide context for the potentially-unfamiliar word *quixotic*:

> Rebecca had never been one to settle into a predictable, ordinary life. Her quixotic personality led her to leave behind a job with a prestigious law firm in Manhattan and move halfway around the world to pursue her dream of becoming a sushi chef in Tokyo.

A reader unfamiliar with the word *quixotic* doesn't have many clues to use in terms of affixes or root meaning. The suffix *–ic* indicates that the word is an adjective, but that is it. In this case, then, a reader would need to look at surrounding information to obtain some clues about the word. Other adjectives in the passage include *predictable* and *ordinary*, things that Rebecca was definitely not, as indicated by "Rebecca had never been one to settle." Thus, a first clue might be that *quixotic* means the opposite of predictable.

The second sentence doesn't offer any other modifier of *personality* other than *quixotic*, but it does include a story that reveals further information about her personality. She had a stable, respectable job, but she decided to give it up to follow her dream. Combining these two ideas together, then—unpredictable and dream-seeking—gives the reader a general idea of what *quixotic* probably means. In fact, the root of the word is the character Don Quixote, a romantic dreamer who goes on an impulsive adventure.

While context clues are useful for making an approximate definition for newly-encountered words, these types of clues also come in handy when encountering common words that have multiple meanings. The word *reservation* is used differently in each the following sentences:

> A. That restaurant is booked solid for the next month; it's impossible to make a reservation unless you know somebody.
>
> B. The hospital plans to open a branch office inside the reservation to better serve Native American patients who cannot easily travel to the main hospital fifty miles away.
>
> C. Janet Clark is a dependable, knowledgeable worker, and I recommend her for the position of team leader without reservation.

All three sentences use the word to express different meanings. In fact, most words in English have more than one meaning—sometimes meanings that are completely different from one another. Thus, context can provide clues as to which meaning is appropriate in a given situation. A quick search in the dictionary reveals several possible meanings for *reservation*:

1. An exception or qualification

2. A tract of public land set aside, such as for the use of American Indian tribes

3. An arrangement for accommodations, such as in a hotel, on a plane, or at a restaurant

Sentence A mentions a restaurant, making the third definition the correct one in this case. In sentence B, some context clues include Native Americans, as well as the implication that a reservation is a place—"inside the reservation," both of which indicate that the second definition should be used here. Finally, sentence C uses *without reservation* to mean "completely" or "without exception," so the first definition can be applied here.

Using context clues in this way can be especially useful for words that have multiple, widely varying meanings. If a word has more than one definition and two of those definitions are the opposite of each other, it is known as an *auto-antonym*—a word that can also be its own antonym. In the case of auto-antonyms, context clues are crucial to determine which definition to employ in a given sentence. For example, the word *sanction* can either mean "to approve or allow" or "a penalty." Approving and penalizing have opposite meanings, so *sanction* is an example of an auto-antonym. The following sentences reflect the distinction in meaning:

A. In response to North Korea's latest nuclear weapons test, world leaders have called for harsher sanctions to punish the country for its actions.

B. The general has sanctioned a withdrawal of troops from the area.

A context clue can be found in sentence A, which mentions "to punish." A punishment is similar to a penalty, so sentence A is using the word *sanction* according to this definition.

Other examples of auto-antonyms include *oversight*—"to supervise something" or "a missed detail," *resign*—"to quit" or "to sign again, as a contract," and *screen*—"to show" or "to conceal." For these types of words, recognizing context clues is an important way to avoid misinterpreting the sentence's meaning.

Affixes

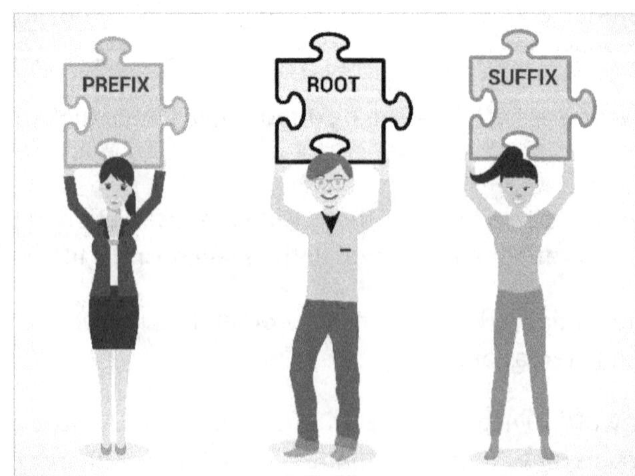

Individual words are constructed from building blocks of meaning. An *affix* is an element that is added to a root or stem word that can change the word's meaning.

For example, the stem word *fix* is a verb meaning *to repair*. When the ending *–able* is added, it becomes the adjective *fixable*, meaning "capable of being repaired." Adding *un–* to the beginning changes the word to *unfixable*, meaning "incapable of being repaired." In this way, affixes attach to the word stem to create a new word and a new meaning. Knowledge of affixes can assist in deciphering the meaning of unfamiliar words.

Affixes are also related to inflection. *Inflection* is the modification of a base word to express a different grammatical or syntactical function. For example, countable nouns such as *car* and *airport* become plural with the addition of *–s* at the end: *cars* and *airports*.

Verb tense is also expressed through inflection. *Regular verbs*—those that follow a standard inflection pattern—can be changed to past tense using the affixes *–ed*, *–d*, or *–ied*, as in *cooked* and *studied*. Verbs can also be modified for continuous tenses by using *–ing*, as in *working* or *exploring*. Thus, affixes are used not only to express meaning but also to reflect a word's grammatical purpose.

A *prefix* is an affix attached to the beginning of a word. The meanings of English prefixes mainly come from Greek and Latin origins. The chart below contains a few of the most commonly used English prefixes.

Prefix	**Meaning**	**Example**
a-	Not	amoral, asymptomatic
anti-	Against	antidote, antifreeze
auto-	self	automobile, automatic
circum-	around	circumference, circumspect
co-, com-, con-	together	coworker, companion
contra-	against	contradict, contrary
de-	negation or reversal	deflate, deodorant
extra-	outside, beyond	extraterrestrial, extracurricular
in-, im-, il-, ir-	not	impossible, irregular
inter-	between	international, intervene
intra-	within	intramural, intranet
mis-	wrongly	mistake, misunderstand
mono-	one	monolith, monopoly
non-	not	nonpartisan, nonsense
pre-	before	preview, prediction
re-	again	review, renew
semi-	half	semicircle, semicolon
sub-	under	subway, submarine
super-	above	superhuman, superintendent
trans-	across, beyond, through	trans-Siberian, transform
un-	not	unwelcome, unfriendly

While the addition of a prefix alters the meaning of the base word, the addition of a *suffix* may also affect a word's part of speech. For example, adding a suffix can change the noun *material* into the verb *materialize* and back to a noun again in *materialization*.

Suffix	Part of Speech	Meaning	Example
-able, -ible	adjective	having the ability to	honorable, flexible
-acy, -cy	noun	state or quality	intimacy, dependency
-al, -ical	adjective	having the quality of	historical, tribal
-en	verb	to cause to become	strengthen, embolden
-er, -ier	adjective	comparative	happier, longer
-est, -iest	adjective	superlative	sunniest, hottest
-ess	noun	female	waitress, actress
-ful	adjective	full of, characterized by	beautiful, thankful
-fy, -ify	verb	to cause, to come to be	liquefy, intensify
-ism	noun	doctrine, belief, action	Communism, Buddhism
-ive, -ative, -itive	adjective	having the quality of	creative, innovative
-ize	verb	to convert into, to subject to	Americanize, dramatize
-less	adjective	without, missing	emotionless, hopeless
-ly	adverb	in the manner of	quickly, energetically
-ness	noun	quality or state	goodness, darkness
-ous, -ious, -eous	adjective	having the quality of	spontaneous, pious
-ship	noun	status or condition	partnership, ownership
-tion	noun	action or state	renovation, promotion
-y	adjective	characterized by	smoky, dreamy

Through knowledge of prefixes and suffixes, a student's vocabulary can be instantly expanded with an understanding of *etymology*—the origin of words. This, in turn, can be used to add sentence structure variety to academic writing.

Syntax

Syntax refers to the arrangement of words, phrases, and clauses to form a sentence. Knowledge of syntax can also give insight into a word's meaning. The section above considered several examples using the word *reservation* and applied context clues to determine the word's appropriate meaning in each sentence. Here is an example of how the placement of a word can impact its meaning and grammatical function:

A. The development team has reserved the conference room for today.

B. Her quiet and reserved nature is sometimes misinterpreted as unfriendliness when people first meet her.

In addition to using *reserved* to mean different things, each sentence also uses the word to serve a different grammatical function. In sentence A, *reserved* is part of the verb phrase *has reserved*, indicating the meaning "to set aside for a particular use." In sentence B, *reserved* acts as a modifier within the noun phrase "her quiet and reserved nature." Because the word is being used as an adjective to describe a personality characteristic, it calls up a different definition of the word—"restrained or lacking familiarity with others." As this example shows, the function of a word within the overall sentence structure can allude to its meaning. It is also useful to refer to the earlier chart about suffixes and parts of speech as another clue into what grammatical function a word is serving in a sentence.

Analyzing Nuances of Word Meaning and Figures of Speech

By now, it should be apparent that language is not as simple as one word directly correlated to one meaning. Rather, one word can express a vast array of diverse meanings, and similar meanings can be expressed through different words. However, there are very few words that express exactly the same meaning. For this reason, it is important to be able to pick up on the nuances of word meaning.

Many words contain two levels of meaning: connotation and denotation as discussed previously in the informational texts and rhetoric section. A word's *denotation* is its most literal meaning—the definition that can readily be found in the dictionary. A word's *connotation* includes all of its emotional and cultural associations.

In literary writing, authors rely heavily on connotative meaning to create mood and characterization. The following are two descriptions of a rainstorm:

> A. The rain slammed against the windowpane and the wind howled through the fireplace. A pair of hulking oaks next to the house cast eerie shadows as their branches trembled in the wind.
>
> B. The rain pattered against the windowpane and the wind whistled through the fireplace. A pair of stately oaks next to the house cast curious shadows as their branches swayed in the wind.

Description A paints a creepy picture for readers with strongly emotional words like *slammed*, connoting force and violence. *Howled* connotes pain or wildness, and *eerie* and *trembled* connote fear. Overall, the connotative language in this description serves to inspire fear and anxiety.

However, as can be seen in description B, swapping out a few key words for those with different connotations completely changes the feeling of the passage. *Slammed* is replaced with the more cheerful *pattered*, and *hulking* has been swapped out for *stately*. Both words imply something large, but *hulking* is more intimidating whereas *stately* is more respectable. *Curious* and *swayed* seem more playful than the language used in the earlier description. Although both descriptions represent roughly the same situation, the nuances of the emotional language used throughout the passages create a very different sense for readers.

Selective choice of connotative language can also be extremely impactful in other forms of writing, such as editorials or persuasive texts. Through connotative language, writers reveal their biases and opinions while trying to inspire feelings and actions in readers:

> 1. Parents won't stop complaining about standardized tests.
>
> 2. Parents continue to raise concerns about standardized tests.

Readers should be able to identify the nuance in meaning between these two sentences. The first one carries a more negative feeling, implying that parents are being bothersome or whiny. Readers of the second sentence, though, might come away with the feeling that parents are concerned and involved in their children's education. Again, the aggregate of even subtle cues can combine to give a specific emotional impression to readers, so from an early age, students should be aware of how language can be used to influence readers' opinions.

Another form of non-literal expression can be found in *figures of speech*. As with connotative language, figures of speech tend to be shared within a cultural group and may be difficult to pick up on for learners outside of that group. In some cases, a figure of speech may be based on the literal denotation of the words it contains, but in other cases, a figure of speech is far removed from its literal meaning. A case in point is *irony*, where what is said is the exact opposite of what is meant:

> The new tax plan is poorly planned, based on faulty economic data, and unable to address the financial struggles of middle class families. Yet legislators remain committed to passing this brilliant proposal.

When the writer refers to the proposal as brilliant, the opposite is implied—the plan is "faulty" and "poorly planned." By using irony, the writer means that the proposal is anything but brilliant by using the word in a non-literal sense.

Another figure of speech is *hyperbole*—extreme exaggeration or overstatement. Statements like, "I love you to the moon and back" or "Let's be friends for a million years" utilize hyperbole to convey a greater depth of emotion, without literally committing oneself to space travel or a life of immortality.

Figures of speech may sometimes use one word in place of another. *Synecdoche*, for example, uses a part of something to refer to its whole. The expression "Don't hurt a hair on her head!" implies protecting more than just an individual hair, but rather her entire body. "The art teacher is training a class of Picassos" uses Picasso, one individual notable artist, to stand in for the entire category of talented artists. Another figure of speech using word replacement is *metonymy*, where a word is replaced with something closely associated to it. For example, news reports may use the word "Washington" to refer to the American government or "the crown" to refer to the British monarch.

Main Ideas

It is very important to know the difference between the topic and the main idea of the text. Even though these two are similar because they both present the central point of a text, they have distinctive differences. A *topic* is the subject of the text; it can usually be described in a one- to two-word phrase and appears in the simplest form. On the other hand, the *main idea* is more detailed and provides the author's central point of the text. It can be expressed through a complete sentence and is often found in the beginning, middle, or end of a paragraph. In most nonfiction books, the first sentence of the passage usually (but not always) states the main idea. Review the passage below to explore the topic versus the main idea.

Cheetahs

> *Cheetahs are one of the fastest mammals on the land, reaching up to 70 miles an hour over short distances. Even though cheetahs can run as fast as 70 miles an hour, they usually only have to run half that speed to catch up with their choice of prey. Cheetahs cannot maintain a fast pace over long periods of time because their bodies will overheat. After a chase, cheetahs need to rest for approximately 30 minutes prior to eating or returning to any other activity.*

In the example above, the topic of the passage is "Cheetahs" simply because that is the subject of the text. The main idea of the text is "Cheetahs are one of the fastest mammals on the land but can only maintain a fast pace for shorter distances." While it covers the topic, it is more detailed and refers to the text in its entirety. The text continues to provide additional details called *supporting details,* which will be discussed shortly.

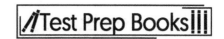

Identifying the Theme or Central Message

The *theme* is the central message of a fictional work, whether that work is structured as prose, drama, or poetry. It is the heart of what an author is trying to say to readers through the writing, and theme is largely conveyed through literary elements and techniques.

In literature, a theme can often be determined by considering the over-arching narrative conflict with the work. Though there are several types of conflicts and several potential themes within them, the following are the most common:

- *Individual against the self*—relevant to themes of self-awareness, internal struggles, pride, coming-of-age, facing reality, fate, free will, vanity, loss of innocence, loneliness, isolation, fulfillment, failure, and disillusionment
- *Individual against nature*— relevant to themes of knowledge vs. ignorance, nature as beauty, quest for discovery, self-preservation, chaos and order, circle of life, death, and destruction of beauty
- *Individual against society*— relevant to themes of power, beauty, good, evil, war, class struggle, totalitarianism, role of men/women, wealth, corruption, change vs. tradition, capitalism, destruction, heroism, injustice, and racism
- *Individual against another individual*— relevant to themes of hope, loss of love or hope, sacrifice, power, revenge, betrayal, and honor

For example, in Hawthorne's *The Scarlet Letter,* one possible narrative conflict could be the individual against the self, with a relevant theme of internal struggles. This theme is alluded to through characterization—Dimmesdale's moral struggle with his love for Hester and Hester's internal struggles with the truth and her daughter, Pearl. It's also alluded to through plot—Dimmesdale's suicide and Hester helping the very townspeople who initially condemned her.

Sometimes, a text can convey a *message* or *universal lesson*—a truth or insight that the reader infers from the text, based on analysis of the literary and/or poetic elements. This message is often presented as a statement. For example, a potential message in Shakespeare's *Hamlet* could be "Revenge is what ultimately drives the human soul." This message can be immediately determined through plot and characterization in numerous ways, but it can also be determined through the setting of Norway, which is bordering on war.

How Authors Develop Theme

Authors employ a variety of techniques to present a theme. They may compare or contrast characters, events, places, ideas, or historical or invented settings to speak thematically. They may use analogies, metaphors, similes, allusions, or other literary devices to convey the theme. An author's use of diction, syntax, and tone can also help convey the theme. Authors will often develop themes through the development of characters, use of the setting, repetition of ideas, use of symbols, and through contrasting value systems. Authors of both fiction and nonfiction genres will use a variety of these techniques to develop one or more themes.

Regardless of the literary genre, there are commonalities in how authors, playwrights, and poets develop themes or central ideas.

Authors often do research, the results of which contributes to the theme. In prose fiction and drama, this research may include real historical information about the setting the author has chosen or include elements that make fictional characters, settings, and plots seem realistic to the reader. In nonfiction, research is critical since the information contained within the work must be accurate and, moreover, accurately represented.

In fiction, authors present a narrative conflict that will contribute to the overall theme. In fiction, this conflict may involve the storyline itself and some trouble within characters that needs resolution. In nonfiction, this conflict may be an explanation or commentary on factual people and events.

Authors will sometimes use character motivation to convey theme, such as in the example from *Hamlet* regarding revenge. In fiction, the characters an author creates will think, speak, and act in ways that effectively convey the theme to readers. In nonfiction, the characters are factual, as in a biography, but authors pay particular attention to presenting those motivations to make them clear to readers.

Authors also use literary devices as a means of conveying theme. For example, the use of moon symbolism in Mary Shelley's *Frankenstein* is significant as its phases can be compared to the phases that the Creature undergoes as he struggles with his identity.

The selected point of view can also contribute to a work's theme. The use of first-person point of view in a fiction or nonfiction work engages the reader's response differently than third person point of view. The central idea or theme from a first-person narrative may differ from a third-person limited text.

In literary nonfiction, authors usually identify the purpose of their writing, which differs from fiction, where the general purpose is to entertain. The purpose of nonfiction is usually to inform, persuade, or entertain the audience. The stated purpose of a nonfiction text will drive how the central message or theme, if applicable, is presented.

Authors identify an audience for their writing, which is critical in shaping the theme of the work. For example, the audience for J.K. Rowling's *Harry Potter* series would be different than the audience for a biography of George Washington. The audience an author chooses to address is closely tied to the purpose of the work. The choice of an audience also drives the choice of language and level of diction an author uses. Ultimately, the intended audience determines the level to which that subject matter is presented and the complexity of the theme.

Supporting Details

Supporting details help readers better develop and understand the main idea. Supporting details answer questions like *who, what, where, when, why,* and *how*. Different types of supporting details include examples, facts and statistics, anecdotes, and sensory details.

Persuasive and informative texts often use supporting details. In persuasive texts, authors attempt to make readers agree with their points of view, and supporting details are often used as "selling points." If authors make a statement, they need to support the statement with evidence in order to adequately persuade readers. Informative texts use supporting details such as examples and facts to inform readers. Review the previous "Cheetahs" passage to find examples of supporting details.

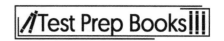

Cheetahs

Cheetahs are one of the fastest mammals on the land, reaching up to 70 miles an hour over short distances. Even though cheetahs can run as fast as 70 miles an hour, they usually only have to run half that speed to catch up with their choice of prey. Cheetahs cannot maintain a fast pace over long periods of time because their bodies will overheat. After a chase, cheetahs need to rest for approximately 30 minutes prior to eating or returning to any other activity.

In the example, supporting details include:

- Cheetahs reach up to 70 miles per hour over short distances.
- They usually only have to run half that speed to catch up with their prey.
- Cheetahs will overheat if they exert at a high speed over longer distances.
- Cheetahs need to rest for 30 minutes after a chase.

Look at the diagram below (applying the cheetah example) to help determine the hierarchy of topic, main idea, and supporting details.

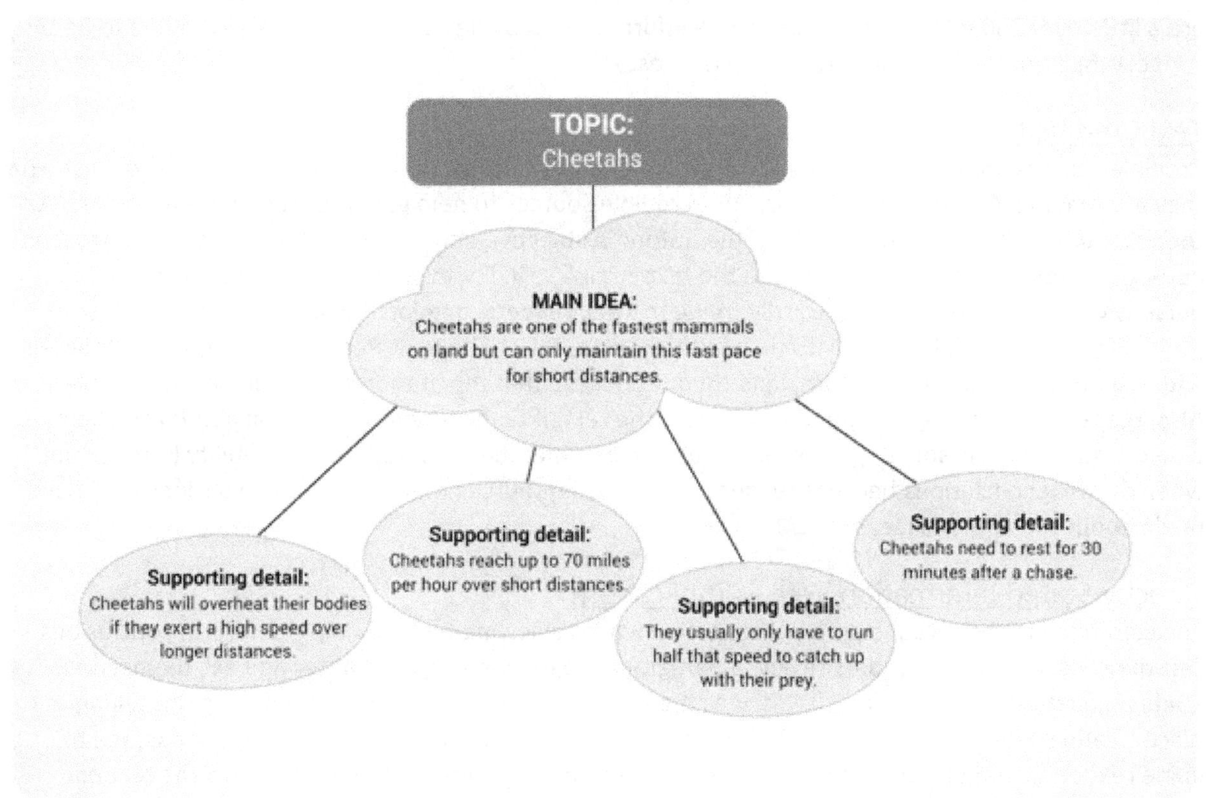

Drawing Conclusions

When drawing conclusions about texts or passages, readers should do two main things: 1) Use the information that they already know and 2) Use the information they have learned from the text or passage. Authors write with an intended purpose, and it is the readers' responsibility to understand and form logical conclusions of authors' ideas. It is important to remember that the readers' conclusions should be supported by information directly from the text. Readers cannot simply form conclusions based off of only information they already know.

There are several ways readers can draw conclusions from authors' ideas and points to consider when doing so, such as text evidence, text credibility, and directly stated information versus implications.

Text Evidence

Text evidence is the information readers find in a text or passage that supports the main idea or point(s) in a story. In turn, text evidence can help readers draw conclusions about the text or passage. The information should be taken directly from the text or passage and placed in quotation marks. Text evidence provides readers with information to support ideas about the text or passage so that they do not just rely on their own thoughts. Details should be precise, descriptive, and factual. Statistics are a great piece of text evidence because they provide readers with exact numbers and not just a generalization. For example, instead of saying "Asia has a larger population than Europe," authors could provide detailed information such as "In Asia, there are over 7 billion people, whereas in Europe there are a little over 750 million." More definitive information provides better evidence to readers to help support their conclusions about texts or passages.

Text Credibility

Credible sources are important when drawing conclusions because readers need to be able to trust what they are reading. Authors should always use credible sources to help gain the trust of their readers. A text is *credible* when it is believable and the author is objective and unbiased. If readers do not trust an author's words, they may simply dismiss the text completely. For example, if an author writes a persuasive essay, he or she is outwardly trying to sway readers' opinions to align with his or her own, providing readers with the liberty to do what they please with the text. Readers may agree or disagree with the author, which may, in turn, lead them to believe that the author is credible or not credible. Also, readers should keep in mind the source of the text. If readers review a journal about astronomy, would a more reliable source be a NASA employee or a plumber? Overall, text credibility is important when drawing conclusions because readers want reliable sources that support the decisions they have made about the author's ideas.

Directly Stated Information Versus Implications

Engaged readers should constantly self-question while reviewing texts to help them form conclusions. Self-questioning is when readers review a paragraph, page, passage, or chapter and ask themselves, "Did I understand what I read?," "What was the main event in this section?," "Where is this taking place?," and so on. Authors can provide clues or pieces of evidence throughout a text or passage to guide readers toward a conclusion. This is why active and engaged readers should read the text or passage in its entirety before forming a definitive conclusion. If readers do not gather all the necessary pieces of evidence, then they may jump to an illogical conclusion.

At times, authors directly state conclusions while others simply imply them. Of course, it is easier if authors outwardly provide conclusions to readers because this does not leave any information open to interpretation. However, implications are things that authors do not directly state but can be assumed based off of information they provided. If authors only imply what may have happened, readers can form a menagerie of ideas for conclusions. For example, in the statement: *Once we heard the sirens, we hunkered down in the storm shelter*, the author does not directly state that there was a tornado, but clues such as "sirens" and "storm shelter" provide insight to the readers to help form that conclusion.

Inferences in a Text

Readers should be able to make *inferences*. Making an inference requires the reader to read between the lines and look for what is *implied* rather than what is directly stated. That is, using information that is known from the text, the reader is able to make a logical assumption about information that is *not* directly stated but is probably true. Read the following passage:

> "Hey, do you wanna meet my new puppy?" Jonathan asked.
>
> "Oh, I'm sorry but please don't—" Jacinta began to protest, but before she could finish, Jonathan had already opened the passenger side door of his car and a perfect white ball of fur came bouncing towards Jacinta.
>
> "Isn't he the cutest?" beamed Jonathan.
>
> "Yes—achoo!—he's pretty—aaaachooo!!—adora—aaa—aaaachoo!" Jacinta managed to say in between sneezes. "But if you don't mind, I—I—achoo!—need to go inside."

Which of the following can be inferred from Jacinta's reaction to the puppy?

a. She hates animals
b. She is allergic to dogs
c. She prefers cats to dogs
d. She is angry at Jonathan

An inference requires the reader to consider the information presented and then form their own idea about what is probably true. Based on the details in the passage, what is the best answer to the question? Important details to pay attention to include the tone of Jacinta's dialogue, which is overall polite and apologetic, as well as her reaction itself, which is a long string of sneezes. Answer choices (a) and (d) both express strong emotions ("hates" and "angry") that are not evident in Jacinta's speech or actions. Answer choice (c) mentions cats, but there is nothing in the passage to indicate Jacinta's feelings about cats. Answer choice (b), "she is allergic to dogs," is the most logical choice—based on the fact that she began sneezing as soon as a fluffy dog approached her. It makes sense to guess that Jacinta might be allergic to dogs. So even though Jacinta never directly states, "Sorry, I'm allergic to dogs!", using the clues in the passage, it is still reasonable to guess that this is true.

Making inferences is crucial for readers of literature, because literary texts often avoid presenting complete and direct information to readers about characters' thoughts or feelings, or they present this information in an unclear way, leaving it up to the reader to interpret clues given in the text. In order to make inferences while reading, readers should ask themselves:

- What details are being presented in the text?
- Is there any important information that seems to be missing?
- Based on the information that the author *does* include, what else is probably true?
- Is this inference reasonable based on what is already known?

Apply Information

A natural extension of being able to make an inference from a given set of information is also being able to apply that information to a new context. This is especially useful in nonfiction or informative writing. Considering the facts and details presented in the text, readers should consider how the same information might be relevant in a different situation. The following is an example of applying an inferential conclusion to a different context:

> Often, individuals behave differently in large groups than they do as individuals. One example of this is the psychological phenomenon known as the bystander effect. According to the bystander effect, the more people who witness an accident or crime occur, the less likely each individual bystander is to respond or offer assistance to the victim. A classic example of this is the murder of Kitty Genovese in New York City in the 1960s. Although there were over thirty witnesses to her killing by a stabber, none of them intervened to help Kitty or contact the police.

Considering the phenomenon of the bystander effect, what would probably happen if somebody tripped on the stairs in a crowded subway station?

a. Everybody would stop to help the person who tripped
b. Bystanders would point and laugh at the person who tripped
c. Someone would call the police after walking away from the station
d. Few, if any, bystanders would offer assistance to the person who tripped

This question asks readers to apply the information they learned from the passage, which is an informative paragraph about the bystander effect. According to the passage, this is a concept in psychology that describes the way people in groups respond to an accident—the more people present, the less likely any one person is to intervene. While the passage illustrates this effect with the example of a woman's murder, the question asks readers to apply it to a different context—in this case, someone falling down the stairs in front of many subway passengers. Although this specific situation is not discussed in the passage, readers should be able to apply the general concepts described in the paragraph. The definition of the bystander effect includes any instance of an accident or crime in front of a large group of people. The question asks about a situation that falls within the same definition, so the general concept should still hold true: in the midst of a large crowd, few individuals are likely to actually respond to an accident. In this case, answer choice (d) is the best response.

Analysis

Relationships Between Ideas

Even if the author includes plenty of information to support his or her point, the writing is only coherent when the information is in a logical order. First, the author should introduce the main idea, whether for a paragraph, a section, or the entire piece. Second, they should present evidence to support the main idea by using transitional language. This shows the reader how the information relates to the main idea and to the sentences around it. The author should then take time to interpret the information, making sure necessary connections are obvious to the reader. Finally, the author can summarize the information in a closing section.

Although most writing follows this pattern, it isn't a set rule. Sometimes authors change the order for effect. For example, the author can begin with a surprising piece of supporting information to grab the reader's attention, and then transition to the main idea. Thus, if a passage doesn't follow the logical order, don't immediately assume it's wrong. However, most writing usually settles into a logical sequence after a nontraditional beginning.

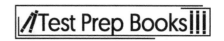

Depending on what the author is attempting to accomplish, certain formats or text structures work better than others. For example, a sequence structure might work for narration but not when identifying similarities and differences between dissimilar concepts. Similarly, a comparison-contrast structure is not useful for narration. It is the author's job to put the right information in the correct format.

Readers should be familiar with the five main literary structures:

1. *Sequence* structure (sometimes referred to as the order structure) is when the order of events proceed in a predictable order. In many cases, this means the text goes through the plot elements: exposition, rising action, climax, falling action, and resolution. Readers are introduced to characters, setting, and conflict in the exposition. In the rising action, there's an increase in tension and suspense. The climax is the height of tension and the point of no return. Tension decreases during the falling action. In the resolution, any conflicts presented in the exposition are solved, and the story concludes. An informative text that is structured sequentially will often go in order from one step to the next.

2. In the *problem-solution* structure, authors identify a potential problem and suggest a solution. This form of writing is usually divided into two paragraphs and can be found in informational texts. For example, cell phone, cable, and satellite providers use this structure in manuals to help customers troubleshoot or identify problems with services or products.

3. When authors want to discuss similarities and differences between separate concepts, they arrange thoughts in a *comparison-contrast* paragraph structure. Venn diagrams are an effective graphic organizer for comparison-contrast structures, because they feature two overlapping circles that can be used to organize similarities and differences. A comparison-contrast essay organizes one paragraph based on similarities and another based on differences. A comparison-contrast essay can also be arranged with the similarities and differences of individual traits addressed within individual paragraphs. Words such as *however*, *but*, and *nevertheless* help signal a contrast in ideas.

4. *Descriptive* writing structure is designed to appeal to the reader's senses. Much like an artist who constructs a painting, good descriptive writing builds an image in the reader's mind by appealing to the five senses: sight, hearing, taste, touch, and smell. However, overly descriptive writing can become tedious; sparse descriptions can make settings and characters seem flat. Good authors strike a balance by applying descriptions only to passages, characters, and settings that are integral to the plot.

5. Passages that use the *cause and effect* structure are simply asking *why* by demonstrating some type of connection between ideas. Words such as *if*, *since*, *because*, *then*, or *consequently* indicate a relationship. By switching the order of a complex sentence, the writer can rearrange the emphasis on different clauses. Saying *If Sheryl is late, we'll miss the dance* is different from saying *We'll miss the dance if Sheryl is late*. One emphasizes Sheryl's tardiness while the other emphasizes missing the dance. Paragraphs can also be arranged in a cause and effect format. Since the format—before and after—is sequential, it is useful when authors wish to discuss the impact of choices. Researchers often apply this paragraph structure to the scientific method.

Comparison and Contrast

One writing device authors use is comparison and contrast. *Comparison* is when authors take objects and show how they are the same. *Contrast* is when authors take objects and show how they differ.

Comparison and contrast essays are mostly written in nonfiction form. There are common words used when authors compare or contrast. The list below will show you some of these words:

Comparison Words and Phrases:

- Similar to
- Alike
- As well as
- Both

Contrast Words and Phrases:

- Although
- On the other hand
- Different from
- However
- As opposed to
- More than
- Less than
- On the contrary

Cause and Effect

Cause and effect is a common writing device. A cause is why something happens. An effect is something that happens because of the cause. Many times, authors use key words to show cause and effect, such as *because, so, therefore, without, now, then,* and *since*. For example: "Because of the sun shower, a rainbow appeared." In this sentence, due to the sun shower (the cause), a rainbow appeared (the effect).

Analogy

An analogyis a comparison between two things. Sometimes the two things are very different from one another. Authors often use analogies to add meaning and make ideas relatable in texts. There are two types of analogies: metaphors and similes. Metaphors compare two things that are not similar. Similes also compare two unlike things but use the words *like* or *as*. For example, "In the library, students are asked to be as quiet as a mouse." Clearly, students and mice are very different. However, when students are asked to be as quiet as a mouse, readers understand that they are being asked to be absolutely silent.

Transitional Words and Phrases

There are approximately 200 transitional words and phrases that are commonly used in the English language. Below are lists of common transition words and phrases used throughout transitions.

Time

- after
- before
- during
- in the middle

Example about to be Given

- for example
- in fact
- for instance

Compare

- likewise
- also

Contrast

- however
- yet
- but

Addition

- and
- also
- furthermore
- moreover

Logical Relationships

- if
- then
- therefore
- as a result
- since

Steps in a Process

- first
- second
- last

Transitional words and phrases are important writing devices because they connect sentences and paragraphs. Transitional words and phrases present logical order to writing and provide more coherent meaning to readers.

Transition words can be categorized based on the relationships they create between ideas:

- *General order*: signaling elaboration of an idea to emphasize a point—e.g., *for example, for instance, to demonstrate, including, such as, in other words, that is, in fact, also, furthermore, likewise, and, truly, so, surely, certainly, obviously, doubtless*
- *Chronological order*: referencing the time frame in which main event or idea occurs—e.g., *before, after, first, while, soon, shortly thereafter, meanwhile*
- *Numerical order/order of importance*: indicating that related ideas, supporting details, or events will be described in a sequence, possibly in order of importance—e.g., *first, second, also, finally,*

another, in addition, equally important, less importantly, most significantly, the main reason, last but not least

- *Spatial order*: referring to the space and location of something or where things are located in relation to each other—e.g., *inside, outside, above, below, within, close, under, over, far, next to, adjacent to*
- *Cause and effect order*: signaling a causal relationship between events or ideas—e.g., *thus, therefore, since, resulted in, for this reason, as a result, consequently, hence, for, so*
- *Compare and contrast order*: identifying the similarities and differences between two or more objects, ideas, or lines of thought—e.g., *like, as, similarly, equally, just as, unlike, however, but, although, conversely, on the other hand, on the contrary*
- *Summary order*: indicating that a particular idea is coming to a close—e.g., *in conclusion, to sum up, in other words, ultimately, above all*

The Author's Purpose

No matter the genre or format, all authors are writing to persuade, inform, entertain, or express feelings. Often, these purposes are blended, with one dominating the rest. It's useful to learn to recognize the author's intent.

Persuasive writing is used to persuade or convince readers of something. It often contains two elements: the argument and the counterargument. The argument takes a stance on an issue, while the counterargument pokes holes in the opposition's stance. Authors rely on logic, emotion, and writer credibility to persuade readers to agree with them. If readers are opposed to the stance before reading, they are unlikely to adopt that stance. However, those who are undecided or committed to the same stance are more likely to agree with the author.

Informative writing tries to teach or inform. Workplace manuals, instructor lessons, statistical reports, and cookbooks are examples of informative texts. Informative writing is usually based on facts and is often void of emotion and persuasion. Informative texts generally contain statistics, charts, and graphs. Though most informative texts lack a persuasive agenda, readers must examine the text carefully to determine whether one exists within a given passage.

Stories or narratives are designed to entertain. When you go to the movies, you often want to escape for a few hours, not necessarily to think critically. Entertaining writing is designed to delight and engage the reader. However, sometimes this type of writing can be woven into more serious materials, such as persuasive or informative writing to hook the reader before transitioning into a more scholarly discussion.

Emotional writing works to evoke the reader's feelings, such as anger, euphoria, or sadness. The connection between reader and author is an attempt to cause the reader to share the author's intended emotion or tone. Sometimes in order to make a piece more poignant, the author simply wants readers to feel the same emotions that the author has felt. Other times, the author attempts to persuade or manipulate the reader into adopting his stance. While it's okay to sympathize with the author, readers should be aware of the individual's underlying intent.

Appealing to the Readers' Emotions

Authors write to captivate the attention of their readers. Oftentimes, authors will appeal to their readers' emotions to convince or persuade their audience, especially in when trying to win weak arguments that lack factual evidence. Authors may tell sob stories or use bandwagon approaches in their writing to tap into the readers' emotions. For example, "Everyone is voting yes" or "He only has two months to live" are statements that can tug at the heartstrings of readers. Authors may use other tactics, such as name-calling or advertising, to lead their readers into believing something is true or false. These emotional pleas are clear signs that the authors do not have a favorable point and that they are trying to distract the readers from the fact that their argument is factually weak.

The Author's Tone

Style, tone, and mood are often thought to be the same thing. Though they're closely related, there are important differences to keep in mind. The easiest way to do this is to remember that style "creates and affects" tone and mood. More specifically, style is how the writer uses words to create the desired tone and mood for their writing.

Tone

Tone refers to the writer's attitude toward the subject matter. Tone is usually explained in terms of a work of fiction. For example, the tone conveys how the writer feels about their characters and the situations in which they're involved. Nonfiction writing is sometimes thought to have no tone at all; however, this is incorrect.

A lot of nonfiction writing has a neutral tone, which is an important tone for the writer to take. A neutral tone demonstrates that the writer is presenting a topic impartially and letting the information speak for itself. On the other hand, nonfiction writing can be just as effective and appropriate if the tone isn't neutral. For instance, take this example involving seat belts:

> Seat belts save more lives than any other automobile safety feature. Many studies show that airbags save lives as well; however, not all cars have airbags. For instance, some older cars don't. Furthermore, air bags aren't entirely reliable. For example, studies show that in 15% of accidents airbags don't deploy as designed, but, on the other hand, seat belt malfunctions are extremely rare. The number of highway fatalities has plummeted since laws requiring seat belt usage were enacted.

In this passage, the writer mostly chooses to retain a neutral tone when presenting information. If the writer would instead include their own personal experience of losing a friend or family member in a car accident, the tone would change dramatically. The tone would no longer be neutral and would show that the writer has a personal stake in the content, allowing them to interpret the information in a different way. When analyzing tone, consider what the writer is trying to achieve in the text and how they *create* the tone using style.

Style

Style can include any number of technical writing choices. A few examples of style choices include:

- Sentence Construction: When presenting facts, does the writer use shorter sentences to create a quicker sense of the supporting evidence, or do they use longer sentences to elaborate and explain the information?
- Technical Language: Does the writer use jargon to demonstrate their expertise in the subject, or do they use ordinary language to help the reader understand things in simple terms?
- Formal Language: Does the writer refrain from using contractions such as *won't* or *can't* to create a more formal tone, or do they use a colloquial, conversational style to connect to the reader?
- Formatting: Does the writer use a series of shorter paragraphs to help the reader follow a line of argument, or do they use longer paragraphs to examine an issue in great detail and demonstrate their knowledge of the topic?

On the test, examine the writer's style and how their writing choices affect the way the text comes across.

Mood

Mood refers to the feelings and atmosphere that the writer's words create for the reader. Like tone, many nonfiction texts can have a neutral mood. To return to the previous example, if the writer would choose to include information about a person they know being killed in a car accident, the text would suddenly carry an emotional component that is absent in the previous example. Depending on how they present the information, the writer can create a sad, angry, or even hopeful mood. When analyzing the mood, consider what the writer wants to accomplish and whether the best choice was made to achieve that end.

Point of View

Point of view is an important writing device to consider. In fiction writing, point of view refers to who tells the story or from whose perspective readers are observing as they read. In nonfiction writing, the *point of view* refers to whether the author refers to himself/herself, his/her readers, or chooses not to mention either. Whether fiction or nonfiction, the author will carefully consider the impact the perspective will have on the purpose and main point of the writing.

- *First-person point of view*: The story is told from the writer's perspective. In fiction, this would mean that the main character is also the narrator. First-person point of view is easily recognized by the use of personal pronouns such as *I, me, we, us, our, my,* and *myself*.
- *Third-person point of view*: In a more formal essay, this would be an appropriate perspective because the focus should be on the subject matter, not the writer or the reader. Third-person

point of view is recognized using the pronouns *he, she, they,* and *it.* In fiction writing, third person point of view has a few variations.

- *Third-person limited* point of view refers to a story told by a narrator who has access to the thoughts and feelings of just one character.
- In *third-person omniscient* point of view, the narrator has access to the thoughts and feelings of all the characters.
- In *third-person objective* point of view, the narrator is like a fly on the wall and can see and hear what the characters do and say but does not have access to their thoughts and feelings.

- *Second-person point of view*: This point of view isn't commonly used in fiction or nonfiction writing because it directly addresses the reader using the pronouns *you, your,* and *yourself.* Second-person perspective is more appropriate in direct communication, such as business letters or emails.

Point of View	Pronouns Used
First person	I, me, we, us, our, my, myself
Second person	You, your, yourself
Third person	He, she, it, they

Understanding the Effect of Word Choice

An author's choice of words—also referred to as *diction*—helps to convey his or her meaning in a particular way. Through diction, an author can convey a particular tone—e.g., a humorous tone, a serious tone—in order to support the thesis in a meaningful way to the reader.

Connotation and Denotation

Connotation is when an author chooses words or phrases that invoke ideas or feelings other than their literal meaning. An example of the use of connotation is the word *cheap,* which suggests something is poor in value or negatively describes a person as reluctant to spend money. When something or someone is described this way, the reader is more inclined to have a particular image or feeling about it or him/her. Thus, connotation can be a very effective language tool in creating emotion and swaying opinion. However, connotations are sometimes hard to pin down because varying emotions can be associated with a word. Generally, though, connotative meanings tend to be fairly consistent within a specific cultural group.

Denotation refers to words or phrases that mean exactly what they say. It is helpful when a writer wants to present hard facts or vocabulary terms with which readers may be unfamiliar. Some examples of denotation are the words *inexpensive* and *frugal. Inexpensive* refers to the cost of something, not its value, and *frugal* indicates that a person is conscientiously watching his or her spending. These terms do not elicit the same emotions that *cheap* does.

Authors sometimes choose to use both, but what they choose and when they use it is what critical readers need to differentiate. One method isn't inherently better than the other; however, one may create a better effect, depending upon an author's intent. If, for example, an author's purpose is to inform, to instruct, and to familiarize readers with a difficult subject, his or her use of connotation may be helpful. However, it may also undermine credibility and confuse readers. An author who wants to create a credible, scholarly effect in his or her text would most likely use denotation, which emphasizes literal, factual meaning and examples.

Technical Language

Test takers and critical readers alike should be very aware of technical language used within informational text. *Technical language* refers to terminology that is specific to a particular industry and is best understood by those specializing in that industry. This language is fairly easy to differentiate, since it will most likely be unfamiliar to readers. It's critical to be able to define technical language either by the author's written definition, through the use of an included glossary—if offered—or through context clues that help readers clarify word meaning.

Figurative Language

Literary texts employ rhetorical devices. Figurative language like simile and metaphor is a type of rhetorical device commonly found in literature. In addition to rhetorical devices that play on the *meanings* of words, there are also rhetorical devices that use the *sounds* of words. These devices are most often found in poetry but may also be found in other types of literature and in non-fiction writing like speech texts.

Alliteration and *assonance* are both varieties of sound repetition. Other types of sound repetition include: anaphora, repetition that occurs at the beginning of the sentences; epiphora, repetition occurring at the end of phrases; antimetabole, repetition of words in reverse order; and antiphrasis, a form of denial of an assertion in a text.

Alliteration refers to the repetition of the first sound of each word. Recall Robert Burns' opening line:

> My love is like a red, red rose

This line includes two instances of alliteration: "love" and "like" (repeated *L* sound), as well as "red" and "rose" (repeated *R* sound). Next, assonance refers to the repetition of vowel sounds, and can occur anywhere within a word (not just the opening sound). Here is the opening of a poem by John Keats:

> When I have fears that I may cease to be
>
> Before my pen has glean'd my teeming brain

Assonance can be found in the words "fears," "cease," "be," "glean'd," and "teeming," all of which stress the long *E* sound. Both alliteration and assonance create a harmony that unifies the writer's language.

Another sound device is *onomatopoeia*, or words whose spelling mimics the sound they describe. Words such as "crash," "bang," and "sizzle" are all examples of onomatopoeia. Use of onomatopoetic language adds auditory imagery to the text.

Readers are probably most familiar with the technique of *pun*. A pun is a play on words, taking advantage of two words that have the same or similar pronunciation. Puns can be found throughout Shakespeare's plays, for instance:

> Now is the winter of our discontent
> Made glorious summer by this son of York

These lines from *Richard III* contain a play on words. Richard III refers to his brother, the newly crowned King Edward IV, as the "son of York," referencing their family heritage from the house of York. However, while drawing a comparison between the political climate and the weather (times of political trouble were the "winter," but now the new king brings "glorious summer"), Richard's use of the word "son" also implies another word with the same pronunciation, "sun"—so Edward IV is also like the sun, bringing light, warmth, and hope to England. Puns are a clever way for writers to suggest two meanings at once.

Some examples of figurative language are included in the following graphic.

	Definition	**Example**
Simile	Compares two things using "like" or "as"	Her hair was like gold.
Metaphor	Compares two things as if they are the same	He was a giant teddy bear.
Idiom	Using words with predictable meanings to create a phrase with a different meaning	The world is your oyster.
Alliteration	Repeating the same beginning sound or letter in a phrase for emphasis	The busy baby babbled.
Personification	Attributing human characteristics to an object or an animal	The house glowered menacingly with a dark smile.
Foreshadowing	Giving an indication that something is going to happen later in the story	I wasn't aware at the time, but I would come to regret those words.
Symbolism	Using symbols to represent ideas and provide a different meaning	The ring represented the bond between us.
Onomatopoeia	Using words that imitate sound	The tire went off with a bang and a crunch.
Imagery	Appealing to the senses by using descriptive language	The sky was painted with red and pink and streaked with orange.
Hyperbole	Using exaggeration not meant to be taken literally	The girl weighed less than a feather.

Figurative language can be used to give additional insight into the theme or message of a text by moving beyond the usual and literal meaning of words and phrases. It can also be used to appeal to the senses of readers and create a more in-depth story.

Facts and Opinions

As mentioned previously, authors write with a purpose. They adjust their writing for an intended audience. It is the readers' responsibility to comprehend the writing style or purpose of the author. When readers understand a writer's purpose, they can then form their own thoughts about the text(s), regardless of whether their thoughts are the same as or different from the author's.

Facts Versus Opinions

Readers need to be aware of the writer's purpose to help discern facts and opinions within texts. A *fact* is a piece of information that is true. It can either prove or disprove claims or arguments presented in texts. Facts cannot be changed or altered. For example, the statement: *Abraham Lincoln was assassinated on April 15, 1865*, is a fact. The date and related events cannot be altered.

Authors not only present facts in their writing to support or disprove their claim(s), but they may also express their opinions. Authors may use facts to support their own opinions, especially in a persuasive text; however, that does not make their opinions facts. An *opinion* is a belief or view formed about something that is not necessarily based on the truth. Opinions often express authors' personal feelings about a subject and use words like *believe, think,* or *feel.* For example, the statement: *Abraham Lincoln was the best president who has ever lived*, expresses the writer's opinion. Not all writers or readers agree or disagree with the statement. Therefore, the statement can be altered or adjusted to express opposing or supporting beliefs, such as "Abraham Lincoln was the worst president who has ever lived" or "I also think Abraham Lincoln was a great president."

When authors include facts and opinions in their writing, readers may be less influenced by the text(s). Readers need to be conscious of the distinction between facts and opinions while going through texts. Not only should the intended audience be vigilant in following authors' thoughts versus valid information, readers need to check the source of the facts presented. Facts should have reliable sources derived from credible outlets like almanacs, encyclopedias, medical journals, and so on.

Rhetorical Strategies

Rhetoric refers to an author's use of particular strategies, appeals, and devices to persuade an intended audience. The more effective the use of rhetoric, the more likely the audience will be persuaded.

Determining an Author's Point of View

A *rhetorical strategy*—also referred to as a *rhetorical mode*—is the structural way an author chooses to present his/her argument. Though the terms noted below are similar to the organizational structures noted earlier, these strategies do not imply that the entire text follows the approach. For example, a cause and effect organizational structure is solely that, nothing more. A persuasive text may use cause and effect as a strategy to convey a singular point. Thus, an argument may include several of the strategies as the author strives to convince his or her audience to take action or accept a different point of view. It's important that readers are able to identify an author's thesis and position on the topic in order to be able to identify the careful construction through which the author speaks to the reader. The following are some of the more common rhetorical strategies:

- *Cause and effect*—establishing a logical correlation or causation between two ideas
- *Classification/division*—grouping similar items together or dividing something into parts
- *Comparison/contrast*—the distinguishing of similarities/differences to expand on an idea
- *Definition*—clarifies abstract ideas, unfamiliar concepts, or distinguishes one idea from another
- *Description*—use of vivid imagery, active verbs, and clear adjectives to explain ideas
- *Exemplification*—the use of examples to explain an idea
- *Narration*—anecdotes or personal experience to present or expand on a concept
- *Problem/Solution*—presentation of a problem or problems, followed by proposed solution(s)

Rhetorical Strategies and Devices

A *rhetorical device* is the phrasing and presentation of an idea that reinforces and emphasizes a point in an argument. A rhetorical device is often quite memorable. One of the more famous uses of a rhetorical device is in John F. Kennedy's 1961 inaugural address: "Ask not what your country can do for you, ask what you can do for your country." The contrast of ideas presented in the phrasing is an example of the rhetorical device of antimetabole.

Some other common examples are provided below, but test takers should be aware that this is not a complete list.

Device	Definition	Example
Allusion	A reference to a famous person, event, or significant literary text as a form of significant comparison	"We are apt to shut our eyes against a painful truth, and listen to the song of that siren till she transforms us into beasts." Patrick Henry
Anaphora	The repetition of the same words at the beginning of successive words, phrases, or clauses, designed to emphasize an idea	"We shall not flag or fail. We shall go on to the end. We shall fight in France, we shall fight on the seas and oceans, we shall fight with growing confidence ... we shall fight in the fields and in the streets, we shall fight in the hills. We shall never surrender." Winston Churchill
Understatement	A statement meant to portray a situation as less important than it actually is to create an ironic effect	"The war in the Pacific has not necessarily developed in Japan's favor." Emperor Hirohito, surrendering Japan in World War II
Parallelism	A syntactical similarity in a structure or series of structures used for impact of an idea, making it memorable	"A penny saved is a penny earned." Ben Franklin
Rhetorical question	A question posed that is not answered by the writer though there is a desired response, most often designed to emphasize a point	"Can anyone look at our reduced standing in the world today and say, 'Let's have four more years of this?'" Ronald Reagan

Rhetorical Appeals

In an argument or persuasive text, an author will strive to sway readers to an opinion or conclusion. To be effective, an author must consider his or her intended audience. Although an author may write text for a general audience, he or she will use methods of appeal or persuasion to convince that audience. Aristotle asserted that there were three methods or modes by which a person could be persuaded. These are referred to as *rhetorical appeals*.

The three main types of rhetorical appeals are shown in the following graphic:

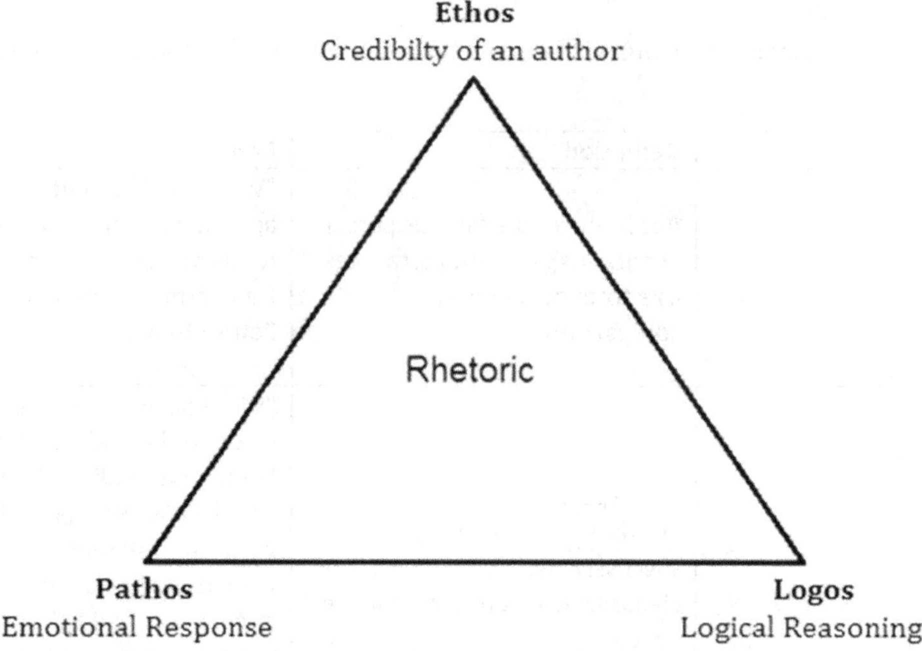

Ethos, also referred to as an *ethical appeal*, is an appeal to the audience's perception of the writer as credible (or not), based on their examination of their ethics and who the writer is, his/her experience or incorporation of relevant information, or his/her argument. For example, authors may present testimonials to bolster their arguments. The reader who critically examines the veracity of the testimonials and the credibility of those giving the testimony will be able to determine if the author's use of testimony is valid to his or her argument. In turn, this will help the reader determine if the author's thesis is valid. An author's careful and appropriate use of technical language can create an overall knowledgeable effect and, in turn, act as a convincing vehicle when it comes to credibility. Overuse of technical language, however, may create confusion in readers and obscure an author's overall intent.

Pathos, also referred to as a *pathetic* or *emotional appeal*, is an appeal to the audience's sense of identity, self-interest, or emotions. A critical reader will notice when the author is appealing to pathos through anecdotes and descriptions that elicit an emotion such as anger or pity. Readers should also beware of factual information that uses generalization to appeal to the emotions. While it's tempting to believe an author is the source of truth in his or her text, an author who presents factual information as universally true, consistent throughout time, and common to all groups is using *generalization*. Authors who exclusively use generalizations without specific facts and credible sourcing are attempting to sway readers solely through emotion.

Logos, also referred to as a *logical appeal*, is an appeal to the audience's ability to see and understand the logic in a claim offered by the writer. A critical reader has to be able to evaluate an author's arguments for validity of reasoning and for sufficiency when it comes to argument.

Evaluation

Bias

Not only can authors state facts or opinions in their writing, they sometimes intentionally or unintentionally show bias or portray a stereotype. A *bias* is when someone demonstrates a prejudice in favor of or against something or someone in an unfair manner. When an author is biased in his or her writing, readers should be skeptical despite the fact that the author's bias may be correct. For example, two athletes competed for the same position. One athlete is related to the coach and is a mediocre athlete, while the other player excels and deserves the position. The coach chose the less talented player who is related to him for the position. This is a biased decision because it favors someone in an unfair way.

Similar to a bias, a *stereotype* shows favoritism or opposition but toward a specific group or place. Stereotypes create an oversimplified or overgeneralized idea about a certain group, person, or place. For example,

> Women are horrible drivers.

This statement basically labels *all* women as horrible drivers. While there may be some terrible female drivers, the stereotype implies that *all* women are bad drivers when, in fact, not *all* women are. While many readers are aware of several vile ethnic, religious, and cultural stereotypes, audiences should be cautious of authors' flawed assumptions because they can be less obvious than the despicable examples that are unfortunately pervasive in society.

Fallacies

A fallacy is a mistaken belief or faulty reasoning, otherwise known as a *logical fallacy.* It is important for readers to recognize logical fallacies because they discredit the author's message. Readers should continuously self-question as they go through a text to identify logical fallacies. Readers cannot simply complacently take information at face value. There are six common types of logical *fallacies:*

1. False analogy
2. Circular reasoning
3. False dichotomy
4. Overgeneralization
5. Slippery slope
6. Hasty generalization

Each of the six logical fallacies are reviewed individually.

False Analogy

A *false analogy* is when the author assumes two objects or events are alike in all aspects despite the fact that they may be vastly different. Authors intend on making unfamiliar objects relatable to convince readers of something. For example, the letters *A* and *E* are both vowels; therefore, *A* = *E*. Readers cannot assume that because *A* and *E* are both vowels that they perform the same function in words or independently. If authors tell readers, *A* = *E*, then that is a false analogy. While this is a simple example, other false analogies may be less obvious.

Circular Reasoning

Circular reasoning is when the reasoning is decided based upon the outcome or conclusion and then vice versa. Basically, those who use circular reasoning start out with the argument and then use false logic to try to prove it, and then, in turn, the reasoning supports the conclusion in one big circular pattern. For example, consider the two thoughts, "I don't have time to get organized" and "My disorganization is costing me time." Which is the argument? What is the conclusion? If there is not time to get organized, will more time be spent later trying to find whatever is needed? In turn, if so much time is spent looking for things, there is not time to get organized. The cycle keeps going in an endless series. One problem affects the other; therefore, there is a circular pattern of reasoning.

False Dichotomy

A *false dichotomy,* also known as a false dilemma, is when the author tries to make readers believe that there are only two options to choose from when, in fact, there are more. The author creates a false sense of the situation because he or she wants the readers to believe that his or her claim is the most logical choice. If the author does not present the readers with options, then the author is purposefully limiting what readers may believe. In turn, the author hopes that readers will believe that his or her point of view is the most sensible choice. For example, in the statement: *you either love running, or you are lazy*, the fallacy lies in the options of loving to run or being lazy. Even though both statements do not necessarily have to be true, the author tries to make one option seem more appealing than the other.

Overgeneralization

An *overgeneralization* is a logical fallacy that occurs when authors write something so extreme that it cannot be proved or disproved. Words like *all, never, most,* and *few* are commonly used when an overgeneralization is being made. For example,

> All kids are crazy when they eat sugar; therefore, my son will not have a cupcake at the birthday party.

Not *all* kids are crazy when they eat sugar, but the extreme statement can influence the readers' points of view on the subject. Readers need to be wary of overgeneralizations in texts because authors may try to sneak them in to sway the readers' opinions.

Slippery Slope

A *slippery slope* is when an author implies that something will inevitably happen as a result of another action. A slippery slope may or may not be true, even though the order of events or gradations may seem logical. For example, in the children's book *If You Give a Mouse a Cookie*, the author goes off on tangents such as "If you give a mouse a cookie, he will ask for some milk. When you give him the milk, he'll probably ask you for a straw." The mouse in the story follows a series of logical events as a result of a previous action. The slippery slope continues on and on throughout the story. Even though the mouse made logical decisions, it very well could have made a different choice, changing the direction of the story.

Hasty Generalization

A *hasty generalization* is when the reader comes to a conclusion without reviewing or analyzing all the evidence. It is never a good idea to make a decision without all the information, which is why hasty generalizations are considered fallacies. For example, if two friends go to a hairdresser and give the hairdresser a positive recommendation, that does not necessarily mean that a new client will have the same experience. Two referrals is not quite enough information to form an educated and well-formed conclusion.

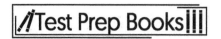

Overall, readers should carefully review and analyze authors' arguments to identify logical fallacies and come to sensible conclusions.

Support in an Argument

Evaluating an Author's Purpose

A reader must be able to evaluate the argument or point the author is trying to make and determine if it is adequately supported. The first step is to determine the main idea. The main idea is what the author wants to say about a specific topic. The next step is to locate the supporting details. An author uses supporting details to illustrate the main idea. These are the details that provide evidence or examples to help make a point. Supporting details often appear in the form of quotations, paraphrasing, or analysis. Test takers should then examine the text to make sure the author connects details and analysis to the main point. These steps are crucial to understanding the text and evaluating how well the author presents his or her argument and evidence. The following graphic demonstrates the connection between the main idea and the supporting details.

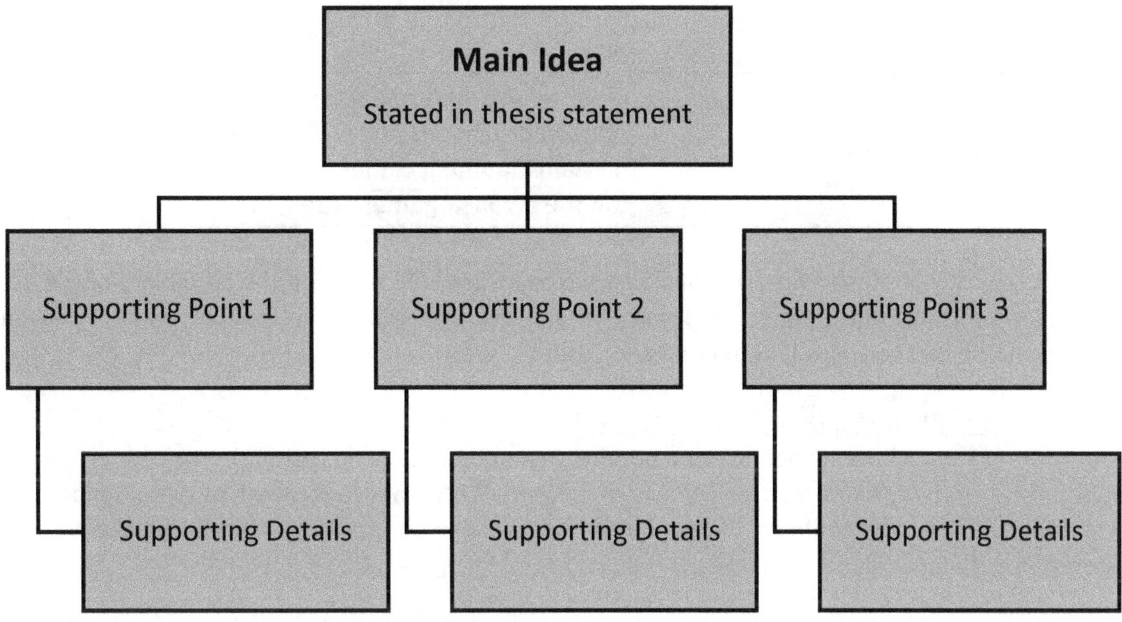

Evaluating Evidence

It is important to evaluate the author's supporting details to be sure that they are credible, provide evidence of the author's point, and directly support the main idea. Critical readers examine the facts used to support an author's argument and check those facts against other sources to be sure the facts are correct. They also check the validity of the sources used to be sure those sources are credible, academic, and/or peer- reviewed. A strong argument uses valid, measurable facts to support ideas.

Identifying False Statements

A reader must also be able to identify any *logical fallacies*—logically-flawed statements—that an author may make as those fallacies impact the validity and veracity of the author's claims.

Some of the more common fallacies are shown in the following chart.

Fallacy	Definition
Slippery Slope	A fallacy that is built on the idea that a particular action will lead to a series of events with negative results
Red Herring	The use of an observation or distraction to remove attention from the actual issue
Straw Man	An exaggeration or misrepresentation of an argument so that it is easier to refute
Post Hoc Ergo Propter Hoc	A fallacy that assumes an event to be the consequence of an earlier event merely because it came after it
Bandwagon	A fallacy that assumes because the majority of people feel or believe a certain way then it must be the right way
Ad Hominem	The use of a personal attack on the person or persons associated with a certain argument rather than focusing on the actual argument itself

Readers who are aware of the types of fallacious reasoning are able to weigh the credibility of the author's statements in terms of effective argument. Rhetorical text that contains a myriad of fallacious statements should be considered ineffectual and suspect.

Counterarguments and Evaluating Arguments

If an author presents a differing opinion or a counterargument in order to refute it, the reader should consider how and why this information is being presented. It is meant to strengthen the original argument and shouldn't be confused with the author's intended conclusion, but it should also be considered in the reader's final evaluation.

Authors can also use bias if they ignore the opposing viewpoint or present their side in an unbalanced way. A strong argument considers the opposition and finds a way to refute it. Critical readers should look for an unfair or one-sided presentation of the argument and be skeptical, as a bias may be present. Even if this bias is unintentional, if it exists in the writing, the reader should be wary of the validity of the argument. Readers should also look for the use of stereotypes, which refer to specific groups. Stereotypes are often negative connotations about a person or place, and should always be avoided. When a critical reader finds stereotypes in a piece of writing, they should be critical of the argument, and consider the validity of anything the author presents. Stereotypes reveal a flaw in the writer's thinking and may suggest a lack of knowledge or understanding about the subject.

In general, readers should always heed attention to whether an author's ideas or stated facts are relevant to the argument or counterargument posed in the reading. Those that are irrelevant can cloud the argument or weaken it. In much the same way, critical readers are able to identify whether statements in a reading strengthen or weaken the author's argument.

Authors want readers to accept their assertions and arguments as true but critical readers evaluate the strength of the argument instead of simply taking it at face value and accepting it as the truth or only point of view. All arguments need two parts: the claim and the supporting evidence or rationale. The claim *is* the argument. It asserts an opinion, idea, point of view, or conclusion. The supporting evidence is the rationale, assumptions, beliefs, as well as the factual evidence in support of the stated claim. The supporting evidence is what gives readers the information necessary to accept or reject the stated claim. Critical readers should assess the argument in its entirety by evaluating the claims and conclusions themselves, the process of reasoning, and the accuracy of the evidence. For example, arguments are weaker and should be skeptically considered when the supporting evidence is highly opinionated, biased, or derived from sources that are not credible. Authors should cite where statistics and other stated facts were found. Lastly, the support for a claim should be pertinent to it and consistent with the other statements and evidence.

The Author's Conclusion and Thesis

An informational text is specifically designed to relate factual information, and although it is open to a reader's interpretation and application of the facts, the structure of the presentation is carefully designed to lead the reader to a particular conclusion or central idea. When reading an informational text, it is important that readers are able to understand its organizational structure as the structure often directly relates to an author's intent to inform and/or persuade the reader.

The first step in identifying the text's structure is to determine the thesis or main idea. The thesis statement and organization of a work are closely intertwined. *A thesis statement* indicates the writer's purpose and may include the scope and direction of the text. It may be presented at the beginning of a text or at the end, and it may be explicit or implicit.

Once a reader has a grasp of the thesis or main idea of the text, he or she can better determine its organizational structure. Test takers are advised to read informational text passages more than once in order to comprehend the material fully. It is also helpful to examine any text features present in the text including the table of contents, index, glossary, headings, footnotes, and visuals. The analysis of these features and the information presented within them, can offer additional clues about the central idea and structure of a text. The following questions should be asked when considering structure:

- How does the author assemble the parts to make an effective whole argument?
- Is the passage linear in nature and if so, what is the timeline or thread of logic?
- What is the presented order of events, facts, or arguments?
- Is the order used effective in contributing to the author's thesis?
- How can the passage be divided into sections?
- How can the sections of the passage be related to each other and to the main idea or thesis?
- What key terms are used to indicate the organization?

Once a reader has determined an author's thesis or main idea, he or she will need to understand how textual evidence supports interpretation of that thesis or main idea. Test takers will be asked direct questions regarding an author's main idea and may be asked to identify evidence that would support those ideas. This will require test takers to comprehend literal and figurative meanings within the text passage, be able to draw inferences from provided information, and be able to separate important evidence from minor supporting detail. It's often helpful to skim test questions and answer options prior to critically reading informational text; however, test takers should avoid the temptation to solely look for the correct answers. Just trying to find the "right answer" may cause test takers to miss important supporting textual evidence. Making mental note of test questions is only helpful as a guide when reading.

After identifying an author's thesis or main idea, a test taker should look at the supporting details that the author provides to back up his or her assertions, identifying those additional pieces of information that help expand the thesis. From there, test takers should examine the additional information and related details for credibility, the author's use of outside sources, and be able to point to direct evidence that supports the author's claims. It's also imperative that test takers be able to identify what is strong support and what is merely additional information that is nice to know, but not necessary. Being able to make this differentiation will help test takers effectively answer questions regarding an author's use of supporting evidence within informational text.

In a conclusion, the writer restates their main idea a final time, often after summarizing the smaller pieces of that idea. If the introduction uses a quote or anecdote to grab the reader's attention, the conclusion often makes reference to it again. Whatever way the writer chooses to arrange the conclusion, the final restatement of the main idea should be clear and simple for the reader to interpret. Finally, conclusions shouldn't introduce any new information.

Practice Questions

Questions 1-4 are based on the following passage:

Smoking is Terrible

Smoking tobacco products is terribly destructive. A single cigarette contains over 4,000 chemicals, including 43 known carcinogens and 400 deadly toxins. Some of the most dangerous ingredients include tar, carbon monoxide, formaldehyde, ammonia, arsenic, and DDT. Smoking can cause numerous types of cancer including throat, mouth, nasal cavity, esophageal, gastric, pancreatic, renal, bladder, and cervical cancer.

Cigarettes contain a drug called nicotine, one of the most addictive substances known to man. Addiction is defined as a compulsion to seek the substance despite negative consequences. According to the National Institute of Drug Abuse, nearly 35 million smokers expressed a desire to quit smoking in 2015; however, more than 85 percent of those who struggle with addiction will not achieve their goal. Almost all smokers regret picking up that first cigarette. You would be wise to learn from their mistake if you have not yet started smoking.

According to the U.S. Department of Health and Human Services, 16 million people in the United States presently suffer from a smoking-related condition and nearly nine million suffer from a serious smoking-related illness. According to the Centers for Disease Control and Prevention (CDC), tobacco products cause nearly six million deaths per year. This number is projected to rise to over eight million deaths by 2030. Smokers, on average, die ten years earlier than their nonsmoking peers.

In the United States, local, state, and federal governments typically tax tobacco products, which leads to high prices. Nicotine users who struggle with addiction sometimes pay more for a pack of cigarettes than for a few gallons of gas. Additionally, smokers tend to stink. The smell of smoke is all-consuming and creates a pervasive nastiness. Smokers also risk staining their teeth and fingers with yellow residue from the tar.

Smoking is deadly, expensive, and socially unappealing. Clearly, smoking is not worth the risks.

1. Which of the following best describes the passage?
    a. Narrative
    b. Persuasive
    c. Expository
    d. Informative

2. Which of the following statements most accurately summarizes the passage?
    a. Almost all smokers regret picking up that first cigarette.
    b. Tobacco is deadly, expensive, and socially unappealing, and smokers would be much better off kicking the addiction.
    c. In the United States, local, state, and federal governments typically tax tobacco products, which leads to high prices.
    d. Tobacco products shorten smokers' lives by ten years and kill more than six million people per year.

3. The author would be most likely to agree with which of the following statements?
   a. Smokers should only quit cold turkey and avoid all nicotine cessation devices.
   b. Other substances are more addictive than tobacco.
   c. Smokers should quit for whatever reason gets them to stop smoking.
   d. People who want to continue smoking should advocate for a reduction in tobacco product taxes.

4. Which of the following represents an opinion statement on the part of the author?
   a. According to the Centers for Disease Control and Prevention (CDC), tobacco products cause nearly six million deaths per year.
   b. Nicotine users who struggle with addiction sometimes pay more for a pack of cigarettes than a few gallons of gas.
   c. They also risk staining their teeth and fingers with yellow residue from the tar.
   d. Additionally, smokers tend to stink. The smell of smoke is all-consuming and creates a pervasive nastiness.

Questions 5-7 are based on the following passage:

George Washington emerged out of the American Revolution as an unlikely champion of liberty. On June 14, 1775, the Second Continental Congress created the Continental Army, and John Adams, serving in the Congress, nominated Washington to be its first commander. Washington fought under the British during the French and Indian War, and his experience and prestige proved instrumental to the American war effort. Washington provided invaluable leadership, training, and strategy during the Revolutionary War. He emerged from the war as the embodiment of liberty and freedom from tyranny.

After vanquishing the heavily favored British forces, Washington could have pronounced himself as the autocratic leader of the former colonies without any opposition, but he famously refused and returned to his Mount Vernon plantation. His restraint proved his commitment to the fledgling state's republicanism. Washington was later unanimously elected as the first American president. But it is Washington's farewell address that cemented his legacy as a visionary worthy of study.

In 1796, President Washington issued his farewell address by public letter. Washington enlisted his good friend, Alexander Hamilton, in drafting his most famous address. The letter expressed Washington's faith in the Constitution and rule of law. He encouraged his fellow Americans to put aside partisan differences and establish a national union. Washington warned Americans against meddling in foreign affairs and entering military alliances. Additionally, he stated his opposition to national political parties, which he considered partisan and counterproductive.

Americans would be wise to remember Washington's farewell, especially during presidential elections when politics hits a fever pitch. They might want to question the political institutions that were not planned by the Founding Fathers, such as the nomination process and political parties themselves.

5. Which of the following statements is logically based on the information contained in the passage above?
   a. George Washington's background as a wealthy landholder directly led to his faith in equality, liberty, and democracy.
   b. George Washington would have opposed America's involvement in the Second World War.
   c. George Washington would not have been able to write as great a farewell address without the assistance of Alexander Hamilton.
   d. George Washington would probably not approve of modern political parties.

6. Which of the following statements is the best description of the author's purpose in writing this passage about George Washington?
    a. To caution American voters about being too political during election times because George Washington would not have agreed with holding elections
    b. To introduce George Washington to readers as a historical figure worthy of study
    c. To note that George Washington was more than a famous military hero
    d. To convince readers that George Washington is a hero of republicanism and liberty

7. In which of the following materials would the author be the most likely to include this passage?
    a. A history textbook
    b. An obituary
    c. A fictional story
    d. A newspaper editorial

Questions 8-12 are based on the following passage:

Christopher Columbus is often credited for discovering America. This is incorrect. First, it is impossible to "discover" somewhere that people already lived; however, Christopher Columbus did explore places in the New World that were previously untouched by Europe, so the term "explorer" would be more accurate. Another correction must be made, as well: Christopher Columbus was not the first European explorer to reach the present-day Americas! Rather, it was Leif Erikson who first came to the New World and contacted the natives, nearly five hundred years before Christopher Columbus.

Leif Erikson, the son of Erik the Red (a famous Viking outlaw and explorer in his own right), was born in either 970 or 980, depending on which historian you seek. His own family, though, did not raise Leif, which was a Viking tradition. Instead, one of Erik's prisoners taught Leif reading and writing, languages, sailing, and weaponry. At age 12, Leif was considered a man and returned to his family. He killed a man during a dispute shortly after his return, and the council banished the Erikson clan to Greenland.

In 999, Leif left Greenland and traveled to Norway where he would serve as a guard to King Olaf Tryggvason. It was there that he became a convert to Christianity. Leif later tried to return home with the intention of taking supplies and spreading Christianity to Greenland; however, his ship was blown off course and he arrived in a strange new land: present day Newfoundland, Canada".

When he finally returned to his adopted homeland Greenland, Leif consulted with a merchant who had also seen the shores of this previously unknown land we now know as Canada. The son of the legendary Viking explorer then gathered a crew of 35 men and set sail. Leif became the first European to touch foot in the New World as he explored present-day Baffin Island and Labrador, Canada. His crew called the land Vinland since it was plentiful with grapes.

During their time in present-day Newfoundland, Leif's expedition made contact with the natives whom they referred to as Skraelings (which translates to "wretched ones" in Norse). There are several secondhand accounts of their meetings. Some contemporaries described trade between the peoples. Other accounts describe clashes where the Skraelings defeated the Viking explorers with long spears, while still others claim the Vikings dominated the natives. Regardless of the circumstances, it seems that the Vikings made contact of some kind. This happened around 1000, nearly five hundred years before Columbus famously sailed the ocean blue.

Eventually, in 1003, Leif set sail for home and arrived at Greenland with a ship full of timber. In 1020, seventeen years later, the legendary Viking died. Many believe that Leif Erikson should receive more credit for his contributions in exploring the New World.

8. Which of the following best describes how the author generally presents the information?
   a. Chronological order
   b. Comparison-contrast
   c. Cause-effect
   d. Conclusion-premises

9. Which of the following is an opinion, rather than historical fact, expressed by the author?
   a. Leif Erikson was definitely the son of Erik the Red; however, historians debate the year of his birth.
   b. Leif Erikson's crew called the land Vinland since it was plentiful with grapes.
   c. Leif Erikson deserves more credit for his contributions in exploring the New World.
   d. Leif Erikson explored the Americas nearly five hundred years before Christopher Columbus.

10. Which of the following most accurately describes the author's main conclusion?
   a. Leif Erikson is a legendary Viking explorer.
   b. Leif Erikson deserves more credit for exploring America hundreds of years before Columbus.
   c. Spreading Christianity motivated Leif Erikson's expeditions more than any other factor.
   d. Leif Erikson contacted the natives nearly five hundred years before Columbus.

11. Which of the following best describes the author's intent in the passage?
   a. To entertain
   b. To inform
   c. To alert
   d. To suggest

12. Which of the following can be logically inferred from the passage?
   a. The Vikings disliked exploring the New World.
   b. Leif Erikson's banishment from Iceland led to his exploration of present-day Canada.
   c. Leif Erikson never shared his stories of exploration with the King of Norway.
   d. Historians have difficulty definitively pinpointing events in the Vikings' history.

Questions 13-17 are based on the chart following a brief introduction to the topic:

The American Civil War was fought from 1861 to 1865. It is the only civil war in American history. While the South's secession was the initiating event of the war, the conflict grew out of several issues like slavery and differing interpretations of individual state rights. General Robert E. Lee led the Confederate Army for the South for the duration of the conflict (although other generals held command positions over individual battles, as you will see next). The North employed a variety of lead generals, but Ulysses S. Grant finished the war as the victorious general. There were more American casualties in the Civil War than any other military conflict in American history.

Civil War Casualties by Battle (approximate)					
Battle	**Date**	**Union General**	**Confederate General**	**Union Casualties**	**Confederate Casualties**
Gettysburg	July 1863	George Meade	Robert E. Lee	23,049	28,063
Chancellorsville	May 1863	Joseph Hooker	Robert E. Lee	17,304	13,460
Shiloh	April 1862	Ulysses S. Grant	Albert Sydney Johnston	13,047	10,669
Cold Harbor	May 1864	Ulysses S. Grant	Robert E. Lee	12,737	4,595
Atlanta	July 1864	William T. Sherman	John Bell Hood	3,722	5,500

13. In which of the following battles were there more Confederate casualties than Union casualties?
    a. The one in May 1864
    b. Chancellorsville
    c. The one in April 1862
    d. Atlanta

14. Which one of the following battles occurred first?
    a. Cold Harbor
    b. Chancellorsville
    c. Gettysburg
    d. Shiloh

15. Robert E. Lee did NOT lead the Confederate forces in which one of the following battles?
    a. Atlanta
    b. The one in May 1863
    c. Cold Harbor
    d. Gettysburg

16. In which of the following battles did the Union casualties exceed the Confederate casualties by the greatest number?
    a. Cold Harbor
    b. Chancellorsville
    c. Atlanta
    d. Shiloh

17. The total number of American casualties suffered at the battle of Gettysburg is about double the total number of casualties suffered at which one of the following battles?
   a. Cold Harbor
   b. Chancellorsville
   c. Atlanta
   d. Shiloh

Question 18-19 are based on the graphic that follows a brief introduction to the topic:

The United States Constitution directs Congress to conduct a census of the population to determine the country's population and demographic information. The United States Census Bureau carries out the survey. In 1790, then Secretary of State Thomas Jefferson conducted the first census, and the most recent U.S. census was in 2010. The next U.S. census will be the first to be issued primarily through the Internet.

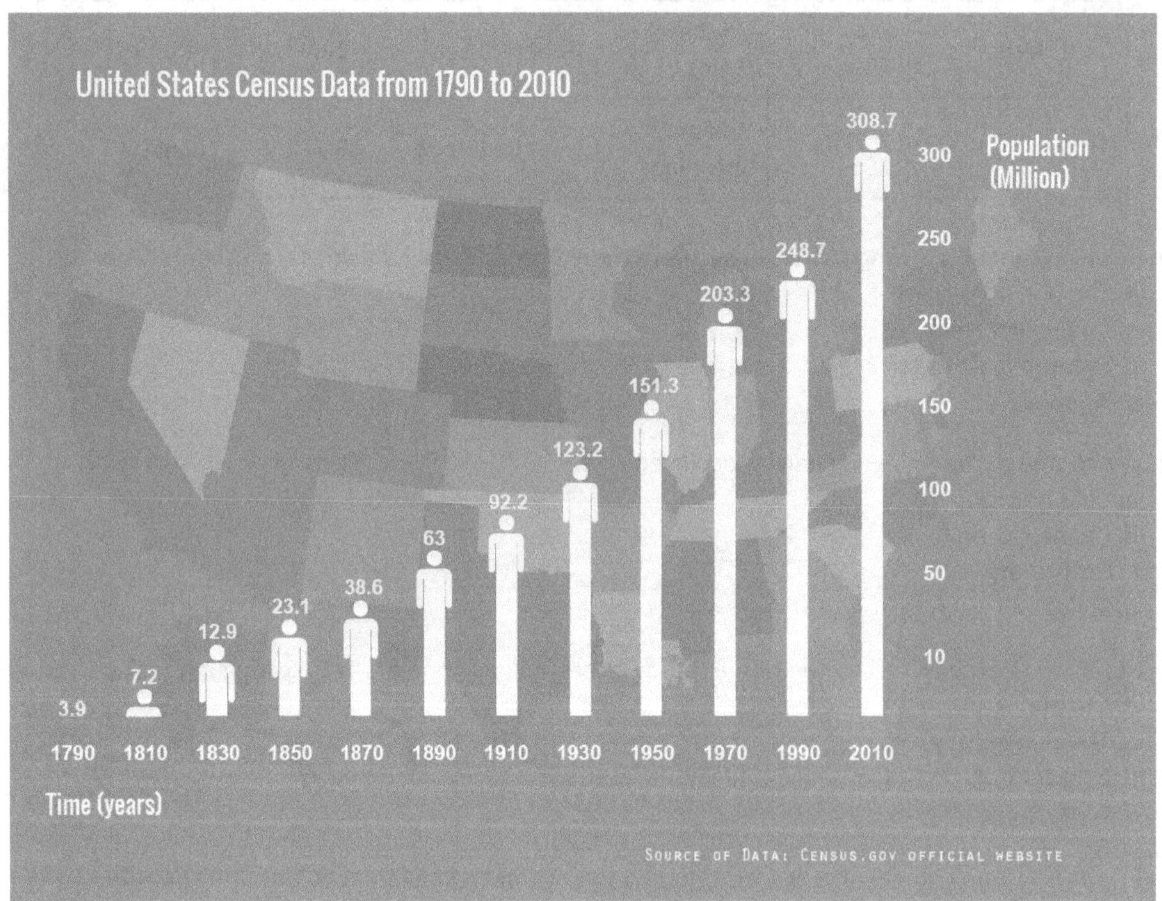

18. In which of the following years was the United States population less than it was in 1930?
   a. 1950
   b. 1970
   c. 1910
   d. 1990

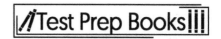

19. In which twenty-year interval did the population increase the most?
    a. From 1930 to 1950
    b. From 1950 to 1970
    c. From 1970 to 1990
    d. From 1990 to 2010

Questions 20-22 are based on the graphic following a brief introduction to the topic:

A food chain is a diagram used by biologists to better understand ecosystems. It represents the interrelationships between different plants and animals. The energy is derived from the sun and converted into stored energy by plants through photosynthesis, which travels up the food chain. The energy returns to the ecosystem after the organisms die and decompose back into the Earth. This process is an endless cycle.

In food chains, living organisms are grouped into categories called producers and consumers, which come in multiple tiers. For example, secondary consumers feed on primary consumers, while tertiary consumers feed on secondary consumers. Apex predators are the animals at the top of the food chain. They are the highest category consumer in an ecosystem, and apex predators do not have natural predators.

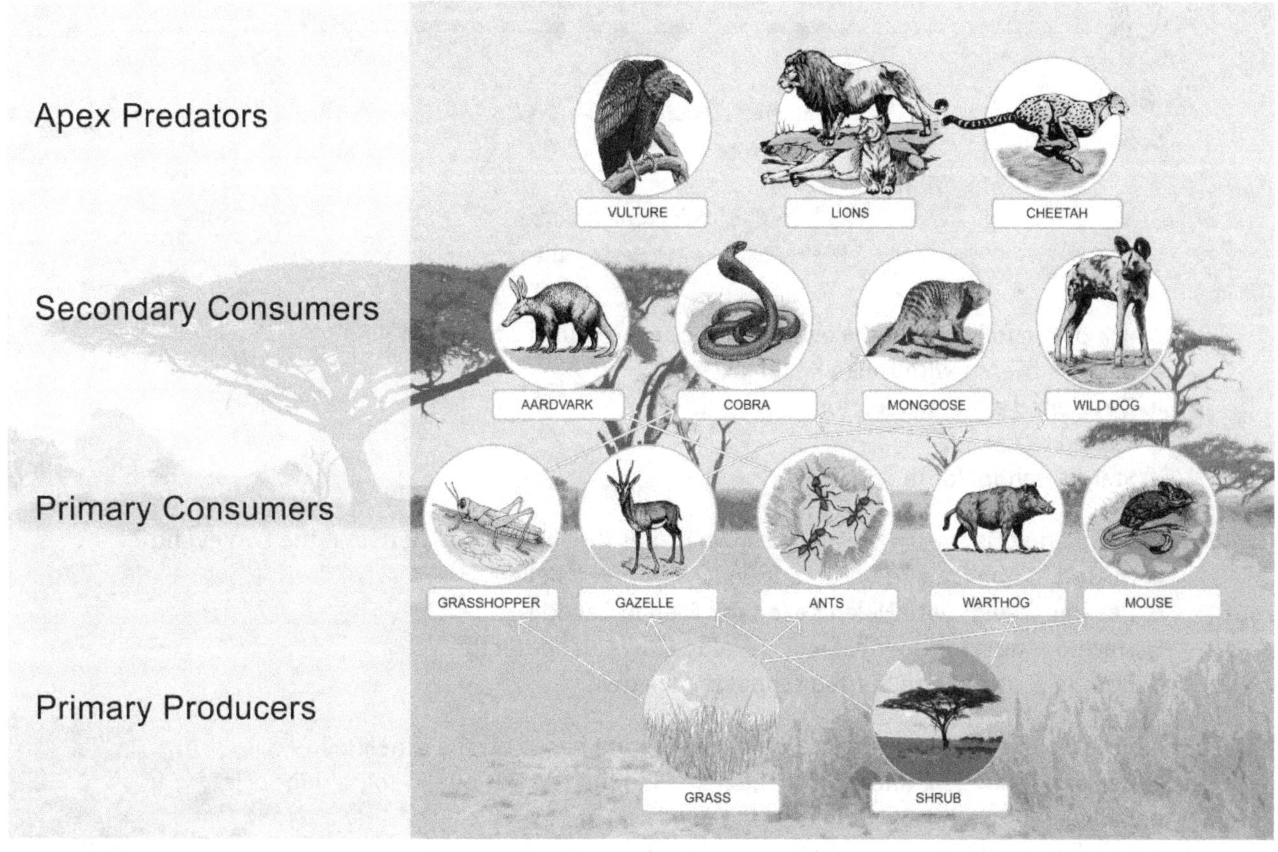

20. Which of the following eats primary producers according to the food chain diagram?
    a. Cobra
    b. Gazelle
    c. Wild dog
    d. Aardvark

21. Which of the following animals has no natural predators according to the food chain diagram?
    a. Vulture
    b. Cobra
    c. Grass
    d. Aardvark

22. Which of the following is something that the mongoose would eat?
    a. Shrub
    b. Aardvark
    c. Vulture
    d. Mouse

Questions 23-26 are based upon the following timeline:

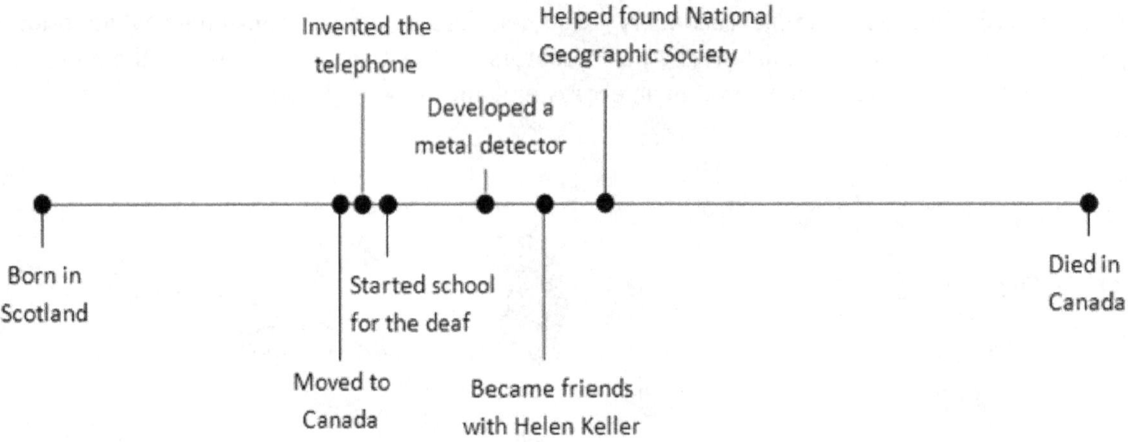

23. Which of the following is the event that occurred fourth on the timeline?
    a. Became friends with Helen Keller
    b. Developed a metal detector
    c. Moved to Canada
    d. Started school for the deaf

24. Of the pairings in the answer choices, which has the longest gap between the two events?
    a. Moved to Canada and Became friends with Helen Keller
    b. Became friends with Helen Keller and Died in Canada
    c. Started school for the deaf and Developed a metal detector
    d. Born in Scotland and Started school for the deaf

25. Which one of the following statements is accurate based on the timeline?
    a. Bell did nothing significant after he helped found the National Geographic Society.
    b. Bell started a school for the deaf in Canada.
    c. Bell lived in at least two countries.
    d. Developing a metal detector allowed Bell to meet Helen Keller.

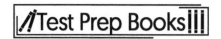

26. Which one of the following events occurred most recently?
    a. Bell's invention of the telephone
    b. Bell's founding the National Geographic Society
    c. Bell's birth
    d. Bell's move to Canada

Questions27-28 are based on the following graph of high school students:

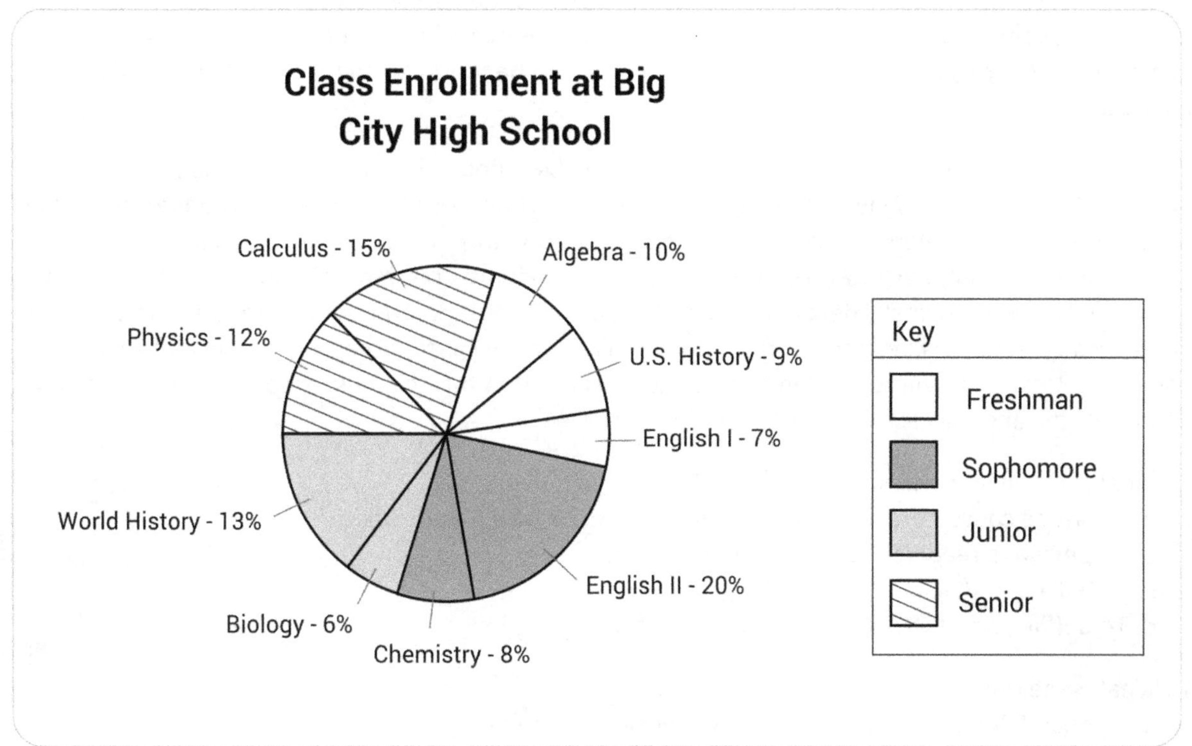

27. Which grade level has the most students in it?
    a. Freshman
    b. Sophomore
    c. Junior
    d. Senior

28. What percent of the school is made up of freshman?
    a. 26%
    b. 27%
    c. 28%
    d. 29%

Questions 29-34 are based on the following passage:

When researchers and engineers undertake a large-scale scientific project, they may end up making discoveries and developing technologies that have far wider uses than originally intended. This is especially true in NASA, one of the most influential and innovative scientific organizations in America. NASA *spinoff technology* refers to innovations originally developed for NASA space projects that are now used in a wide range of different commercial fields. Many consumers are unaware that products they are buying are based on NASA research! Spinoff technology proves that it is worthwhile to invest in science research because it could enrich people's lives in unexpected ways.

The first spinoff technology worth mentioning is baby food. In space, where astronauts have limited access to fresh food and fewer options about their daily meals, malnutrition is a serious concern. Consequently, NASA researchers were looking for ways to enhance the nutritional value of astronauts' food. Scientists found that a certain type of algae could be added to food, improving the food's neurological benefits. When experts in the commercial food industry learned of this algae's potential to boost brain health, they were quick to begin their own research. The nutritional substance from algae then developed into a product called life's DHA, which can be found in over 90% of infant food sold in America.

Another intriguing example of a spinoff technology can be found in fashion. People who are always dropping their sunglasses may have invested in a pair of sunglasses with scratch resistant lenses—that is, it's impossible to scratch the glass, even if the glasses are dropped on an abrasive surface. This innovation is incredibly advantageous for people who are clumsy, but most shoppers don't know that this technology was originally developed by NASA. Scientists first created scratch resistant glass to help protect costly and crucial equipment from getting scratched in space, especially the helmet visors in space suits. However, sunglasses companies later realized that this technology could be profitable for their products, and they licensed the technology from NASA.

29. What is the main purpose of this article?
    a. To advise consumers to do more research before making a purchase
    b. To persuade readers to support NASA research
    c. To tell a narrative about the history of space technology
    d. To define and describe instances of spinoff technology

30. What is the organizational structure of this article?
    a. A general definition followed by more specific examples
    b. A general opinion followed by supporting arguments
    c. An important moment in history followed by chronological details
    d. A popular misconception followed by counterevidence

31. Why did NASA scientists research algae?
    a. They already knew algae was healthy for babies.
    b. They were interested in how to grow food in space.
    c. They were looking for ways to add health benefits to food.
    d. They hoped to use it to protect expensive research equipment.

32. What does the word "neurological" mean in the second paragraph?
    a. Related to the body
    b. Related to the brain
    c. Related to vitamins
    d. Related to technology

33. Why does the author mention space suit helmets?
    a. To give an example of astronaut fashion
    b. To explain where sunglasses got their shape
    c. To explain how astronauts protect their eyes
    d. To give an example of valuable space equipment

34. Which statement would the author probably NOT agree with?
    a. Consumers don't always know the history of the products they are buying.
    b. Sometimes new innovations have unexpected applications.
    c. It is difficult to make money from scientific research.
    d. Space equipment is often very expensive.

Questions 35-40 are based on the following passage:

This excerpt is an adaptation of Robert Louis Stevenson's The Strange Case of Dr. Jekyll and Mr. Hyde.

> "Did you ever come across a protégé of his—one Hyde?" He asked.
>
> "Hyde?" repeated Lanyon. "No. Never heard of him. Since my time."
>
> That was the amount of information that the lawyer carried back with him to the great, dark bed on which he tossed to and fro until the small hours of the morning began to grow large. It was a night of little ease to his toiling mind, toiling in mere darkness and besieged by questions.
>
> Six o'clock struck on the bells of the church that was so conveniently near to Mr. Utterson's dwelling, and still he was digging at the problem. Hitherto it had touched him on the intellectual side alone; but now his imagination also was engaged, or rather enslaved; and as he lay and tossed in the gross darkness of the night in the curtained room, Mr. Enfield's tale went by before his mind in a scroll of lighted pictures. He would be aware of the great field of lamps in a nocturnal city; then of the figure of a man walking swiftly; then of a child running from the doctor's; and then these met, and that human Juggernaut trod the child down and passed on regardless of her screams. Or else he would see a room in a rich house, where his friend lay asleep, dreaming and smiling at his dreams; and then the door of that room would be opened, the curtains of the bed plucked apart, the sleeper recalled, and, lo! There would stand by his side a figure to whom power was given, and even at that dead hour he must rise and do its bidding. The figure in these two phrases haunted the lawyer all night; and if at anytime he dozed over, it was but to see it glide more stealthily through sleeping houses, or move the more swiftly, and still the more smoothly, even to dizziness, through wider labyrinths of lamplighted city, and at every street corner crush a child and leave her screaming. And still the figure had no face by which he might know it; even in his dreams it had no face, or one that baffled him and melted before his eyes; and thus there it was that there sprung up and grew apace in the lawyer's mind a singularly strong, almost an inordinate, curiosity to behold the features of the real Mr. Hyde. If he could but once set eyes on him, he thought the mystery would lighten and perhaps roll altogether away, as was the habit of mysterious things when well examined. He might see a reason for his friend's strange preference or bondage, and even for the startling clauses of the will. And at least it would be a face worth seeing: the face of a man who was without bowels of mercy: a face which had but to show itself to raise up, in the mind of the unimpressionable Enfield, a spirit of enduring hatred.
>
> From that time forward, Mr. Utterson began to haunt the door in the by street of shops. In the morning before office hours, at noon when business was plenty of time scarce, at night under the face of the full city moon, by all lights and at all hours of solitude or concourse, the lawyer was to be found on his chosen post.

"If he be Mr. Hyde," he had thought, "I should be Mr. Seek."

35. What is the purpose of the use of repetition in the following passage?

It was a night of little ease to his toiling mind, toiling in mere darkness and besieged by questions.

a. It serves as a demonstration of the mental state of Mr. Lanyon.
b. It is reminiscent of the church bells that are mentioned in the story.
c. It mimics Mr. Utterson's ambivalence.
d. It emphasizes Mr. Utterson's anguish in failing to identify Hyde's whereabouts.

36. What is the setting of the story in this passage?

a. In the city
b. On the countryside
c. In a jail
d. In a mental health facility

37. What can one infer about the meaning of the word "Juggernaut" from the author's use of it in the passage?

a. It is an apparition that appears at daybreak.
b. It scares children.
c. It is associated with space travel.
d. Mr. Utterson finds it soothing.

38. What is the definition of the word *haunt* in the following passage?

From that time forward, Mr. Utterson began to haunt the door in the by street of shops. In the morning before office hours, at noon when business was plenty of time scarce, at night under the face of the full city moon, by all lights and at all hours of solitude or concourse, the lawyer was to be found on his chosen post.

a. To levitate
b. To constantly visit
c. To terrorize
d. To daunt

39. The phrase *labyrinths of lamplighted city* contains an example of what?

a. Hyperbole
b. Simile
c. Juxtaposition
d. Alliteration

40. What can one reasonably conclude from the final comment of this passage?

"If he be Mr. Hyde," he had thought, "I should be Mr. Seek."

a. The speaker is considering a name change.
b. The speaker is experiencing an identity crisis.
c. The speaker has mistakenly been looking for the wrong person.
d. The speaker intends to continue to look for Hyde.

Questions 41-44 are based on the following passage:

Dana Gioia argues in his article that poetry is dying, now little more than a limited art form confined to academic and college settings. Of course, poetry remains healthy in the academic setting, but the idea of poetry being limited to this academic subculture is a stretch. New technology and social networking alone have contributed to poets and other writers' work being shared across the world. YouTube has emerged to be a major asset to poets, allowing live performances to be streamed to billions of users. Even now, poetry continues to grow and voice topics that are relevant to the culture of our time. Poetry is not in the spotlight as it may have been in earlier times, but it's still a relevant art form that continues to expand in scope and appeal.

Furthermore, Gioia's argument does not account for live performances of poetry. Not everyone has taken a poetry class or enrolled in university—but most everyone is online. The Internet is a perfect launching point to get all creative work out there. An example of this was the performance of Buddy Wakefield's *Hurling Crowbirds at Mockingbars*. Wakefield is a well-known poet who has published several collections of contemporary poetry. One of my favorite works by Wakefield is *Crowbirds*, specifically his performance at New York University in 2009. Although his reading was a campus event, views of his performance online number in the thousands. His poetry attracted people outside of the university setting.

Naturally, the poem's popularity can be attributed both to Wakefield's performance and the quality of his writing. *Crowbirds* touches on themes of core human concepts such as faith, personal loss, and growth. These are not ideas that only poets or students of literature understand, but all human beings: "You acted like I was hurling crowbirds at mockingbars / and abandoned me for not making sense. / Evidently, I don't experience things as rationally as you do" (Wakefield 15-17). Wakefield weaves together a complex description of the perplexed and hurt emotions of the speaker undergoing a separation from a romantic interest. The line "You acted like I was hurling crowbirds at mockingbars" conjures up an image of someone confused, seemingly out of their mind . . . or in the case of the speaker, passionately trying to grasp at a relationship that is fading. The speaker is looking back and finding the words that described how he wasn't making sense. This poem is particularly human and gripping in its message, but the entire effect of the poem is enhanced through the physical performance.

At its core, poetry is about addressing issues/ideas in the world. Part of this is also addressing the perspectives that are exiguously considered. Although the platform may look different, poetry continues to have a steady audience due to the emotional connection the poet shares with the audience.

41. Which one of the following best explains how the passage is organized?
    a. The author begins with a long definition of the main topic, and then proceeds to prove how that definition has changed over the course of modernity.
    b. The author presents a puzzling phenomenon and uses the rest of the passage to showcase personal experiences in order to explain it.
    c. The author contrasts two different viewpoints, then builds a case showing preference for one over the other.
    d. The passage is an analysis of another theory in which the author has no stake in.

42. The author of the passage would likely agree most with which of the following?
   a. Buddy Wakefield is a genius and is considered at the forefront of modern poetry.
   b. Poetry is not irrelevant; it is an art form that adapts to the changing time while containing its core elements.
   c. Spoken word is the zenith of poetic forms and the premier style of poetry in this decade.
   d. Poetry is on the verge of vanishing from our cultural consciousness.

43. Which one of the following words, if substituted for the word *exiguously* in the last paragraph, would LEAST change the meaning of the sentence?
   a. Indolently
   b. Inaudibly
   c. Interminably
   d. Infrequently

44. Which of the following is most closely analogous to the author's opinion of Buddy Wakefield's performance in relation to modern poetry?
   a. Someone's refusal to accept that the Higgs Boson will validate the Standard Model.
   b. An individual's belief that soccer will lose popularity within the next fifty years.
   c. A professor's opinion that poetry contains the language of the heart, while fiction contains the language of the mind.
   d. A student's insistence that psychoanalysis is a subset of modern psychology.

Questions 45-48 are based upon the following passage:

This excerpt is adaptation from Mineralogy --- Encyclopedia International, Grolier

Mineralogy is the science of minerals, which are the naturally occurring elements and compounds that make up the solid parts of the universe. Mineralogy is usually considered in terms of materials in the Earth, but meteorites provide samples of minerals from outside the Earth.

A mineral may be defined as a naturally occurring, homogeneous solid, inorganically formed, with a definite chemical composition and an ordered atomic arrangement. The qualification *naturally occurring* is essential because it is possible to reproduce most minerals in the laboratory. For example, evaporating a solution of sodium chloride produces crystal indistinguishable from those of the mineral halite, but such laboratory-produced crystals are not minerals.

A *homogeneous solid* is one consisting of a single kind of material that cannot be separated into simpler compounds by any physical method. The requirement that a mineral be solid eliminates gases and liquids from consideration. Thus, ice is a mineral (a very common one, especially at high altitudes and latitudes) but water is not. Some mineralogists dispute this restriction and would consider both water and native mercury (also a liquid) as minerals.

The restriction of minerals to *inorganically formed* substances eliminates those homogenous solids produced by animals and plants. Thus, the shell of an oyster and the pearl inside, though both consist of calcium carbonate indistinguishable chemically or physically from the mineral aragonite, are not usually considered minerals.

The requirement of a *definite chemical composition* implies that a mineral is a chemical compound, and the composition of a chemical compound is readily expressed by a formula. Mineral formulas may be simple or complex, depending upon the number of elements present and the proportions in which they are combined.

Minerals are crystalline solids, and the presence of an *ordered atomic arrangement* is the criterion of the crystalline state. Under favorable conditions of formation, the ordered atomic arrangement is expressed in the external crystal form. In fact, the presence of an ordered atomic arrangement and crystalline solids was deduced from the external regularity of crystals by a French mineralogist, Abbé R. Haüy, early in the 19th century.

45. According to the text, an object or substance must have all EXCEPT which of the following criteria to be considered a mineral?

a. Be naturally-occurring
b. Be a homogeneous solid
c. Be organically-formed
d. Have a definite chemical composition

46. What is the definition of the word "homogeneous" as it appears in the following sentence?

"A homogeneous solid is one consisting of a single kind of material that cannot be separated into simpler compounds by any physical method."

a. Made of similar substances
b. Differing in some areas
c. Having a higher atomic mass
d. Lacking necessary properties

47. The suffix *-logy* refers to which of the following?

a. The properties of
b. The chemical makeup of
c. The study of
d. The classification of

48. The author included the counterargument in the following passage to achieve which following effect?

The requirement that a mineral be solid eliminates gases and liquids from consideration. Thus, ice is a mineral (a very common one, especially at high altitudes and latitudes) but water is not. Some mineralogists dispute this restriction and would consider both water and native mercury (also a liquid) as minerals.

a. To complicate the subject matter
b. To express a bias
c. To point to the fact that there are differing opinions in the field of mineralogy concerning the characteristics necessary to determine whether a substance or material is a mineral
d. To create a new subsection of minerals

Answer Explanations

1. B: Narrative, Choice *A*, means a written account of connected events. Think of narrative writing as a story. Choice *C*, expository writing, generally seeks to explain or describe some phenomena, whereas Choice *D*, informative writing, may be an appealing choice since this passage is informative in some ways, but informative texts should be very objective in their language. In contrast, this passage is definitely persuasive writing, which hopes to change someone's beliefs based on an appeal to reason or emotion. The author is aiming to convince the reader that smoking is terrible. The author uses health, price, and beauty in his or her argument against smoking, so Choice *B*, persuasive, is the correct answer. Persuasive is another term for argumentative.

2. B: The author is clearly opposed to tobacco. He cites disease and deaths associated with smoking. He points to the monetary expense and aesthetic costs. Choices *A* and *C* are wrong because they do not summarize the passage, but rather are each just a premise. Choice *D* is wrong because, while these statistics are a premise in the argument, they do not represent a summary of the piece. Choice *B* is the correct answer because it states the three critiques offered against tobacco and expresses the author's conclusion.

3. C: We are looking for something the author would agree with, so it will almost certainly be anti-smoking or an argument in favor of quitting smoking. Choice *A* is wrong because the author does not speak against means of cessation. Choice *B* is wrong because the author does not reference other substances but does speak of how addictive nicotine, a drug in tobacco, is. Choice *D* is wrong because the author certainly would not encourage reducing taxes to encourage a reduction of smoking costs, thereby helping smokers to continue the habit. Choice *C* is correct because the author is definitely attempting to persuade smokers to quit smoking.

4. D: Here, we are looking for an opinion of the author's rather than a fact or statistic. Choice *A* is wrong because quoting statistics from the Centers of Disease Control and Prevention is stating facts, not opinions. Choice *B* is wrong because it expresses the fact that cigarettes sometimes cost more than a few gallons of gas. It would be an opinion if the author said that cigarettes were not affordable. Choice *C* is incorrect because yellow stains are a known possible adverse effect of smoking. Choice *D* is correct as an opinion because smell is subjective. Some people might like the smell of smoke, they might not have working olfactory senses, and/or some people might not find the smell of smoke akin to "pervasive nastiness," so this is the expression of an opinion. Thus, Choice *D* is the correct answer.

5. D: Although Washington was from a wealthy background, the passage does not say that his wealth led to his republican ideals, so Choice *A* is not supported. Choice *B* also does not follow from the passage. Washington's warning against meddling in foreign affairs does not mean that he would oppose wars of every kind, so Choice *B* is wrong. Choice *C* is also unjustified since the author does not indicate that Alexander Hamilton's assistance was absolutely necessary. Choice *D* is correct because the farewell address clearly opposes political parties and partisanship. The author then notes that presidential elections often hit a fever pitch of partisanship. Thus, it follows that George Washington would not approve of modern political parties and their involvement in presidential elections.

6. C: The author finishes the passage by applying Washington's farewell address to modern politics, so the purpose probably includes this application. Choice *A* does focus on modern politics, but it is incorrect. The passage does not state that it is the election process itself that George Washington would oppose; in fact, it mentions that he was also elected. Choice *B* is wrong because George Washington is already a well-established historical figure; furthermore, the passage does not seek to introduce him. Choice *D* is wrong because the author is not convincing readers. Persuasion does not correspond to the passage. Choice *C* states the primary purpose.

7. D: Choice *A* is wrong because the last paragraph is not appropriate for a history textbook, which should be strictly objective and research-based. Choice *B* is false because the piece is not a notice or announcement of Washington's death. Choice *C* is clearly false because it is not fiction, but a historical writing. Choice *D* is correct. The passage is most likely to appear in a newspaper editorial because it cites information relevant and applicable to the present day, a popular format in editorials.

8. D: The passage does not proceed in chronological order since it begins by pointing out Leif Erikson's explorations in America so Choice *A* does not work. Although the author compares and contrasts Erikson with Christopher Columbus, this is not the main way the information is presented; therefore, Choice *B* does not work. Neither does Choice *C* because there is no mention of or reference to cause and effect in the passage. However, the passage does offer a conclusion (Leif Erikson deserves more credit) and premises (first European to set foot in the New World and first to contact the natives) to substantiate Erikson's historical importance. Thus, Choice *D* is correct.

9. C: Choice *A* is wrong because it describes facts: Leif Erikson was the son of Erik the Red and historians debate Leif's date of birth. These are not opinions. Choice *B* is wrong; that Erikson called the land Vinland is a verifiable fact as is Choice *D* because he did contact the natives almost 500 years before Columbus. Choice *C* is the correct answer because it is the author's opinion that Erikson deserves more credit. That, in fact, is his conclusion in the piece, but another person could argue that Columbus or another explorer deserves more credit for opening up the New World to exploration. Rather than being an incontrovertible fact, it is a subjective value claim.

10. B: Choice *A* is wrong because the author aims to go beyond describing Erikson as a mere legendary Viking. Choice *C* is wrong because the author does not focus on Erikson's motivations, let alone name the spreading of Christianity as his primary objective. Choice *D* is wrong because it is a premise that Erikson contacted the natives 500 years before Columbus, which is simply a part of supporting the author's conclusion. Choice *B* is correct because, as stated in the previous answer, it accurately identifies the author's statement that Erikson deserves more credit than he has received for being the first European to explore the New World.

11. B: Choice *A* is wrong because the author is not in any way trying to entertain the reader. Choice *D* is wrong because he goes beyond a mere suggestion; "suggest" is too vague. Choice *C* is wrong for the same reason. Although the author is certainly trying to alert the readers of Leif Erikson's unheralded accomplishments, the nature of the writing does not indicate the author would be satisfied with the reader merely knowing of Erikson's exploration. Rather, the author would want the reader to be informed about it, which is more substantial (Choice *B*).

12. D: Choice *A* is wrong because the author never addresses the Vikings' state of mind or emotions. Choice *B* is wrong because the author does not elaborate on Erikson's exile and whether he would have become an explorer if not for his banishment. Choice *C* is wrong because there is not enough information to support this premise. It is unclear whether Erikson informed the King of Norway of his finding. Although it is true that the King did not send a follow-up expedition, he could have simply chosen not to expend the resources after receiving Erikson's news. It is not possible to logically infer whether Erikson told him. Choice *D* is correct because there are two examples—Leif Erikson's date of birth and what happened during the encounter with the natives—of historians having trouble pinning down important dates in Viking history.

13. D: The question asks which of the battles in the chart that are listed in this question had more Confederate casualties than Union casualties. There were more Confederate casualties than Union casualties at the Battles of Gettysburg and Atlanta. Of the two, only Atlanta is listed as an answer choice out of the battles explicitly listed or referred to by their dates. Thus, *D*, Atlanta, is the correct answer.

14. D: The question is asking you to find where the dates are located in the table and to identify the earliest battle. Answer *D*, Shiloh, occurred in April 1862 and no other battle listed on the table happened until May 1863. Choice *C*, Gettysburg, is listed first but did not occur first.

15. A: Robert E. Lee led the Confederate army in all battles listed on the table, except Shiloh and Atlanta. Looking at the dates and corresponding battles, as well as the battle explicitly listed, Shiloh is not listed as a choice; therefore Atlanta, Choice *A* is the correct answer.

16. A: This question is asking you to compare the Union and Confederate casualties and find the one listed where the Union casualties most exceeded the Confederate ones. At Cold Harbor, there were approximately 8,142 more Union casualties than Confederate. At Chancellorsville, there were approximately 3,844 more Union casualties. At Atlanta, the number of Confederate casualties exceeded the Union number, so it can be the correct answer. At Shiloh, there were approximately 2,378 more Union casualties. Thus, the number of Union casualties most greatly exceeding the Confederate number was at Cold Harbor, making Choice *A*, Cold Harbor, the correct answer.

17. D: To calculate the total American casualties, the Union and Confederate casualties need to be combined since it was a civil war with Americans on both sides. There were approximately 51,112 (Union + Confederate losses) American casualties at Gettysburg; thus, the correct answer will be a battle with approximately 25,556 casualties, which is half of that number. Shiloh is the closest with a total of 23,716 casualties, making Choice *D* the correct answer.

18. C: The correct answer is Choice *C*, 1910. There are two ways to arrive at the correct answer. You could find the four answer choices on the graph, or you could have identified that the population never dips at any point. Thus, the correct answer needs to be the only answer choice that is earlier in time than the others, which is Choice *C*.

19. D: The population increased the most between 1990 and 2010. The question is asking you to identify the rate of change for each interval. Between 1790 to 1810, the population increased by about 3.3 million. Between 1930 and 1950, the population increased by approximately 28 million. Between 1950 and 1970, the population increased by approximately 52 million. Between 1970 and 1990, the population increased by approximately 45 million. Between 1990 and 2010, the population increased by approximately 60 million. Thus, *D* is the correct answer. The slope is also the steepest in this interval, which represents its higher increase.

20. B: Primary producers make up the base of the food chain, so the correct answer will be in the level just above—a primary consumer. The cobra, wild dog, and aardvark are all secondary consumers. The gazelle is a primary consumer, so Choice *B* is the correct answer.

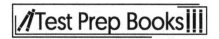

21. A: According to the passage preceding the food chain, the apex predators do not have natural predators. So, the question is really asking which of the answer choices is an apex predator. The cobra and aardvark are both secondary consumers. Grass is a primary producer. The vulture is an apex predator; thus, a vulture has no natural predators, making Choice A the correct answer.

22. D: A mongoose is a secondary consumer; thus, the mongoose consumes primary consumers. The shrub is a primary producer. The aardvark is a secondary consumer. The vulture is an apex predator. The mouse is a primary consumer, so Choice *D* is the correct answer.

23. D: This question is testing whether you realize how a timeline illustrates information in chronological order from left to right. "Started school for the deaf" is fourth on the timeline from the left, which means that it is the fourth event on the timeline. Thus, Choice *D* is the correct answer.

24. B: This question is asking you to determine the length of time between the pairs of events listed as answer choices. Events in timelines are arranged proportional to time. To determine the answer to this question, one must find the largest space between two events. Visually, this can be seen between the events of befriending Helen Keller and dying in Canada. Thus, Choice *B* is the correct answer.

25. C: This question is testing whether you can discern accurate conclusions from a timeline. Although the incorrect answer choices can seem correct, they cannot be confirmed from the information presented on the timeline. Choice *A* is incorrect; while it may be reasonable to assume that the timeline documents all major life events, we do not know for certain that Bell did not engage in any notable activities after founding the National Geographic Society. Choice *B* is incorrect because the timeline does not confirm that the school was in Canada; Bell actually started it in the United States. Choice *D* is incorrect because nothing on the timeline shows causation between the two events. Choice *C* is the only verifiable statement based on the timeline. Thus, *C* is the correct answer.

26. D: The founding of the National Geographic Society is the event listed farthest to the right of the events in the answer choices. This means it occurred most recently. Thus, *B* is the correct answer.

27. B: The sophomore class is made up of English II and Chemistry and encompasses 28% of the students. Freshman only make up 26% of the students, while Seniors make up 27%, and Juniors make up 19%.

28. A: To find this, add up the percent of Algebra, US History, and English I. This comes up to 26%.

29. D: To define and describe instances of spinoff technology. This is an example of a purpose question—*why* did the author write this? The article contains facts, definitions, and other objective information without telling a story or arguing an opinion. In this case, the purpose of the article is to inform the reader. The only answer choice that is related to giving information is answer Choice *D*—to define and describe.

30. A: A general definition followed by more specific examples. This organization question asks readers to analyze the structure of the essay. The topic of the essay is about spinoff technology; the first paragraph gives a general definition of the concept, while the following two paragraphs offer more detailed examples to help illustrate this idea.

31. C: This reading comprehension question can be answered based on the second paragraph—scientists were concerned about astronauts' nutrition and began researching useful nutritional supplements. Therefore, they were looking for ways to add health benefits to food. Choice *A,* in particular, is not true because it reverses the order of discovery (first, NASA identified algae for astronaut use, and then it was further developed for use in baby food).

32. B: This vocabulary question could be answered based on the reader's prior knowledge; but even for readers who have never encountered the word "neurological" before, the passage does provide context clues. The very next sentence talks about "this algae's potential to boost brain health," which is a paraphrase of "neurological benefits." From this context, readers should be able to infer that "neurological" is related to the brain.

33. D: This purpose question requires readers to understand the relevance of the given detail. In this case, the author mentions "costly and crucial equipment" before mentioning space suit visors, which are given as an example of something that is very valuable. Choice *A* is not correct because fashion is only related to sunglasses, not to NASA equipment. Choice *B* can be eliminated because it is simply not mentioned in the passage. While Choice *C* seems like it could be a true statement, it is also not relevant to what is being explained by the author. Instead, the purpose is to give an example of valuable space equipment.

34. C: The author would likely disagree with the statement: It is difficult to make money from scientific research. The article gives several examples of how businesses have been able to capitalize on NASA research, so it is unlikely that the author would agree with this statement. Evidence for the other answer choices can be found in the article: For Choice *A*, the author mentions that "many consumers are unaware that products they are buying are based on NASA research"; Choice *B* is a general definition of spinoff technology; Choice *D* is mentioned in the final paragraph.

35. D: It emphasizes Mr. Utterson's anguish in failing to identify Hyde's whereabouts. Context clues indicate that Choice *D* is correct because the passage provides great detail of Mr. Utterson's feelings about locating Hyde. Choice *A* does not fit because there is no mention of Mr. Lanyon's mental state. Choice *B* is incorrect; although the text does make mention of bells, Choice *B* is not the *best* answer overall. Choice *C* is incorrect because the passage clearly states that Mr. Utterson was determined, not unsure.

36. A: In the city. The word *city* appears in the passage several times, thus establishing the location for the reader.

37. B: It scares children. The passage states that the Juggernaut causes the children to scream. Choices *A* and *D* don't apply because the text doesn't mention either of these instances specifically. Choice *C* is incorrect because there is nothing in the text that mentions space travel.

38. B: To constantly visit. The mention of *morning*, *noon*, and *night* make it clear that the word *haunt* refers to frequent appearances at various locations. Choice *A* doesn't work because the text makes no mention of levitating. Choices *C* and *D* are not correct because the text makes mention of Mr. Utterson's anguish and disheartenment because of his failure to find Hyde but does not make mention of Mr. Utterson's feelings negatively affecting anyone else.

39. D: This is an example of alliteration. Choice *D* is the correct answer because of the repetition of the *L*-words. Hyperbole is an exaggeration, so Choice *A* doesn't work. No comparison or contrast is being made, so no simile or juxtaposition is being used, thus eliminating Choices *B* and *C*.

40. D: The speaker intends to continue to look for Hyde. Choices *A* and *B* are not possible answers because the text doesn't refer to any name changes or an identity crisis, despite Mr. Utterson's extreme obsession with finding Hyde. The text also makes no mention of a mistaken identity when referring to Hyde, so Choice *C* is also incorrect.

41. C: The author contrasts two different viewpoints, then builds a case showing preference for one over the other. Choice *A* is incorrect because the introduction does not contain an impartial definition, but rather, an opinion. Choice *B* is incorrect. There is no puzzling phenomenon given, as the author doesn't mention any peculiar cause or effect that is in question regarding poetry. Choice *D* does contain another's viewpoint at the beginning of the passage; however, to say that the author has no stake in this argument is incorrect; the author uses personal experiences to build their case.

42. B: Choice *B* accurately describes the author's argument in the text: that poetry is not irrelevant. While the author does praise, and even value, Buddy Wakefield as a poet, the author never heralds him as a genius. Eliminate Choice *A*, as it is an exaggeration. Not only is Choice *C* an exaggerated statement, but the author never mentions spoken word poetry in the text. Choice *D* is wrong because this statement contradicts the writer's argument.

43. D: *Exiguously* means not occurring often, or occurring rarely, so Choice *D* would LEAST change the meaning of the sentence. Choice *A*, *indolently*, means unhurriedly, or slow, and does not fit the context of the sentence. Choice *B*, *inaudibly*, means quietly or silently. Choice *C*, *interminably*, means endlessly, or all the time, and is the opposite of the word *exiguously*.

44. D: A student's insistence that psychoanalysis is a subset of modern psychology is the most analogous option. The author of the passage tries to insist that performance poetry is a subset of modern poetry, and therefore, tries to prove that modern poetry is not "dying," but thriving on social media for the masses. Choice *A* is incorrect, as the author is not refusing any kind of validation. Choice *B* is incorrect; the author's insistence is that poetry will *not* lose popularity. Choice *C* mimics the topic but compares two different genres, while the author does no comparison in this passage.

45. C: The text mentions all of the listed properties of minerals except the instance of minerals being organically-formed. Objects or substances must be naturally-occurring, must be a homogeneous solid, and must have a definite chemical composition in order to be considered a mineral.

46. A: Choice *A* is the correct answer because the prefix *homo-* means same. Choice *B* is incorrect because "differing in some areas" would be linked to the root word *hetero-*, meaning different or other.

47: C: Choice *C* is the correct answer because *-logy* refers to the study of a particular subject matter.

48: C: Choice *C* is the correct answer because the counterargument is necessary to point to the fact that researchers don't always agree with findings. Choices *A* and *B* are incorrect because the counterargument isn't overcomplicated or expressing bias, but simply stating an objective dispute. Choice *D* is incorrect because the counterargument is not used to persuade readers to create a new subsection of minerals.

Quantitative Reasoning

Basic Math

Fractions

This section starts with a review of a few basic terms for describing numbers.

Recall that *integers*, or whole numbers, are numbers that are used to count things; the integers also include negative numbers and zero. This means such numbers as -9, -2, 0, 4, and 14 are integers. However, the integers do not include fractions or numbers that have nonzero digits after the decimal point.

One integer is a *factor* of another integer if it divides it evenly into the second integer. For example, 4 is a factor of 8 because 4 divides evenly into 8. Integers for which 2 is a factor are called *even*; otherwise, they are called *odd*.

A *prime number* is an integer that is greater than one whose only factors are itself and one. The list of the first few prime numbers includes 2, 3, 5, 7, 11, 13, 17, and 19.

A *composite number* is any integer greater than one that is not a prime number.

The basic form of a fraction is $\frac{x}{y}$, where *x* and *y* are integers. By the definition of a fraction, $x \div y = \frac{x}{y}$. In the expression $\frac{x}{y}$, *x* is called the *numerator*, and *y* is called the denominator. The denominator can be any value except zero.

When working with fractions, the numerator and denominator can be multiplied or divided by the same number (other than zero) without changing the value of the fraction. This means $\frac{x}{y} = \frac{a \times x}{a \cdot y} = \frac{x \div a}{y \div a}$, as long as *a* and *y* are not zero; for example,

$$\frac{2}{5} = \frac{2 \cdot 2}{5 \cdot 2} = \frac{4}{10}$$

If *x* and *y* are integers that do not share any common factors, then the fraction is said to be *simplified*. In the example, $\frac{2}{5}$ is simplified, but $\frac{4}{10}$ is not.

With many fraction problems, the fractions may need to be rewritten so they all share the same denominator. This process is called *finding a common denominator* for the fractions. Given two fractions $\frac{a}{b}$ and $\frac{c}{d}$, multiply the numerator and the denominator of the left fraction by *d*, and multiply the numerator and the denominator of the right fraction by *b*. This operation results in the two fractions

$$\frac{a \times d}{b \times d} \text{ and } \frac{c \times b}{d \times b}$$

which share the common denominator $b \times d$.

The *reciprocal* or *multiplicative inverse* of the fraction $\frac{x}{y}$ is the fraction $\frac{y}{x}$.

As with integers, there are 4 basic arithmetic operations that can be performed with fractions: addition, subtraction, multiplication, and division.

To add fractions together, first rewrite them so they share a common denominator. Next, add the numerators together to get a new numerator. The denominator is the least common denominator.

Example: $\frac{2}{3} + \frac{5}{6} = \frac{4}{6} + \frac{5}{6} = \frac{9}{6} = \frac{3}{2}$.

In the last step, the fraction has been simplified by dividing the numerator and denominator by 3.

To subtract fractions, as with addition, first rewrite the fractions so they share a common denominator. Next, subtract the numerators to get a new numerator. The denominator remains the common denominator that was found.

Example: $\frac{2}{3} - \frac{5}{6} = \frac{4}{6} - \frac{5}{6} = -\frac{1}{6}$.

To multiply fractions, there is no need to find a common denominator. Instead, simply multiply the numerators to get the new numerator, and multiply the denominators to get the new denominator.

Example: $\frac{2}{3} \times \frac{5}{6} = \frac{2\times5}{3\times6} = \frac{10}{18} = \frac{5}{9}$.

In the last step, the fraction has been simplified by dividing the numerator and denominator by 2.

When multiplying fractions, it is sometimes possible to make the problem simpler by doing the following operation first: cancel factors that appear in the numerator of one fraction and in the denominator of the other fraction, and then multiply.

Example: $\frac{1}{3} \times \frac{12}{5} = \frac{3\times4}{3\times5} = 1 \times \frac{4}{5} = \frac{4}{5}$.

To divide fractions, multiply the first fraction by the reciprocal of the second fraction.

Example: $\frac{1}{3} \div \frac{5}{6} = \frac{1}{3} \times \frac{6}{5} = \frac{6}{15} = \frac{2}{5}$.

In the last step, the fraction has been simplified by dividing the numerator and denominator by 3.

A *proper fraction* has a smaller numerator than denominator. A *mixed number* has a larger numerator than denominator. It is possible to rewrite such mixed numbers as a combination of integers and proper fractions, if an answer in that format is desired.

For example, $\frac{6}{5} = \frac{5}{5} + \frac{1}{5} = 1 + \frac{1}{5}$, and can be written as $1\frac{1}{5}$.

Another operation closely related to multiplication is the *exponential*. This operation is written as x^n. In this expression, *x* is called the *base*, and *n* is called the *exponent*. When *n* is a positive integer, this indicates that *x* is multiplied by itself *n* times. For example

$$2^3 = 2 \times 2 \times 2 = 8$$

If the exponent is a negative integer, this means that the reciprocal of *x* is multiplied by itself *n* times.

For example, $3^{-2} = (\frac{1}{3})^2 = \frac{1}{3} \times \frac{1}{3} = \frac{1}{9}$.

When the exponent is zero, the result is always equal to one, even if the base is zero.

A *perfect square* is a whole number that is the square of another whole number. For example, 16 and 36 are perfect squares because 16 is the square of 4 and 36 is the square of 6.

When the exponent is 2, the operation is called *squaring* the base. When the exponent is 3, the operation is called *cubing* the base.

An exponent of $\frac{1}{n}$ for a positive integer *n* is also called an nth root, and can be written as $x^{\frac{1}{n}} = \sqrt[n]{x}$. The symbol on the right is also called a *radical*, and if the *n* is left blank next to the radical, it is assumed to be

$$2: \sqrt{x} = x^{\frac{1}{2}}$$

By definition, the nth root of *x* is the number that, when raised to the *n*-th power, results in *x*. That is, $(x^{\frac{1}{n}})^n = x$.

Here are the basic rules for working with exponents.

For any numbers a, b, m, n:

- $a^1 = a$.
- $1^a = 1$.
- $a^0 = 1$.
- $a^m \times a^n = a^{m+n}$.
- $a^m \div a^n = a^{m-n}$
- $(a^m)^n = a^{m \times n}$.
- $(a \cdot b)^m = a^m \cdot b^m$.
- $(a \div b)^m = a^m \div b^m = a^m \cdot b^{-m}$.

Using these rules, it is possible to determine the value of an exponential expression with any fractional exponent:

$$x^{\frac{m}{n}} = (x^{\frac{1}{n}})^m = (\sqrt[n]{x})^m$$

Note that for even roots of negative numbers, the result is an *imaginary number.*

The *order of operations* is a rule concerning the order in which to perform each operation in a mathematical expression. The rule is to do the operations in the following order.

1. Parentheses
2. Exponents
3. Multiplication
4. Division
5. Addition
6. Subtraction

Parentheses take top priority. The operations inside the parentheses are performed first.

To help remember this order, many students like to use the mnemonic PEMDAS. Some students associate this mnemonic with a phrase to help them, such as "Pirates Eat Many Donuts at Sea."

When working with radicals, it is often desirable to avoid having radicals in the denominator of the final answer. This operation is called *rationalizing the denominator*. To do this, multiply the numbers on the top and bottom by enough of the same radicals so the product in the denominator eliminates the radicals. This operation is best illustrated by an example. Consider $\frac{1}{\sqrt[3]{3}}$. To remove the radical from the denominator, multiply by $\frac{\sqrt[3]{3}^2}{\sqrt[3]{3}^2}$, as follows:

$$\frac{1}{\sqrt[3]{3}} = \frac{\sqrt[3]{3}^2}{\sqrt[3]{3}^2} \times \frac{1}{\sqrt[3]{3}} = \frac{\sqrt[3]{3}^2}{\sqrt[3]{3}^3} = \frac{\sqrt[3]{3}^2}{3}$$

One additional operation that is very useful when discussing certain probabilities is the *factorial*. The factorial $n!$ is defined for non-negative integers in the following manner: $0! = 1$, otherwise $n! = 1 \cdot 2 \cdot 3 \cdot \ldots \cdot n$.

Percentages

A percentage can be thought as a fraction with a denominator of 100. Thus, $22\% = \frac{22}{100}$. The word "percent" comes from a Latin phrase that means "by the hundred."

To convert a fraction to a percentage, the fraction is rewritten so that the denominator is 100.

Example: $\frac{2}{5} = \frac{40}{100} = 40\%$.

To convert a percentage to a fraction, the percentage is written over a denominator of 100, and then the result is simplified.

For example, $20\% = \frac{20}{100} = \frac{1}{5}$.

Decimals

A *decimal number* is a way of writing a number that uses a *decimal point* to show the part of the number that is a proper fraction. For example, 11.4 means 11 plus $\frac{4}{10} = 0.4$. The decimal point is indicated with a period in the United States (in some countries, a comma is used instead).

The *decimal place* of a digit in a decimal number describes the location of the digit relative to the decimal point, that is, how far to the right of the decimal point a digit appears. The first spot to the right of the decimal point is the *tenths* spot and indicates how many tenths are in the number. The second spot is the hundredths spot and indicates how many hundredths are in the number, and so on.

It is possible to convert a decimal to a percentage by multiplying the given percentage by 100, which just moves the decimal point to the right two places: $0.45 = 45\%$. To perform the opposite procedure and convert from a percentage to a decimal, divide the number by 100, which moves the decimal point to the left by two places: $11\% = 0.11$.

When working with decimals, it is sometimes easier to write a number by multiplying by a power of 10. A power of 10 can be written as 10^n, where *n* is an integer. The process of multiplying a decimal by 10^n shifts the decimal point *n* places to the right if *n* is positive, and *n* places to the left if *n* is negative. If necessary, extra zeros are used as placeholders.

For example, $2.5 \times 10^3 = 2500, 3.5 \times 10^{-2} = 0.035$.

When the non-decimal part of the first number is a single digit, this is known as *scientific notation*. Often, the number is rounded to only include a certain number of nonzero digits in scientific notation. For example, 2,503 might be rounded to 2.5×10^3.

A decimal number that is equal to some fraction is called a *rational number*. Rational numbers always have decimal expressions. Either the expressions *terminate*, meaning that beyond some point all their digits are zero, or the expressions *repeat*, meaning that their digits eventually repeat a pattern as they continue to the right. For example, $\frac{4}{3}$ has a decimal expression of 1.3333... where the 3 continues repeating infinitely. This number can be written by putting a bar over the digits that repeat: $1.\overline{3}$ indicates the 3 repeats infinitely. The number $1.1\overline{27}$ indicates that the 27 repeats infinitely, 1.127272727....

Decimal numbers that are not equal to any fraction are called *irrational*.

The *real numbers* are all the rational and irrational numbers.

Unit Conversions

Units express measured quantities. The idea is to compare a quantity to some fixed, standard quantity. For example, when measuring a distance, one can measure the distance in a multiple of a foot, which is a fixed, standard distance. One could also measure the distance as a multiple of a meter, which is another fixed, standard distance. Such standards exist for all kinds of physical quantities. When working with physical quantities, it is essential to keep track of which units are involved and to indicate the units in the answer

Converting between two different units requires knowledge of the ratio between the fixed standards. Given a quantity *x* in units *A*, to express the quantity in units of *B*, multiply *x* by the number of units of type *B* per unit of type *A*. For example, the ratio between centimeters (cm) and inches (in) is 2.54 cm/in, meaning there are 2.54 centimeters in every inch. To convert a distance of 4 inches to centimeters, the equation is $4 \times 2.54 = 10.16$. Therefore, the distance of 4 inches can also be expressed as 10.16 centimeters.

One way to help keep track of this is to think of the units as cancelling one another. If the units are written alongside the quantities, then one writes the previous example as $4 \text{ in} \times 2.54 \text{ cm/in} = 10.16\text{cm}$. The "inches" have cancelled one another. This quantity can also be written as

$$4 \text{ in} \times \frac{2.54 \text{ cm}}{1 \text{ in}} = 10.16 \text{ cm}$$

When converting between areas or volumes, if the ratio of the lengths is already known, one can use that ratio to find the area or volume. For example, there are 100 centimeters in every meter (m); that is, the conversion between lengths is 100 cm/m. If a problem requires converting 4 cubic meters, or 4 m^3, into centimeters, then, to cancel the 3 factors of the meter unit and get 3 factors of the centimeter unit, multiply by 100 cm/m 3 times:

$$4\ \text{m}^3 \times 100\frac{\text{cm}}{\text{m}} \times 100\frac{\text{cm}}{\text{m}} \times 100\frac{\text{cm}}{\text{m}} = 4{,}000{,}000\ \text{cm}^3$$

As this example shows, keeping track of the units involved is very important.

The conversion ratio from units *B* to units *A* is always the reciprocal of the conversion from *A* to *B*. The conversion from inches to centimeters is 2.54 cm/in, and the conversion from centimeters to inches is $\frac{1}{2.54}$ in/cm.

Log Base 10

A *logarithm* is the reverse operation of exponentiation. In this section, only logarithms with a base of 10 are considered. This operation can be written as $\log_{10} x$, although for base 10, sometimes the number is omitted and the logarithm is simply written as $\log x$. The basic definition of the logarithm with a base of 10 of the number *x*, when used as an exponent for 10, results in *x*. In other words, $10^{\log x} = x$. The obverse is also true: $\log 10^n = n$. The following are the rules for simplifying logarithms with a base of 10.

1. $\log_{10} 1 = 0$
2. $\log_{10} 10^p = p$
3. $\log_{10} MN = \log_{10} M + \log_{10} N$
4. $\log_{10} \frac{M}{N} = \log_{10} M - \log_{10} N$
5. $\log_{10} M^p = p \log_{10} M$

Ratios

A *ratio* expresses a proportional relationship between 2 quantities. It is generally written as $a{:}\,b$, which can be read as "*a* to *b*." A ratio behaves very much like a fraction. For example, one can multiply both sides of a ratio by the same constant without changing the relationship represented by that ratio. For example, 2:3 and 4:6 both express the same ratios. As with fractions, it is often desirable to express the final answer in a form in which the two sides of the ratio do not share any common factors.

Suppose an office building has 20 offices and 35 employees. The ratio of offices to employees is 20:35. To simplify this ratio, divide both sides by 5, resulting in a ratio of 4:7. This ratio means that in this building, there are 4 offices for every 7 employees.

For another example of applying ratios, suppose that in a school there are 50 girls and 65 boys. The ratio of girls to boys in this school is 50:65. Dividing both sides by 5 results in a ratio of 10:13. This means that in this school, there are 10 girls for every 13 boys.

Algebra

Expressions, Equations, and Inequalities

In algebra, letters are used to symbolize quantities. If these quantities are known and fixed so that they cannot change, then they are called *constants*. If the quantity is not known, or if it is any value from of a set of arbitrary values from some domain, then it is called a *variable*. Any letters can be chosen to represent a constant or a variable. Usually letters from the beginning of the alphabet, like *a*, *b*, and *c*, are used to represent constants, and letters from the end of the alphabet are used to represent variables, such as *x*, *y*, and *z*.

An *expression* is any mathematical statement involving constants, variables, numbers, and operations between them. Therefore, $x + 3$ is an expression, and so is $x^2 - 3x$. Expressions are the basic building blocks of statements that can be made in mathematics.

An *equation* is a mathematical statement that states 2 expressions are equal to one another. For example:

$$2x^3 - 3 = -x^2.$$

Given an equation, both sides of the equation can be multiplied or divided (by a nonzero quantity) by the same constant and get another true equation. Both sides of the equation can also be added or subtracted by the same quantity to get another true equation.

An *inequality* is a mathematical statement in which one expression is stated to be greater than, greater than or equal to, less than, or less than or equal to a second expression. In a *strict inequality*, such as $3 < x$, the two sides cannot equal one another. In *non-strict inequalities*, such as $4x \geq x^2$, the two sides can equal one another.

When working with inequalities, it is possible to add or subtract the same quantity to or from both sides and get another true inequality. However, when multiplying or dividing, some care must be used. When multiplying or dividing both sides by a positive value, the result is another true inequality. However, when multiplying or dividing by a negative quantity, the direction of the inequality must be reversed in order to get another true inequality. For example, given that $x < y$, when multiplying both sides by -1, the inequality must be reversed to the other direction, to get $-x > -y$.

Solving an equation is a common problem in algebra. A problem gives some equation(s) involving one or more variables and requires finding the variable(s) that will make the equation(s) true. To solve the equation, one generally tries to simplify the equation(s) involved until they are in a form in which one can read off the possible values for the variable. It is also often useful to use the following rule: if $ab = 0$, then either $a = 0$ or $b = 0$, or possibly both.

Similarly, to solve an inequality, one must find all possible values of the variable(s) that make the inequality true. The process of solving inequalities is very similar to solving equations. Specific techniques for solving equations are discussed below.

Evaluating Algebraic Expressions

Given an expression involving constants and variables, it is important to be able to evaluate these expressions for given values for the constants and variables. To do this, substitute the constants and variables with the numerical values given for them. This operation is perhaps most easily understood by looking at a few examples.

Consider the expression $3x^2 - x$. Suppose a problem asks for this expression to be evaluated when $x = 2$. To do so, replace each instance of *x* with the value *2*. The expression becomes $3 \times 2^2 - 2$. The next step is to apply the order of operations. First, simplify the exponent: $3 \times 4 - 2$. Then, apply the multiplication $12 - 2$. The last step is to subtract, which results in 10.

When one is substituting values into the expressions, and one is working with negative values, it is important to ensure that the *entire* value is substituted in for the variable or constant. Consider the example of evaluating $3x^2 - x$, but this time, for the case when $x = -2$. To do this properly, one must ensure that the entire given quantity gets squared and subtracted.

The result is $3(-2)^2 - (-2)$. This result simplifies to $3 \times 4 + 2 = 14$.

It is, of course, possible to evaluate expressions with multiple variables and constants. For example,

$$ax + b$$

when

$$a = 2, b = 3, x = \frac{1}{2}$$

As in the previous examples, replace each constant and variable with the given numerical quantity, which results in $2 \times \frac{1}{2} + 3$. The next step is to apply the order of operations. First, the multiplication is done, with the result of $1 + 3$. The last step is to add, which results in 4.

Sometimes, a problem may require one to simplify an expression that has several constants and variables, and to give values only for certain constants or variables. Consider the expression

$$ax^2 + a^2x$$

Suppose it is given that $a = 2$. Since there is no given quantity for x, x is simply left as a variable, while all the instances of a in this expression are replaced with 2. The result of that replacement is

$$2x^2 + 2^2x = 2x^2 + 4x$$

As discussed below, there are many instances where this kind of simplification is utilized in solving algebraic equations and inequalities.

Representing Verbal Quantitative Situations as Algebraic Expressions or Equations

When dealing with a word problem (that is, a "verbal quantitative situation"), the first step is to translate the problem into an appropriate mathematical expression, equation, or inequality. This requires the use of both mathematical knowledge and critical reasoning about the problem itself. The general process is to begin by labeling each quantity involved with a constant or a variable, and then write down the relationships between them.

For example, suppose a problem deals with a situation in which shirts at a store cost $10 each, plus 5% sales tax, and the problem asks for an expression for the amount, in dollars, that a person will spend on an arbitrary number of shirts. In other words, the number of shirts purchased is a variable that can be labeled as x. Now for each shirt, the person spends $10, plus 5% of $10 in sales tax. 5% of $10 is $0.05 \times 10 = 0.5$ dollars. The expression is the total money spent on shirts, which is $10x + 0.5x$, which simplifies to $10.5x$.

Now, suppose there is a problem in which a person is buying fruit; apples cost $1 each, and oranges cost $2 each. Suppose the problem asks for an expression for the total money spent on fruit, assuming the buyer buys only apples and oranges. Begin solving this problem by giving a label to each quantity. Let x

represent the number of apples purchased and y represent the number of oranges purchased. For each apple, the buyer spends \$1, and for each orange they spend \$2.

Therefore, the total amount spent, in dollars, is $1x + 2y = x + 2y$.

Using Linear Equations and Inequalities

A *linear equation* with one variable is an equation with a single variable that can be simplified to the form $ax + b = 0$. Thus, $ax + b = c$ is also a linear equation, since one could subtract the c from both sides to get zero on the right side so long as a, b, and c are held constant.

A *linear inequality* is just like a linear equation, except that it involves an inequality sign instead of an equals sign.

As previously mentioned, solving an equation means finding the values of the variable that make the equation true. The general approach is to try to isolate the variable on one side. For linear equations, this means to first move all the constants to one side and the variables to the other side. Then, divide both sides by the coefficient of the variable.

Thus, consider the equation

$$2x + 1 = -4x + 7$$

Begin solving this equation by subtracting 1 from each side, which results in

$$2x = -4x + 6$$

The next step is to add $4x$ to each side, which gives the equation $6x = 6$. Now, divide both sides by 6, which yields $x = 1$.

A linear equation with one variable always has a single solution, provided that the coefficient of x is not zero.

Solving linear inequalities proceeds in almost exactly the same fashion. However, it is important to keep in mind that multiplying or dividing by a negative number reverses the inequality. Consider the example

$$-2x > x + 6.$$

To solve this inequality, start by subtracting x from both sides. This results in the inequality

$$-3x > 6$$

The next step is to divide both sides by -3. However, this division reverses the inequality, which results in the new inequality $x < -2$.

Absolute Value in Equations and Inequalities

The absolute value of a number is the positive distance of a number from zero. If the number is positive, it is simply that number itself; if the number is negative, its absolute value is that number multiplied by negative one (-1). Therefore, the absolute value is always a non-negative quantity. The absolute value of x is written as $|x|$.

When dealing with equations that have an absolute value, one must split the solution into two cases: the case in which the quantity involved is non-negative, and the case in which it is negative.

Consider the equation

$$3x = |x| + 8$$

This equation can be split into two equations, each with a condition on x. First, if $x \geq 0$, the equation becomes

$$3x = x + 8, \text{ or } 2x = 8$$

which has the solution $x = 4$. This number is greater than or equal to zero, so it is a valid solution. The second case is if $x < 0$. Then the equation becomes

$$3x = -x + 8, \text{ or } 4x = 8$$

which has the solution $x = 2$. However, care is needed at this point, because of the extra conditions on x that were made when splitting the original equation into two. This second equation is only equivalent to the original equation when $x < 0$. Therefore, $x = 2$ is, in fact, *not* a solution to the original equation. The only solution to the original equation is $x = 4$.

Sometimes, the absolute value might be taken of a more complicated expression, for example, consider the equation

$$|2x - 1| = 5$$

Again, this equation can be split into two cases: first, if

$$2x - 1 \geq 0$$

This case is equivalent to saying $x \geq \frac{1}{2}$. In this case, the original equation becomes

$$2x - 1 = 5$$

This simplifies to the equation $2x = 6$, or $x = 3$. Since $3 \geq \frac{1}{2}$, this is a valid solution to the original equation. The second case is when

$$2x - 1 < 0$$

that is, when $x < \frac{1}{2}$. In this case, the equation becomes

$$-(2x - 1) = 5, \text{ or } 2x - 1 = -5$$

Continuing the process of solving this equation results in

$$2x = -4, x = -2$$

Since $-2 < \frac{1}{2}$, this is a valid solution to the original equation. Therefore, this equation has two real solutions: $x = 3$ and $x = -2$.

An absolute value inequality has two different forms. The first form is the inequality $|x| < a$. The value of x is less than *a*, but x is also greater than -*a*. For example, the inequality $|3x + 1| < 4$ can be rewritten as

$$3x + 1 < 4 \text{ and } -4 < 3x + 1$$

The two inequalities can be combined into one compound inequality:

$$-4 < 3x + 1 < 4$$

The inequality can be solved by first subtracting, with a result of

$$-5 < 3x < 3$$

The last step is to divide all values by 3, which yields $-\frac{5}{3} < x < 1$ as the solution set.

The second form is the inequality $|x| > a$. The value of x is greater than *a*, but x is also less than -*a*. For example, the inequality

$$|3x + 1| > 4$$

can be rewritten as

$$3x + 1 > 4 \text{ or } 3x + 1 < -4$$

Both inequalities can be solved by subtracting 1, with a result of

$$3x > 3 \text{ or } 3x < -5$$

The last step is to divide all values by 3, which yields $x < -\frac{5}{3}$ or $x > 1$ as the solution set.

Using Equations and Inequalities Involving Rational Expressions

A *rational expression* is an expression that has the form $\frac{p(x)}{q(x)}$, where $p(x)$ and $q(x)$ are both polynomials. To solve equations or inequalities involving rational expressions, the expression is typically rewritten to get rid of the denominator; as a result, the problem becomes an equation or inequality involving polynomials. One can then apply the techniques mentioned above to complete the solution.

For example, consider the problem $\frac{3x+2}{x-4} = 2$. One can start by multiplying both sides of the equation by $x - 4$. This results in the equation

$$3x + 2 = 2x - 8$$

Now this equation can be solved like any other linear equation. Subtracting $2x$ from both sides and subtracting 2 from both sides gives the solution $x = -10$.

Similarly, when dealing with inequalities, start by multiplying to eliminate the denominator. This multiplication introduces only one complication, namely, determining whether the direction of the inequality is changed. The direction might be changed on only a portion of the domain. Consider the inequality $\frac{3x+2}{x-4} < 2$. The first step is to multiply both sides by $x - 4$, but care is needed regarding when this multiplication changes the direction of the inequality. When $x - 4 \geq 0$, the result is the inequality

$$3x + 2 < 2x - 8$$

but when $x - 4 < 0$, the direction of the inequality changes, and the result is

$$3x + 2 > 2x - 8$$

Case 1: $x - 4 \geq 0$, $3x + 2 < 2x - 8$. Then, $x \geq 4$ and $x < -10$. Clearly, this cannot be true, so there are no solutions from this case.

Case 2: $x - 4 < 0$, $3x + 2 > 2x - 8$. Then, $x < 4$ and $x > -10$. This case has the solutions $-10 < x < 4$, which are the only solutions since there were not any solutions from the first case.

Solving Quadratic Equations and Inequalities

Algebraic expressions are built by adding and subtracting together *monomials*. A monomial is a variable raised to some whole number power, multiplied by a constant (called the *coefficient*): ax^n, where *a* is any constant and *n* is a whole number. A constant by itself is also a monomial.

A *polynomial* is a sum of monomials. If the highest power of x in the polynomial is 1, the polynomial is called *linear*. If the highest power of x is 2, it is called *quadratic*.

If the equation has the form $ax^2 - b = 0$, then it can be solved by adding *b* to both sides and dividing both sides by *a* to get $x^2 = \frac{b}{a}$. Then, the square root of both sides can be calculated. However, when taking the square root, it is necessary to remember that squaring a number gives the same result for both that number and its negative. When taking the square root of both sides, it is necessary to use a $\pm$ symbol to account for this fact: $x = \pm\sqrt{\frac{b}{a}}$. These are two separate solutions, unless *b* happens to be zero.

If a quadratic equation does not have a constant, that is, if the constant term is zero, it takes the form $ax^2 + bx = 0$. In this case, the x can be factored out to get $x(ax + b) = 0$. From this, the solution of this equation is $x = 0$ and the solution to the linear equation is $ax + b = 0$.

Given a quadratic expression that has been written in the form

$$x^2 + bx + c$$

one can attempt to factor the expression as $(x + A)(x + B)$ where $A + B = b$, and $AB = c$. It is sometimes possible to guess such a pair of numbers by looking at the positive and negative factors for *c*. In the expression

$$x^2 - 5x + 6$$

the factors of 6 are 1, 2, and 3. By experimenting a bit, it may be noticed that

$$(-2)(-3) = 6, \text{ and } -2 - 3 = -5$$

This means the expression can be rewritten as

$$x^2 - 5x + 6 = (x - 2)(x + 3)$$

To solve the equation

$$x^2 - 5x + 6 = 0$$

one could rewrite this equation as

$$(x - 2)(x + 3) = 0$$

The solutions of this equation are the solutions to $x - 2 = 0$ and $x - 3 = 0$, so the solutions are $x = 2, 3$.

If, during this procedure, the two terms obtained after factoring are the same, then the equation has only a single root, called a *double root*, and the equation has only one solution. For example, consider

$$x^2 - 4x + 4 = 0$$

Applying the above procedure, this equation can be factored into

$$(x - 2)(x - 2) = 0$$

This equation has only the one solution, $x = 2$, which is a double root.

In general, however, it may not be possible to easily guess a pair of numbers, *A, B*, that enable these kinds of expressions to be factored. In these cases, more general methods for solving quadratic equations are needed, methods that are sometimes a little longer than the ones given above. The two methods that follow always work for any quadratic equation.

The first approach that can always solve a quadratic equation is called *completing the square*. Suppose that a problem asks for the solutions to the equation

$x^2 + 2bx + c = 0$

(if necessary, divide by the coefficient of the squared term first to get the equation into this form). Then, some quantity can be added to both sides of the equation in order to make the left side have the form

$$x^2 + 2xb + b^2$$

Specifically, $b^2 - c$ would need to be added to both sides.

Here is an example to show how this works: Suppose the equation is

$$x^2 + 6x - 1 = 0$$

If the constant on the left side were 9, then this equation could be factored, since

$$x^2 + 6x + 9 = (x + 3)^2$$

Now, in order to get the constant on the left to be 9, 10 must be added to both sides. This gives the equation

$$x^2 + 6x + 9 = 10$$

It is now possible to factor the left side, which gives the equation

$$(x + 3)^2 = 10$$

At this point, the square root can be taken on both sides (but remember, this introduces a $\pm$), with a result of

$$x + 3 = \pm\sqrt{10}$$

Finally, subtract 3 from both sides to get two solutions: $x = -3 \pm \sqrt{10}$.

It is actually possible to perform the process of completing the square in a very general way to give a formula for the solutions to any quadratic equations. This formula is called the *quadratic formula*, and it can be used to solve any quadratic equation. However, because of its length, it can be easier to solve some quadratic equations by simply factoring them manually, rather than using the formula.

Here is a brief review of the derivation of the quadratic formula, since this can help in memorizing it. The derivation starts with the most general form of a quadratic equation,

$$ax^2 + bx + c = 0$$

First, divide both sides by a in order to begin the process of completing the square. This division results in the new equation

$$x^2 + \frac{b}{a}x + \frac{c}{a} = 0$$

Next, subtract $\frac{c}{a}$ on both sides to get

$$x^2 + \frac{b}{a}x = -\frac{c}{a}$$

and then add the quantity $(\frac{b}{2a})^2$ to both sides in order to complete the square. This gives

$$x^2 + \frac{b}{a}x + (\frac{b}{2a})^2 = (\frac{b}{2a})^2 - \frac{c}{a}$$

The left side is now the square of a single linear term, so it can now be factored. Performing this factoring and simplifying the right side results in

$$(x + \frac{b}{2a})^2 = \frac{b^2 - 4ac}{4a}$$

Next, take square roots on both sides to get

$$x + \frac{b}{2a} = \pm\frac{\sqrt{b^2 - 4ac}}{2a}$$

At last, it is possible to solve for x, which gives the quadratic formula:

$$x = \frac{-b \pm \sqrt{b^2 - 4ac}}{2a}$$

It is not necessary to remember how to derive this formula, but the formula itself should be memorized. Knowing where the formula comes from can help in remembering it, however. Note that if

$$b^2 - 4ac = 0$$

then the equation has only a single solution, and it is a double root.

To solve an inequality involving a quadratic term, one needs to use the fact that the value of a quadratic expression only changes sign when it passes through zero. So, once it is known when the two sides of an inequality are equal to one another, it is possible to tell when one side is bigger than the other by checking in between each of the places where they are equal.

For example, consider solving the inequality

$$x^2 - 1 > 3$$

Start by solving the equation

$$x^2 - 1 = 3$$

This is equivalent to $x^2 = 4$, or $x = \pm 2$. To determine when the inequality holds, then, one must only check the inequality for

$$x < -2,\ -2 < x < 2, \text{ and } x > 2$$

By substituting -3 for x, the inequality becomes

$$(-3)^2 - 1 > 3, \text{ or } 8 > 3$$

which is true. So, this inequality is true for $x < -2$. Similarly, substituting 3 for x gives

$$(3)^2 - 1 > 3, \text{ or } 8 > 3$$

which is true. So, this inequality is true for $x > 2$. However, checking the inequality by substituting zero for x gives the inequality $-1 > 3$, which is not true. So, the inequality is false for $-2 < x < 2$. It is also not true for $x = \pm 2$, since this is a strict inequality. Therefore, this inequality is true for $x < -2$ and $x > 2$.

Radicals in Equations and Inequalities

When an equation or an inequality involves radicals, all the radicals must be moved to one side. Then, both sides can be raised to the appropriate power to get rid of the radicals. Remember that the quantity inside a square root must be non-negative. When dealing with inequalities, remember that multiplying both sides by a negative quantity reverses the direction of the inequality.

For example, consider:

$$\sqrt{x+1} - 2 = 2$$

The first step is to isolate the radical, so add 2 to both sides. This addition results in:

$$\sqrt{x+1} = 4$$

Square both sides, and the result is:

$$x + 1 = 16, \text{ or } x = 15$$

When dealing with multiple radicals, proceed by first isolating one radical, squaring both sides to remove it, and then repeating this process to remove the remaining radicals. Consider the equation:

$$\sqrt{3x-1} + 1 = \sqrt{x+1} + 2$$

Start by subtracting 1 from both sides, isolating the radical on the left, which results in:

$$\sqrt{3x-1} = \sqrt{x+1} + 1$$

Then, square both sides:

$$3x - 1 = \left(\sqrt{x+1} + 1\right)^2 = x + 1 + 2\sqrt{x+1} + 1$$

or

$$3x - 1 = x + 2\sqrt{x+1} + 2$$

Isolate the radical on the right:

$$2x - 3 = 2\sqrt{x+1}$$

Next, square both sides, which results in:

$$4x^2 - 12x + 9 = 4x + 4$$

This problem can now be solved by using the quadratic formula.

The process to solve is similar for inequalities. For example, with:

$$\sqrt{x+1} - 2 > 2$$

the first step is to isolate the radical, so add 2 to both sides. This results in:

$$\sqrt{x+1} > 4$$

Then square both sides, which results in $x + 1 > 16$, or $x > 15$.

Another example is:

$$\sqrt{x+1} - 2 < 2$$

There are two inequalities. The first inequality is the original problem. The first step is to isolate the radical, so add 2 to both sides. This addition results in:

$$\sqrt{x+1} < 4$$

Square both sides, which result in

$$x + 1 < 16, \text{ or } x < 15$$

The second inequality is the radical, which has to be greater than or equal to zero since the radical must not be negative. In this case, the inequality is:

$$\sqrt{x+1} \geq 0$$

Square both sides; the result is:

$$x + 1 \geq 0 \text{ or } x \geq -1$$

The solution set for the inequality is $-1 \leq x < 15$.

Equations and Inequalities with Multiple Variables

A *system of equations* is a collection of equations all of which must hold true at the same time. Here are some basic rules to keep in mind when working with a system of equations.

- A single equation can be changed by doing the same operation to both sides, just as one could do if there were only one equation.
- *Substitution*: If one of the equations gives an expression for one of the variables in terms of other variables and constants, it is possible to substitute the expression into the other equations and replace the variable. This means the other equations will have one less variable in them.
- *Elimination*: If there are 2 equations of the form $a = b, c = d$, then it is possible to form a new equation $a + c = b + d$, or $a - c = b - d$. One of the variables is eliminated from an equation.

In general, solving a system of equations involves using substitution and elimination to find the possible values for one variable, and then substituting those values into the original equations and using them to continue to solve for the possible values of the other variables.

The simplest system of equations is a *linear* system of two equations. This means there are two equations in the form:

$$ax + by = c$$

$$dx + ey = f$$

To solve linear systems of two equations, either substitution or elimination can be used. Both methods will be used to solve a system of equations. Consider the following system of equations and solve by elimination first:

$$2x - 3y = 2$$
$$4x + 4y = 3$$

Start by multiplying the first equation on both sides by -2, which changes it into:

$$-4x + 6y = -4$$

Next, add this equation to the second equation, which will eliminate the x term:

$$4x + 4y - 4x + 6y = 3 - 4$$

simplifies to $10y = -1$. This equation can be solved for y, resulting in $y = -\frac{1}{10}$. Now, substitute this value for y into either of the original equations to solve for x. Substituting the result in the first equation results in:

$$2x - 3\left(-\frac{1}{10}\right) = 2$$

This equation can be solved like any linear equation with one variable; first the equation becomes:

$$2x + \frac{3}{10} = 2$$

then $2x = \frac{17}{10}$, and finally, $x = \frac{17}{20}$. So, this system of equations has the solution $x = \frac{17}{20}, y = -\frac{1}{10}$.

Start with the system of equations, and solve by substitution:

$$2x - 3y = 2,$$

$$4x + 4y = 3.$$

This time, solve the first equation to get an expression for y in terms of x. To do so, subtract $2x$ from both sides of the first equation, giving:

$$-3y = 2 - 2x$$

Next, divide both sides by -3, to get:

$$y = \frac{2}{3}x - \frac{2}{3}$$

Next, substitute this value in the second equation for y; the second equation then become:

$$4x + 4\left(\frac{2}{3}x - \frac{2}{3}\right) = 3$$

Since this equation only involves the variable x, it is possible to solve it to find the x-value, and then substitute this value for x back into $y = \frac{2}{3}x - \frac{2}{3}$ to find y.

The approach used to solve the equation does not affect the final answer. Some students are more comfortable using substitution and some students prefer to use elimination. It is best to be familiar with both approaches, because sometimes there is an obvious elimination or an easy substitution to be made.

Note that if one of the equations in the system of two equations can be made to look identical to another equation in the system, then it is redundant. The set of solutions is then all pairs that satisfy the other equation. For instance, in the system of equations

$$4x - 2y = 2, -8x + 4y = -4$$

it is possible to make the second equation into the first equation by dividing both sides by -4. This means the solution set is all pairs satisfying:

$$4x - 2y = 2, \text{ or } y = 2x - 1$$

To see whether one equation in a pair of linear equations is redundant, the simplest way is to rewrite each equation is in the form $ax + by = c$. The equations are redundant if one is a constant multiple of the other when written in this form, and the two together are called a *dependent system*. If the equations are not redundant, they are called *independent*.

It is also possible for two equations to be *inconsistent*. This happens when the system can be made into the form:

$$ax + by = c, ax + by = d$$

with *c* and *d* being different numbers. Another way to determine that the system is inconsistent is if, while trying to solve the system, one ends up with a contradictory equation, such as $3 = -2$.

In general, for a pair of linear equations with two variables, there is always a single solution if they are consistent but independent. There is a complete line of solutions if they are redundant. Finally, there are no solutions if they are inconsistent.

Solving a linear system of three equations with three variables can be very similar to the solution of the case with two equations and two variables. Once again, the goal is to eliminate variables, using the method of adding equations to eliminate variables, or substituting expressions for one variable into another equation. However, this time there are three equations and three variables to keep track of.

Consider the following system:

$$2x - y + 3z = 6$$

$$x + y + 2z = -1$$

$$3x - 2y + z = -1$$

Adding the first two equations will eliminate the y term, obtaining the new equation:

$$3x + 5z = 5$$

Multiply the second equation by 2; the result in:

$$2x + 2y + 4z = -2$$

Add this result to the third equation, and the y term is eliminated there as well, to get:

$$5x + 5z = -3$$

Subtract $3x + 5z = 5$ from this equation to get:

$$2x = -8, \text{ or } x = -4$$

Now, substitute this value for *x* in:

$$5x + 5z = -3$$

This equation becomes:

$$-20 + 5z = -3, \text{ or } z = \frac{17}{5}$$

Substitute both these values in the first, original equation to obtain

$$-8 - y + \frac{51}{5} = 6, \text{ or } y = -\frac{19}{5}$$

The solution to this system is $x = -4, y = -\frac{19}{5}, z = \frac{17}{5}$.

Functions

A *function* is defined as a relationship between inputs and outputs where there is only one output value for a given input. Take for example an equation that says that

$$y = 3x^2 - 1$$

Y is a function of x, since, for each value of x, there is a unique value of *y* that satisfies the equation.

One useful way to express this is to use *function notation*, in which the function itself is given a label. The letters that are used to label functions can, of course, be anything, but conventionally, functions are labeled with the letters *f*, *g*, and *h*. To emphasize the fact that the function *f* takes the variable x as its input, one can write $f(x)$, which is read "*f* of x." If there is a formula for how to compute the value of y from x, this can be expressed by setting $f(x)$ equal to this formula. In the case of the above example, this would be the equation:

$$f(x) = 3x^2 - 1$$

As another example, the following function is in function notation:

$$f(x) = 3x - 4$$

The $f(x)$ represents the output value for an input of x. If $x = 2$, the equation becomes:

$$f(2) = 3(2) - 4$$

$$f(2) = 6 - 4$$

$$f(2) = 2$$

The input of 2 yields an output of 2, forming the ordered pair $(2, 2)$. The following set of ordered pairs corresponds to the given function: $(2, 2), (0, -4), (-2, -10)$.

The set of values that x is allowed to take in $f(x)$ is called the *domain* of the function, and the set of possible outputs is called the *range* of the function. By definition, each member of the domain is paired with only one member of the range.

Unless a problem specifies otherwise, it is usually assumed the domain is all real numbers other than those for which the expression for $f(x)$ is not defined. For example, consider the function $f(x) = \frac{1}{x-2}$, the value $x = 2$ cannot be part of the domain (because the denominator would be zero). Unless the problem specifies a more restricted domain, the domain of this function is all real numbers except $x = 2$.

Functions can be represented multiple ways:

Multiple Representations of a Function

Mapping

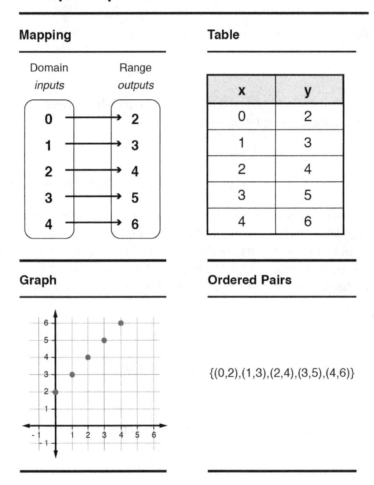

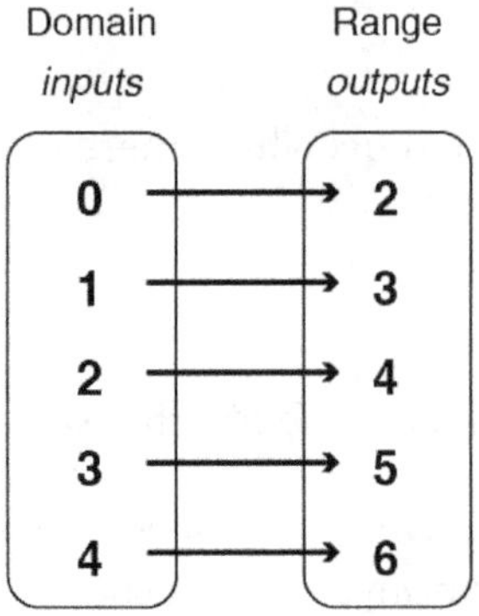

Domain *inputs* → Range *outputs*

0 → 2
1 → 3
2 → 4
3 → 5
4 → 6

Table

x	y
0	2
1	3
2	4
3	5
4	6

Graph

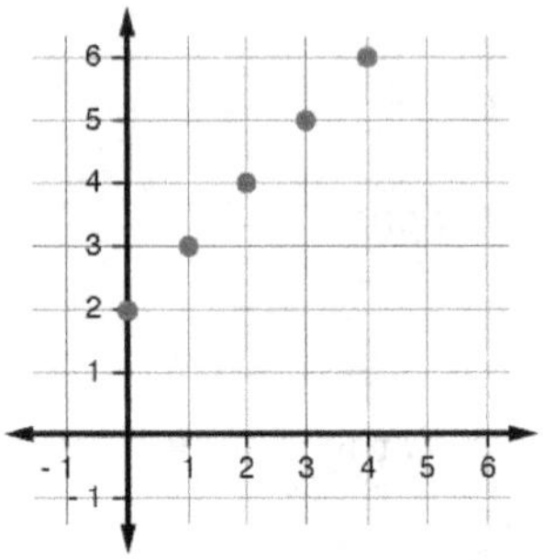

Ordered Pairs

{(0,2),(1,3),(2,4),(3,5),(4,6)}

Interval Notation

The domain of a function, as well as the range, is often expressed by using interval notation. Consider the function $f(x) = \sqrt{1 - x^2}$. This function is defined only when $|x| \leq 1$, or $-1 \leq x \leq 1$. This function can be expressed in interval notation as $x \in [-1, 1]$. Here are some other examples of interval notation.

$x > a$ can be written as $x \in (a, \infty)$.

$x \leq b$ can be written as $x \in (-\infty, b)$.

$x < a$ or $x \geq b$ can be written as $x \in (-\infty, a) \cup [b, \infty)$.

Square brackets indicate non-strict inequalities, and curved parentheses indicate strict inequalities.

If a variable y is a function of x, then x is called the *independent variable* and y is the *dependent variable*. These names come from the fact that in such a problem one often begins with some value of x and then determines how y depends upon that starting value.

To denote the value a function takes for some specific value of x, write that value in place of x in the function notation. Thus, $f(3)$ indicates the value that this function will take when x is equal to 3. If

$$f(x) = 3x^2 - 1, \text{then } f(3) = 3 \cdot 3^2 - 1 = 26.$$

Evaluating functions is exactly like evaluating expressions: substitute the given value into the expression for the function, and perform the indicated arithmetic operations using the order of operations.

Performing Algebraic Operations on Functions

Given a pair of functions $f(x)$ and $g(x)$, it is possible to form new functions by performing arithmetic operations between the functions. For example, one can get the new function:

$$(f + g)(x) = f(x) + g(x)$$

If the functions are $f(x)$ and $g(x)$, then it is possible to compute an expression for $(f + g)(x)$ by adding together those functions. For example, suppose that:

$$f(x) = 4x - 2 \text{ and } g(x) = x^2 - 2x$$

Then the expression for:

$$(f + g)(x) = (4x - 2) + (x^2 - 2x)$$

$$x^2 + 2x - 2$$

Similarly, one can subtract functions:

$$(f - g)(x) = f(x) - g(x)$$

When finding an expression for such subtraction of functions, it is very important to make sure to subtract the *entire* second function from the first function. With the functions from the previous paragraph, the subtraction is:

$$(f - g)(x) = (4x - 2) - (x^2 - 2x) = -x^2 + 6x - 2$$

Multiplying functions is accomplished similarly:

$$(f \times g)(x) = f(x) \times g(x)$$

Once again, when working out the formula for such a product, make sure to multiply both expressions completely. Using the same f and g, the result is

$$(f \times g)(x) = (4x - 2)(x^2 - 2x)$$

$$4x^3 - 8x^2 - 2x^2 + 4x = 4x^3 - 10x^2 + 4x$$

Finally, it is possible to divide functions. By definition:

$$(f/g)(x) = f(x)/g(x)$$

With the above examples:

$$(f/g)(x) = \frac{(4x-2)}{(x^2-2x)}$$

Determining Compositions of Functions

There is another way in which two functions can be combined, which is not an arithmetic operation. This is by *composing* two functions. Given two functions f and g, the composition of g with f is written $g^\circ f$, and it is defined by the equation:

$$(g^\circ f)(x) = g(f(x))$$

In other words, first apply the function f to x, and then apply g to the result.

The domain of such a function is some subset of the domain of f. Specifically, it is those values in the domain of f, such that the result when f yields something in the domain of g.

As a first example, consider the case where:

$$f(x) = 4x - 2 \text{ and } g(x) = x^2 - 2x$$

Suppose a problem asks for $g^\circ f$. To do this, one must substitute $f(x)$ for x in the formula for g. This substitution results in:

$$f(x)^2 - 2f(x)$$

Now, this can be plugged in the formula for f, which gives:

$$(g^\circ f)(x) = (4x-2)^2 - 2(4x-2)$$

This can now be simplified to give

$$16x^2 - 16x + 4 - 8x - 4 = 16x^2 - 24x$$

In this case, because both functions have a domain consisting of all real numbers, the composition has a domain of all real numbers as well.

Here is an example where care is needed regarding the domains. Consider the case where

$$g(x) = \sqrt{x-1}, f(x) = \frac{x}{2}$$

Computing $(g^\circ f)(x)$ by using the same approach first gives

$$\sqrt{f(x)-1}, \text{ and then } \sqrt{\frac{x}{2}-1}$$

The domain of f consisted of all real numbers, but this new function is defined only when $\frac{x}{2} - 1 \geq 0$, that is, when $x \geq 2$, or $x \in [2, \infty)$.

Determining Inverses of Functions

A function f is called "one to one" if, in the equation $y = f(x)$, there is a unique value of y for each unique value of x. In other words, f is one to one if, whenever $f(x_1) = f(x_2)$, it is the case that $x_1 = x_2$.

If a function f is one to one, then it is possible to define an *inverse function* for f. This is a function written as $f^{-1}(x)$, which is defined so that

$$f^{-1}(f(x)) = x$$

One way to find an inverse function is the following. Given a function f, write out the equation $x = f(y)$, and then solve for y. If f is one to one, the result is an equation of the form $y = g(x)$. The expression on the right side of this equation yields the formula for the inverse of f.

Here is an example of this procedure. Suppose that

$$f(x) = \frac{3x}{4} - 2$$

To find the inverse of f, apply the method given in the previous paragraph. Start by writing out the equation:

$$x = \frac{3y}{4} - 2$$

Now solve for y, which gives

$$\frac{3y}{4} = x - 2, \text{ or } y = \frac{4x}{3} + \frac{8}{3}$$

$$\text{So, } f^{-1}(x) = \frac{4x}{3} + \frac{8}{3}$$

Functions that are not one to one for all real numbers may be one to one on a restricted portion of their domain. For example, $f(x) = x^2$ is not one to one, because:

$$f(-a) = a^2 = f(a)$$

However, if the domain is restricted to non-negative x, then f is one to one, and it is possible to find an inverse: $x = y^2$ gives us $y = \pm\sqrt{x}$. This gives two possible values, which does not define a function. However, one may now use the fact that the original f only took values of x that were non-negative. This means that one does not need to consider the $-\sqrt{x}$ possibility. Therefore:

$$f^{-1}(x) = \sqrt{x}$$

Determining Maximum and Minimum Points

Finding the maximum and minimum points of general functions requires the use of calculus. However, for functions such as quadratics, it is possible to write down a general formula for the maximum or minimum point of the function.

Every quadratic function can be written in the form:

$$ax^2 + bx + c$$

The graph of a quadratic function $y = ax^2 + bx + c$ is defined as a *parabola*. Parabolas are vaguely U-shaped. If a is positive, then the U-shape opens upwards; if a is negative, the U-shape opens downwards. Parabolas that open upwards have a minimum point; parabolas that open downwards have a maximum point.

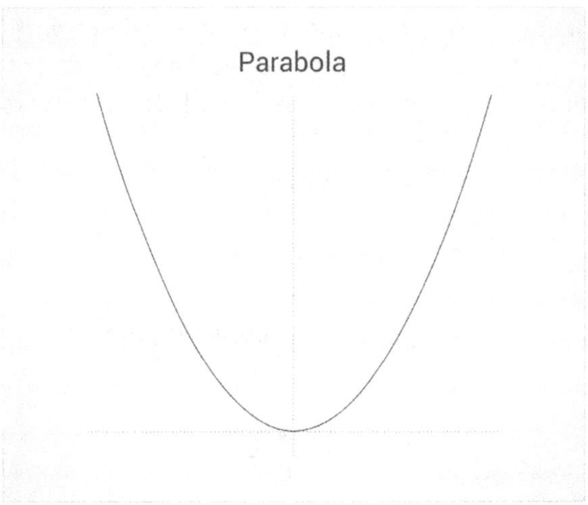

This high or low point is called the *vertex*. Note that a parabola is always symmetric about a vertical line (axis of symmetry). In the graphic above, the axis of symmetry is the line $x = 0$. To graph a parabola, its vertex and at least two points on each side of the axis of symmetry need to be determined.

Given a quadratic function in standard form:

$$y = ax^2 + bx + c$$

the axis of symmetry for its graph is the line $x = -\frac{b}{2a}$. For the quadratic function:

$$y = 2x^2 + 8x - 3$$

$$a = 2 \text{ and } b = 8$$

The axis of symmetry can be calculated as follows: $x = -\frac{8}{2(2)}$, so $x = -2$ is the axis of symmetry. The vertex for the parabola has an *x*-coordinate of $-\frac{b}{2a}$. To find the *y*-coordinate for the vertex of the previous example, the calculated *x*-coordinate needs to be substituted into the original function. Because the axis of symmetry passes through the vertex, the x-coordinate is -2.

The y-coordinate is:

$$y = 2(-2)^2 + 8(-2) - 3 = -11$$

The vertex is $(-2, -11)$. To complete the graph, two different *x*-values need to be selected and substituted into the quadratic function to obtain the corresponding *y*-values. This will give two points on the parabola. These two points and the axis of symmetry are used to determine the two points corresponding to these. The corresponding points are the same distance from the axis of symmetry (on the other side) and contain the same *y*-coordinate. Plotting the vertex and four other points on the parabola allows for constructing the curve.

When finding minimum or maximum values, the y or f(x) value is the only value needed for the answer. Whether that value represents the minimum or maximum, depends on if the parabola opens upwards or downwards. For example, the height of a baseball is given, in feet, by $h(t) = -32t^2 + 16t + 4$. Suppose the problem asks for the highest height the baseball will reach. Clearly it does have some maximum point because the coefficient of t^2 is negative. The time value (t) in this example represents the x-coordinate of the vertex. This value needs to be found first using the formula $-\frac{b}{2a}$ where:

$$a = -32, b = 16, c = 4$$

The value of t is:

$$-\frac{16}{2(-32)} = \frac{1}{4}$$

Substituting this value into the expression gives the maximum height of the baseball:

$$h(t) = -32t^2 + 16t + 4$$

$$h\left(\frac{1}{4}\right) = -32\left(\frac{1}{4}\right)^2 + 16\left(\frac{1}{4}\right) + 4$$

$$h\left(\frac{1}{4}\right) = -2 + 4 + 4$$

$$h\left(\frac{1}{4}\right) = 6$$

Probability and Statistics

In general, probability and statistics deal with relationships between quantities, which may not be exact. For example, a graduating student's salary tends to be higher when that student has a higher GPA, but this correlation need not always be the case. People who exercise regularly tend to live longer than those who do not, but once again, this is not always the case. Probability is the way in which one measures these types of tendencies. Statistics, which is closely related, can be broken into two main parts: descriptive statistics and inferential statistics. Descriptive statistics is the process of analyzing the tendencies of a given population, and inferential statistics is the process of using such an analysis of a sample group to make inferences about the population as a whole. Descriptive statistics includes such things as computing the average score on a test administered to a class. Inferential statistics includes such things as polling a few hundred people in a city to find out their salaries, and then trying to use this information to determine the likely salaries of other people in the city.

Measures of Central Tendency

Given a set X of data points $\{x_1, x_2, x_3, \ldots x_n\}$, one would like to have some way to describe the general tendencies of these data. One of the first questions that can be asked is where the "center" of the data lies. There are a few different ways to measure this. Each describes a slightly different notion of the "center."

The first measure the central tendency of a data set is the arithmetic *mean*, or the average, of the data. The definition of the mean is the following: first add up all the data points, and then divide by the total number of data points in our data set. A convenient way to write this out is to use *summation notation*. To be precise, the mean of the data set *X* is written as

$$\bar{X} = \frac{x_1 + x_2 + x_3 + \cdots + x_n}{n} = \frac{1}{n}\sum_{i=1}^{n} x_i$$

As an example, consider a test given to five students. Suppose the scores on the test were 55, 65, 65, 75, 80, 85, 90, 100. Then, the average test score is the following:

$$\frac{(55+65+65+75+80+85+90+100)}{8} = 76.875.$$

The mean is particularly useful for describing the central tendency when the distribution of data is close to normal, which means that the frequency of different outcomes among our data has a single peak and that the data is approximately equally distributed on both sides of that peak. However, the mean can be somewhat less useful in situations when the data are divided into several different groups that are widely separated, or when there are some *outliers*, which are data points that are very far from the rest of the data. For an example of widely separated data groups, consider a group of six people. Suppose three of these people make $20,000 per year, and three make $100,000 per year. Then the average income of these six people, in dollars, is

$$\frac{3 \cdot 20000 + 3 \cdot 100000}{6} = 60{,}000$$

However, none of the people actually makes anything close to $60,000 per year. For an example of how outliers can throw off data, consider a group of nine students who take a test. Suppose four get a score of 90, four get a score of 100, and one gets a score of 0. Then the average is

$$\frac{4 \cdot 90 + 4 \cdot 100 + 0}{9} = 84.\bar{4}$$

However, the average of the top five students is 95. So, this outlier strongly affects the mean.

Another measurement of central tendency that can be defined is the *median*. Given a data set *X* consisting of data points $x_1, x_2, x_3, \ldots x_n$, the median is defined as the value of the data point in the center, in the sense that half the data lies before it and half lies after it. Therefore, if *n* is odd, the median is defined as $x_{\frac{n+1}{2}}$. However, if *n* is even, the median is defined as $\frac{1}{2}\left(x_{\frac{n}{2}} + x_{\frac{n}{2}+1}\right)$, which is the mean of the two data points closest to the middle of the data points. Consider a group of 5 people whose ages are 19, 21, 22, 22, and 25. The median age of this group is 22.

Although outliers can have a substantial effect upon the mean of a data set, they usually do not change the median very much. For example, consider the following list of numbers: 2, 4, 5, 6, 6, 7. This list has a mean of 5 and a median of 5.5. Now suppose the last number in the list is changed to 99, so that the list is now 2, 4, 5, 6, 6, 99. This list has an average of $20.\bar{3}$, but the median is still 5.5.

One final measure of central tendency that is defined for *X* is the *mode*. The mode is defined as the data point that appears most frequently in the data set; if two or more data points are tied for the most frequent appearance, each is defined as a mode. This means a data set might have multiple modes. For instance, in the following list of numbers, 55, 60, 65, 65, 70, 80, 85, 85, 90, 95, there are two modes: 65 and 85.

Variation

The next problem in statistics is how to measure the degree to which the data are spread out. Given a data set *X* with data points $\{x_1, x_2, x_3, \dots x_n\}$, the *variance* of *X* is defined as:

$$\frac{\sum_{i=1}^{n}(x_i - \bar{X})^2}{n}$$

(recall that $\bar{X}$ indicates the mean). In other words, the variance of *X* is the mean of the squares of the differences between each data point and the mean of *X*.

Given a data set *X* with data points $\{x_1, x_2, x_3, \dots x_n\}$, define the *standard deviation* of *X* as:

$$\sigma_X = \sqrt{\frac{\sum_{i=1}^{n}(x_i - \bar{X})^2}{n}}$$

In other words, the standard deviation is the positive square root of the variance. The symbol for the standard deviation is the Greek lowercase letter *sigma*.

The variance and the standard deviation are both measures of how much the data points are spread out. A low variance or standard deviation means that the data are clumped up closely, and a large variance or standard deviation generally means that the data are either very spread out or that there are a substantial number of outliers.

Consider an example of computing the variance and the standard deviation. Suppose a problem asks for the standard deviation for the data set {2, 3, 3, 4}. Begin by computing the mean, which is:

$$\frac{2+3+3+4}{4} = \frac{12}{4} = 3$$

Now, continue by computing the variance, which is, in summation notation:

$$\frac{1}{4}\sum_{i=1}^{4}(x_i - \bar{X})^2 \frac{1}{4}((2-3)^2 + (3-3)^2 + (3-3)^2 + (4-3)^2)$$

$$\frac{1}{4}(1^2 + 0^2 + 0^2 + 1^2)$$

$$\frac{2}{4}$$

$$\frac{1}{2}$$

Therefore, the variance is $\frac{1}{2}$. To find the standard deviation, take the square root:

$$\sqrt{\frac{1}{2}} = \frac{1}{\sqrt{2}} \times \frac{\sqrt{2}}{\sqrt{2}} = \frac{\sqrt{2}}{\sqrt{4}} = \frac{\sqrt{2}}{2}$$

One last measurement of the variation of a data set is the *range*. The range is the difference between the largest and the smallest values in the set.

Graphical Forms of Data

In some cases, it can be very useful to visualize statistical data by graphical means. Statistical data are typically visualized by making a graph where the horizontal axis represents the possible values that the data can take, and the vertical axis represents the frequency with which the data takes that value. These graphs are called *frequency plots*.

Suppose there is a situation in which the data takes the values 1, 2, 3, 4, and 5. Suppose there are 4 instances of 1, 5 instances of 2, 7 instances of 3, 5 instances of 4, and 6 instances of 5. A frequency plot for this situation might look like the following:

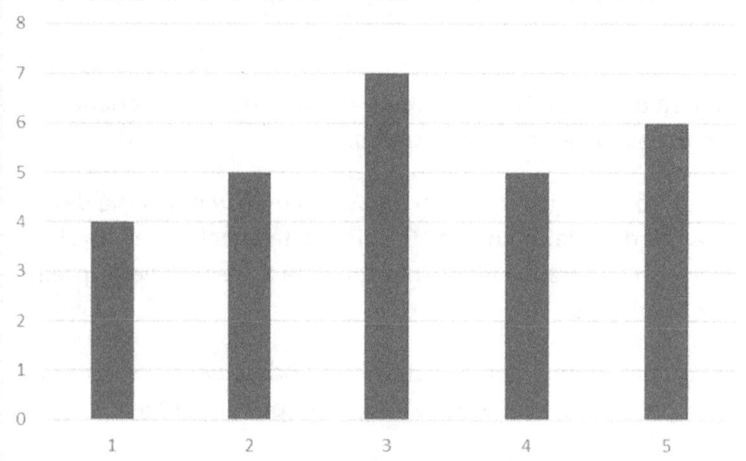

From the frequency plot, it is possible to immediately read off the modes of the data: the modes are the values that have the tallest columns. In this case, the mode is 3. Given a frequency plot, it is possible to easily read off the number of data points that take a given value by checking the height of the column for that value. For this reason, frequency plots are convenient ways of quickly displaying the data.

To determine the median, note that there is a total of 27 data points here, so the median is the thirteenth data point. The thirteenth data point in this case has a value of 3, so the median is 3.

To find the mean, use the formula given above. In this case, the formula results in the following:

$$\frac{1}{27}(4 \times 1 + 5 \times 2 + 7 \times 3 + 5 \times 4 + 6 \times 5) = \frac{85}{27} = 3.15$$

Interpreting Displays of Data

A set of data can be visually displayed in various forms to allow for quick identification of characteristics of the set. Histograms, such as the one shown below, display the number of data points (vertical axis) that fall into given intervals (horizontal axis) across the range of the set. The histogram below displays the heights of black cherry trees in a certain city park. Each rectangle represents the number of trees with heights between a given five-point span. For example, the furthest bar to the right indicates that two trees are between 85 and 90 feet. Histograms can describe the center, spread, shape, and any unusual characteristics of a data set.

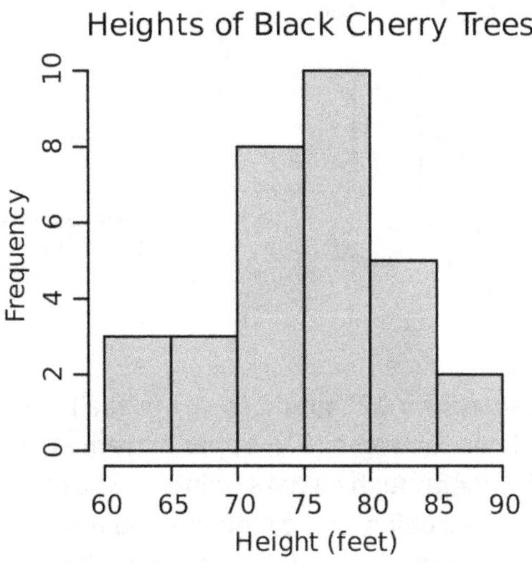

A box plot, also called a box-and-whisker plot, divides the data points into four groups and displays the five-number summary for the set, as well as any outliers. The five-number summary consists of:

- The lower extreme: the lowest value that is not an outlier
- The higher extreme: the highest value that is not an outlier
- The median of the set: also referred to as the second quartile or Q_2
- The first quartile or Q_1: the median of values below Q_2
- The third quartile or Q_3: the median of values above Q_2

To construct a box (or box-and-whisker) plot, the five-number summary for the data set is calculated as follows: the second quartile (Q_2) is the median of the set. The first quartile (Q_1) is the median of the values below Q_2. The third quartile (Q_3) is the median of the values above Q_2. The upper extreme is the highest value in the data set if it is not an outlier (greater than 1.5 times the interquartile range: Q_3- Q_1). The lower extreme is the least value in the data set if it is not an outlier (more than 1.5 times lower than the interquartile range). To construct the box-and-whisker plot, each value is plotted on a number line, along with any outliers. The box consists of Q_1 and Q_3 as its top and bottom and Q_2 as the dividing line inside the box. The whiskers extend from the lower extreme to Q_1 and from Q_3 to the upper extreme.

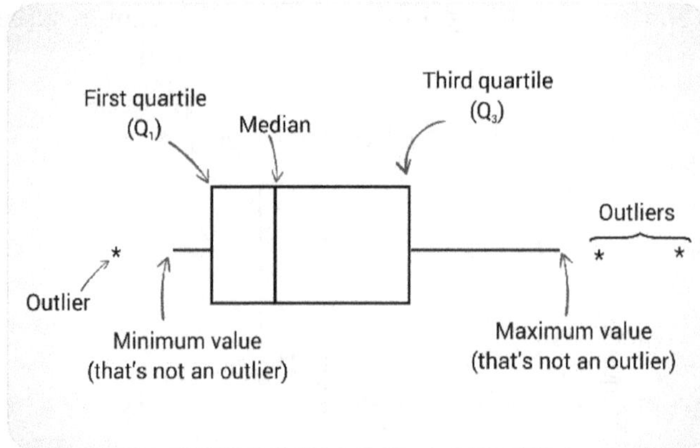

Suppose the box plot displays IQ scores for 12th grade students at a given school. The five-number summary of the data consists of: lower extreme (67); upper extreme (127); Q_2 or median (100); Q_1 (91); Q_3 (108); and outliers (135 and 140). Although all data points are not known from the plot, the points are divided into four quartiles each, including 25% of the data points. Therefore, 25% of students scored between 67 and 91, 25% scored between 91 and 100, 25% scored between 100 and 108, and 25% scored between 108 and 127. These percentages include the normal values for the set and exclude the outliers. This information is useful when comparing a given score with the rest of the scores in the set.

A scatter plot is a mathematical diagram that visually displays the relationship or connection between two variables. The independent variable is placed on the x-axis, or horizontal axis, and the dependent variable is placed on the y-axis, or vertical axis. When visually examining the points on the graph, if the points model a linear relationship, or a line of best-fit can be drawn through the points with the points relatively close on either side, then a correlation exists. If the line of best-fit has a positive slope (rises from left to right), then the variables have a positive correlation. If the line of best-fit has a negative slope (falls from left to right), then the variables have a negative correlation. If a line of best-fit cannot be drawn, then no correlation exists. A positive or negative correlation can be categorized as strong or weak, depending on how closely the points are graphed around the line of best-fit.

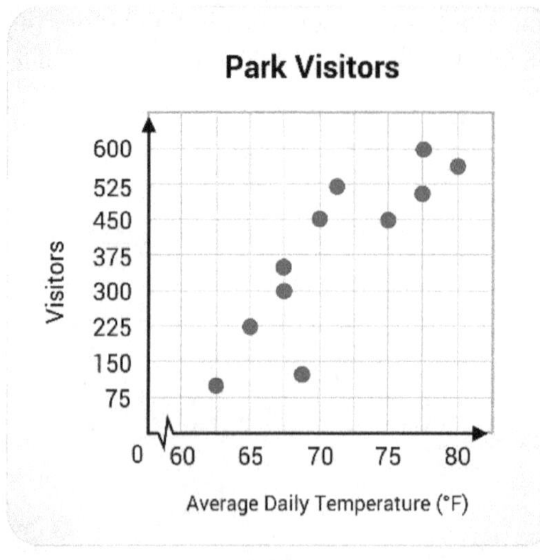

Probability

Given a set of possible outcomes *X*, a *probability distribution* on *X* is defined to be a function that assigns a probability to each possible outcome. If the set *X* consists of $\{x_1, x_2, x_3, \dots x_n\}$, and the probability distribution is the function *p*, then the following must be true of *p*:

1. $0 \leq p(x_i) \leq 1$, for any *i*.
2. $\sum_{i=1}^{n} p(x_i) = 1$.

The first rule says that *p* must always take a value between zero and one. The second rule says that the total probability for all the possible outcomes in *X* is one.

If $p(x_i)$ is a constant function, then this is called a *uniform probability distribution*, and $p(x_i) = \frac{1}{n}$, where *n* is the total number of possible outcomes. A good example of this is a fair 6-sided die, in which the possible outcomes are 1, 2, 3, 4, 5, and 6, and the probability of each of these 6 outcomes is $\frac{1}{6}$.

To determine the probability of an outcome occurring from a range *A* of possible outcomes, write this probability as $P(A)$. To compute this, add up the probabilities for each outcome in *A*. To use the example of a fair 6-sided die, consider the problem of finding the probability of getting a 2 or a lower number when the die is rolled. The possible rolls are 1, 2, 3, 4, 5, and 6. So to get a 2 or lower, one must roll a 1 or a 2. Each probability is $\frac{1}{6}$; add the probablities together to get:

$$p(1) + p(2) = \frac{1}{6} + \frac{1}{6} = \frac{1}{3}$$

Below are a few types of probability distributions that are standard and have standard names.

The binomial distribution: This distribution describes the probability of getting *k* successes in *n* trials, where each trial can either succeed or fail. Suppose the probability of a single trial's being a success is *p*. Then, the probability of getting *k* successes in *n* trials is:

$$\frac{n!}{k!\,(n-k)!} p^k (1-p)^{n-k}$$

A Poisson distribution: This describes the probability of getting *k* events in a fixed interval of time. Suppose the average number of events during this time interval is λ. Then, the probability of getting *k* events during this time interval is given by:

$$\frac{\lambda^k e^{-\lambda}}{k!}$$

Conditional Probabilities

In some cases, it may be known that the outcome lies within the subset of possibilities *B*, and a problem asks for the probability that the outcome will be inside another subset of possibilities *A*. This kind of problem concerns a *conditional probability*. A conditional probability is written as $P(A|B)$, which is read as "the probability of *A* given *B*." The formula for this quantity in general is:

$$P(A|B) = \frac{P(A \cap B)}{P(B)}$$

In the case of uniform probability distributions, it is possible to simplify this formula somewhat. It is standard notation to write $|A|$ to indicate the total number of outcomes in A. Then, if one is dealing with a uniform probability distribution, it is possible to write:

$$P(A|B) = \frac{|A \cap B|}{|B|}$$

(remember, $A \cap B$ means "A intersect B," and is the set of all outcomes that lie in both A and B). So, in this case there is no need to know how many total outcomes there might be; all that one needs to know is the total in B and the total in $A \cap B$.

To understand why this works, suppose that a set of outcomes X is $\{x_1, x_2, x_3, \dots x_n\}$, so that $|X| = n$, and the probability distribution on X is a uniform probability distribution p. Then $p(x_i) = \frac{1}{n}$ for each x_i. Then, from the definition of a uniform probability distribution:

$$P(A) = |A| \cdot \frac{1}{n} = \frac{|A|}{n}$$

Similar formulas are obtained for:

$$P(B) = \frac{|B|}{n} \text{ and } (A \cap B) = \frac{|A \cap B|}{n}$$

Substituting this formula into the formula for conditional probabilities results in:

$$(A|B) = \frac{P(A \cap B)}{P(B)}$$

$$\frac{\frac{|A \cap B|}{n}}{\frac{|B|}{n}} = \frac{|A \cap B|}{|B|}$$

because the n's cancel out.

As an application of this principle, suppose a fair die is rolled. It is known that the roll's value lies between 1 and 4, inclusive, but the number of sides that the die has is not known (not all dice are 6-sided). Suppose the problem asks for the probability that the roll was higher than 2. In this case, the total number of sides of the die is unimportant, and, because this is a fair die, the probability distribution is uniform across all possibilities. Therefore, it is possible to apply the formula $\frac{|A \cap B|}{|B|}$. In this particular problem, B is {1, 2, 3, 4} and $A \cap B$ is {3, 4}. Therefore:

$$\frac{|A \cap B|}{|B|} = \frac{2}{4} = \frac{1}{2}$$

Conditional probability is very important in probability because often the likelihood of one outcome can change substantially after some additional information about the outcome is given. For example, if someone wants to know the probability that a student will pass a test, they could look at the statistics about how many students usually pass that test. However, if they also know that the student in question has spent a lot of time studying, then they know it is much more likely the student will pass (although nothing is guaranteed).

In many cases, changing the order of the conditional probabilities greatly affects the outcome. Consider determining the probability that a person with heart trouble is a person who has exercised regularly, versus the probability of a person who does regular exercise coming down with heart trouble. As another example, given a person who has received a military medal, it is certain that the person served in the military. However, given that a person served in the military, the probability of their receiving a military medal may not be very high.

In some special cases, however, the order in which the conditional probabilities are taken does not change the final probability. Consider the situation in which the probability of A does not change when B is given, that is, the situation where

$$P(A|B) = P(A)$$

In this case, A and B are said to be *independent*. The fact

$$P(A|B) = \frac{P(A \cap B)}{P(B)} = P(A)$$

means that if A and B are independent

$$P(A \cap B) = P(A)P(B)$$

From the equation

$$P(A \cap B) = P(A)P(B)$$

one can perform this computation in reverse to also show that

$$P(A|B) = P(A), \text{ and } P(B|A) = P(B)$$

Therefore, when A is independent of B, B is also independent of A.

A situation in which one would expect the outcomes to be independent is in rolling a pair of dice. Suppose that one rolls 2 dice: a white die and a black die. Then, one would expect that the number that is obtained from the white die should not depend upon the number that is obtained from the black die, or vice versa. The same principle applies to a situation in which one rolls a single die repeatedly. A similar situation applies to flipping a coin repeatedly: whether the next flip is heads or tails does not depend upon the results of previous flips.

Of course, this can be counterintuitive, because in cases as rolling a die or flipping a coin, there is occasionally a series of surprising results, for example, a person might get 5 tails in a row while flipping a coin. But if the probability distribution is already known, then this occurrence is simply random. In fact, if a person keeps flipping a coin or rolling a die for a long while, it is very likely that some unlikely series of outcomes will sometimes occur.

A similar mistake in reasoning about probabilities is the idea that a low-probability outcome is necessarily surprising. Of course, getting a low-probability outcome in a single try would be surprising, but in reality, there are so many things going on at all times that there are almost certain to be a few low-probability occurrences. A good illustration of this phenomenon can be seen in lotteries. The odds of a given person's winning the lottery are low. On the other hand, the odds that some person will win the lottery each week are reasonably high, and people are not surprised when they find out that somebody has won. For a similar reason, one should, in general, not be too surprised by the occurrence of some seemingly-unlikely events.

Statistical Concepts

Statistics involves making decisions and predictions about larger sets of data based on smaller data sets. The information from a small subset can help predict what happens in the entire set. The smaller data set is called a *sample* and the larger data set for which the decision is being made is called a *population.* The three most common types of data-gathering techniques are sample surveys, experiments, and observational studies. *Sample surveys* involve collecting data from a random sample of people from a desired population. The measurement of the variable is only performed on this set of people. To have accurate data, the sampling must be unbiased and random. For example, surveying students in an advanced calculus class on how much they enjoy math classes is not a useful sample if the population should be all college students based on the research question. There are many methods to form a random sample, and all adhere to the fact that every sample that could be chosen has a predetermined probability of being chosen. Once the sample is chosen, statistical experiments can then be carried out to investigate real-world problems.

An *experiment* is the method in which a hypothesis is tested using a trial-and-error process. A cause and the effect of that cause are measured, and the hypothesis is accepted or rejected. Experiments are usually completed in a controlled environment where the results of a control population are compared to the results of a test population. The groups are selected using a randomization process in which each group has a representative mix of the population being tested. Finally, an *observational study* is similar to an experiment. However, this design is used when there cannot be a designed control and test population because of circumstances (e.g., lack of funding or unrealistic expectations). Instead, existing control and test populations must be used, so this method has a lack of randomization.

A statistical question is answered by collecting data with variability. Data consists of facts and/or statistics (numbers), and variability refers to a tendency to shift or change. Data is a broad term, inclusive of things like height, favorite color, name, salary, temperature, gas mileage, and language. Questions requiring data as an answer are not necessarily statistical questions. If there is no variability in the data, then the question is not statistical in nature. Consider the following examples: what is Mary's favorite color? How much money does your mother make? What was the highest temperature last week? How many miles did your car get on its last tank of gas? How much taller than Bob is Ed?

None of the above are statistical questions because each case lacks variability in the data needed to answer the question. The questions on favorite color, salary, and gas mileage each require a single piece of data, whether a fact or statistic. Therefore, variability is absent. Although the temperature question requires multiple pieces of data (the high temperature for each day), a single, distinct number is the answer. The height question requires two pieces of data, Bob's height and Ed's height, but no difference in variability exists between those two values. Therefore, this is not a statistical question. Statistical questions typically require calculations with data.

Consider the following statistical questions:

How many miles per gallon of gas does the 2016 Honda Civic get? To answer this question, data must be collected. This data should include miles driven and gallons used. Different cars, different drivers, and different driving conditions will produce different results. Therefore, variability exists in the data. To answer the question, the mean value could be determined.

Are American men taller than Chinese men? To answer this question, data must be collected. This data should include the heights of American men and the heights of Chinese men. All American men are not the same height and all Chinese men are not the same height. Some American men are taller than some Chinese men and some Chinese men are taller than some American men. Therefore, variability exists in the data. To answer the question, the median values for each group could be determined and compared.

Interpreting Statistical Information

To make decisions concerning populations, data must be collected from a sample. The sample must be large enough to be able to make conclusions. A common way to collect data is via surveys and polls. Every survey and poll must be designed so that there is no bias. An example of a biased survey is one with loaded questions, which are either intentionally worded or ordered to obtain a desired response. Once the data is obtained, conclusions should not be made that are not justified by statistical analysis. One must make sure the difference between correlation and causation is understood. Correlation implies there is an association between two variables, but it does not imply causation.

Population Mean and Proportion

Both the population mean and proportion can be calculated using data from a sample. The *population mean (μ)* is the average value of the parameter for the entire population. Due to size constraints, finding the exact value of μ is impossible, so the mean of the sample population is used as an estimate instead. The larger the sample size, the closer the sample mean gets to the population mean. An alternative to finding μ is to find the *proportion* of the population, which is the part of the population with the given characteristic. The proportion can be expressed as a decimal, fraction, or percentage, and can be given as a single value or a range of values. Because the population mean and proportion are both estimates, there's a *margin of error*, which is the difference between the actual value and the expected value.

T-Tests

A *randomized experiment* is used to compare two treatments by using statistics involving a *t-test,* which tests whether two data sets are significantly different from one another. To use a t-test, the test statistic must follow a normal distribution. The first step of the test involves calculating the *t* value, which is given as:

$$t = \frac{\overline{x_1} - \overline{x_2}}{s_{\bar{x}_1 - \bar{x}_2}}$$

where $\bar{x}_1$ and $\bar{x}_2$ are the averages of the two samples. Also:

$$s_{\bar{x}_1 - \bar{x}_2} = \sqrt{\frac{s_1^2}{n_1} + \frac{s_2^2}{n_2}}$$

where $s_1$and s_2 are the standard deviations of each sample and $n_1$and n_2 are their respective sample sizes. The *degrees of freedom* for two samples are calculated as:

$$df = \frac{(n_1 - 1) + (n_2 - 1)}{2}$$

rounded to the lowest whole number. Also, a significance level α must be chosen; the typical value is $\alpha = 0.05$. Once everything is compiled, the decision is made to use either a *one-tailed test* or a *two-*

tailed test. If there's an assumed difference between the two treatments, a one-tailed test is used. If no difference is assumed, a two-tailed test is used.

Analyzing Test Results

Once the type of test is determined, the t-value, significance level, and degrees of freedom are applied to the published table showing the *t* distribution. The row is associated with degrees of freedom and each column corresponds to the probability. The t-value can be exactly equal to one entry or lie between two entries in a row. For example, consider a t-value of 1.7 with degrees of freedom equal to 30. This *test statistic* falls between the *p* values of 0.05 and 0.025. For a one-tailed test, the corresponding *p* value lies between 0.05 and 0.025. For a two-tailed test, the *p* values need to be doubled, so the corresponding *p* value falls between 0.1 and 0.05. Once the probability is known, this range is compared to α. If $p < \alpha$, the hypothesis is rejected. If $p > \alpha$, the hypothesis isn't rejected. In a two-tailed test, this scenario means the hypothesis is accepted that there's no difference in the two treatments. In a one-tailed test, the hypothesis is accepted, indicating that there's a difference in the two treatments.

Sample Statistics

A *point estimate* is a single value used to approximate a population parameter. The sample proportion is the best point estimate of the population proportion. It is used because it is an *unbiased estimator,* meaning that it is a statistic that targets the value of the population parameter by assuming the mean of the sampling distribution is equal to the mean of the population distribution. Other unbiased estimators include the mean and variance. *Biased estimators* do not target the value of the population parameter, and such values include median, range, and standard deviation. A *confidence interval* consists of a range of values that is utilized to approximate the true value of a population parameter. The *confidence level* is the probability that the confidence interval does contain the population parameter, assuming the estimation process is repeated many times.

Population Inferences Using Distributions

Samples are used to make inferences about a population. The sampling distribution of a sample mean is a distribution of all sample means for a fixed sample size, *n*, which is part of a population. Depending on different criteria, either a binomial, normal, or geometric distribution can be used to determine probabilities. A normal distribution uses a continuous random variable, and is bell-shaped and symmetric. A binomial distribution uses a discrete random variable, has a finite number of trials, and only has two possible outcomes: a success and a failure. A geometric distribution is very similar to a binomial distribution; however, the number of trials does not have to be finite.

Linear Regression

Regression lines are a way to calculate a relationship between the independent variable and the dependent variable. A straight line means that there's a linear trend in the data. Technology can be used to find the equation of this line (e.g., a graphing calculator or Microsoft Excel®). In either case, all of the data points are entered, and a line is "fit" that best represents the shape of the data. Other functions used to model data sets include quadratic and exponential models.

Regression lines can be used to estimate data points not already given. For example, if an equation of a line is found that fit the temperature and beach visitor data set, its input is the average daily temperature and its output is the projected number of visitors. Thus, the number of beach visitors on a 100-degree day can be estimated. The output is a data point on the regression line, and the number of daily visitors is expected to be greater than on a 96-degree day because the regression line has a positive slope.

Plotting and Analyzing Residuals

Once the function is found that fits the data, its accuracy can be calculated. Therefore, how well the line fits the data can be determined. The difference between the actual dependent variable from the data set and the estimated value located on the regression line is known as a *residual*. Therefore, the residual is known as the predicted value $\hat{y}$ minus the actual value y. A residual is calculated for each data point and can be plotted on the scatterplot. If all the residuals appear to be approximately the same distance from the regression line, the line is a good fit. If the residuals seem to differ greatly across the board, the line isn't a good fit.

Interpreting the Regression Line

The formula for a regression line is $y = mx + b$, where m is the slope and b is the y-intercept. Both the slope and y-intercept are found in the *Method of Least Squares*, which is the process of finding the equation of the line through minimizing residuals. The slope represents the rate of change in y as x gets larger. Therefore, because y is the dependent variable, the slope actually provides the predicted values given the independent variable. The y-intercept is the predicted value for when the independent variable equals zero. In the temperature example, the y-intercept is the expected number of beach visitors for a very cold average daily temperature of zero degrees.

The *correlation coefficient (r)* measures the association between two variables. Its value is between -1 and 1, where -1 represents a perfect negative linear relationship, 0 represents no relationship, and 1 represents a perfect positive linear relationship. A *negative linear relationship* means that as x-values increase, y values decrease. A *positive linear relationship* means that as x-values increase, y-values increase. The formula for computing the correlation coefficient is:

$$r = \frac{n\sum xy - (\sum x)(\sum y)}{\sqrt{n(\sum x^2) - (\sum x)^2}\sqrt{n(\sum y^2) - (y)^2}}$$

n is the number of data points

Both Microsoft Excel® and a graphing calculator can evaluate this easily once the data points are entered. A correlation greater than 0.8 or less than -0.8 is classified as "strong," while a correlation between -0.5 and 0.5 is classified as "weak."

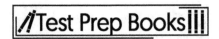

Here is an example of a data set and its regression line:

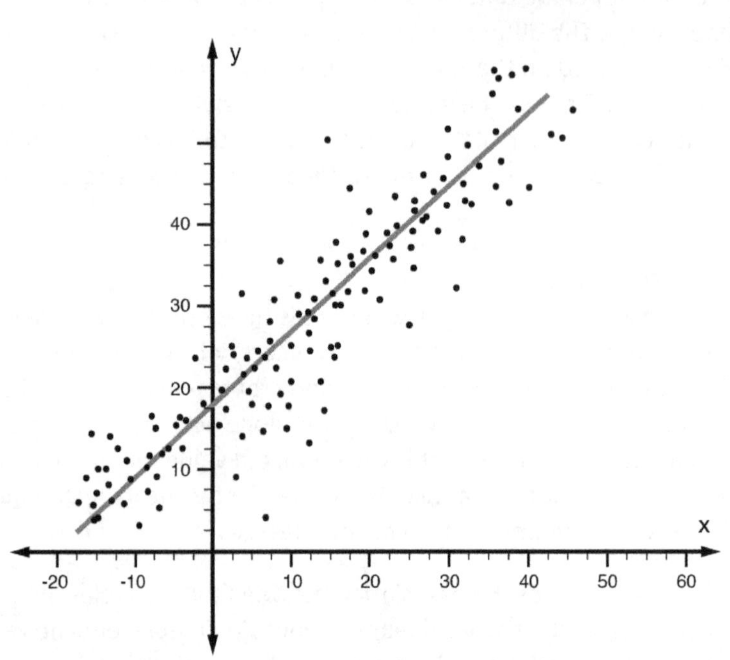

Regression models are highly used for forecasting, and linear regression techniques are the simplest models. If the nonlinear data follows the shape of exponential, logarithmic, or power functions, those types of functions can be used to more accurately model the data rather than lines.

Here is an example of both an exponential regression and a logarithmic regression model:

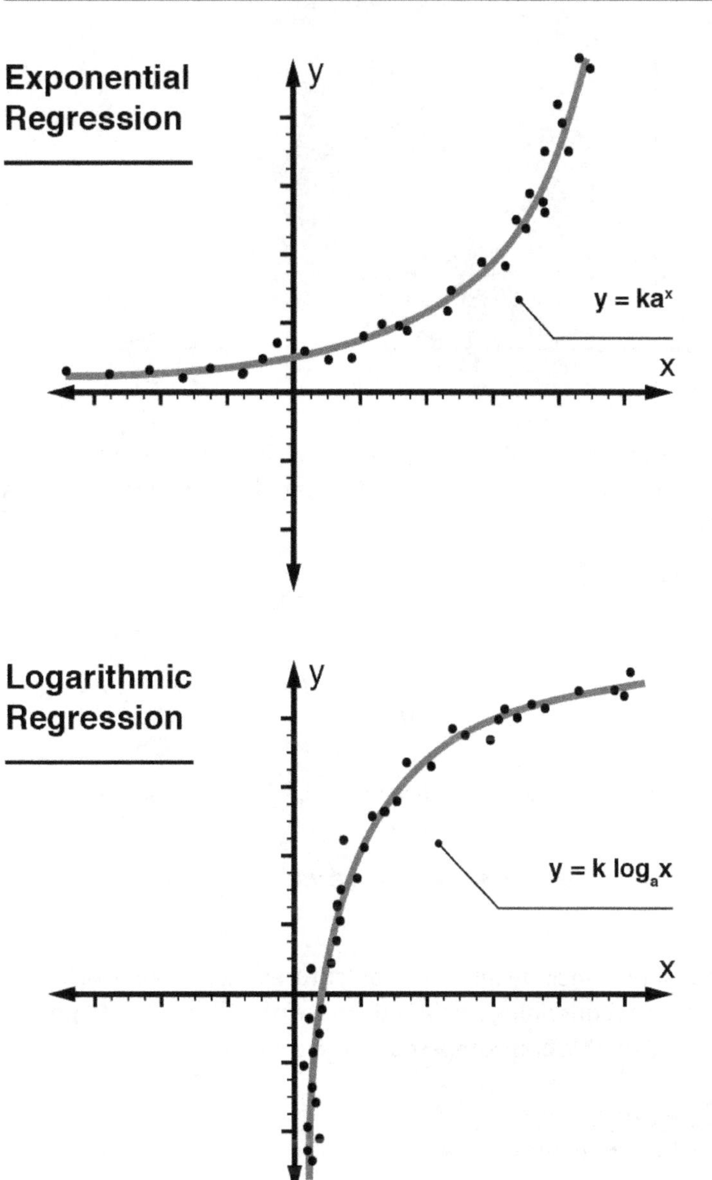

A set of data can be described in terms of its center, spread, shape and any unusual features. The center of a data set can be measured by its mean, median, or mode. The spread of a data set refers to how far the data points are from the center (mean or median). The spread can be measured by the range or the quartiles and interquartile range. A data set with data points clustered around the center will have a small spread. A data set covering a wide range will have a large spread.

When a data set is displayed as a histogram or frequency distribution plot, the shape indicates if a sample is normally distributed, symmetrical, or has measures of skewness or kurtosis. When graphed, a data set with a normal distribution will resemble a bell curve.

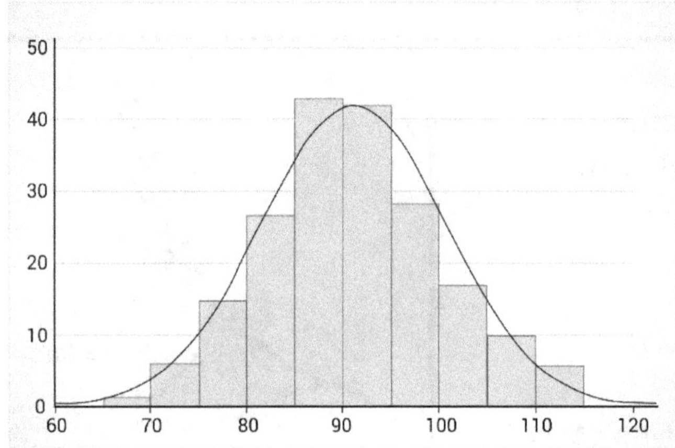

If the data set is symmetrical, each half of the graph when divided at the center is a mirror image of the other. If the graph has fewer data points to the right, the data is skewed right. If it has fewer data points to the left, the data is skewed left.

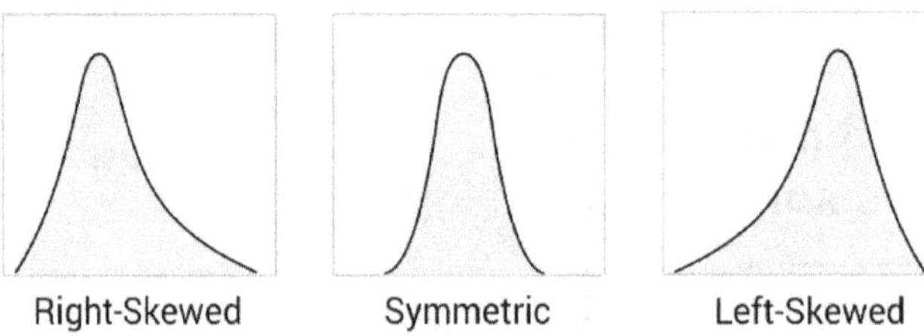

Kurtosis is a measure of whether the data is heavy-tailed with a high number of outliers, or light-tailed with a low number of outliers.

A description of a data set should include any unusual features such as gaps or outliers. A gap is a span within the range of the data set containing no data points. An outlier is a data point with a value either extremely large or extremely small when compared to the other values in the set.

Correlation Versus Causation

Correlation and causation have two different meanings. If two values are correlated, there is an association between them. However, correlation doesn't necessarily mean that one variable causes the other. *Causation* (or "cause and effect") occurs when one variable causes the other. Average daily temperature and number of beachgoers are correlated and have causation. If the temperature increases, the change in weather causes more people to go to the beach. However, alcoholism and smoking are correlated but don't have causation. The more someone drinks, the more likely they are to smoke, but drinking alcohol doesn't cause someone to smoke.

Precalculus

Functions

Graphing and Identifying Domains, Ranges, Intercepts, and Zeros of Exponential Functions

The logarithmic function with base b is denoted $y = \log_b x$. Its base must be greater than 0 and not equal to 1, and the domain is all $x > 0$. The exponential function with base b is denoted $y = b^x$. Exponential and logarithmic functions with base b are inverses. By definition, if $y = \log_b x, x = b^y$. Because exponential and logarithmic functions are inverses, the graph of one is obtained by reflecting the other over the line $y = x$. A common base used is e, and in this case $y = e^x$ and its inverse $y = \log_e x$ is commonly written as the natural logarithmic function $y = \ln x$.

Here is the graph of both functions:

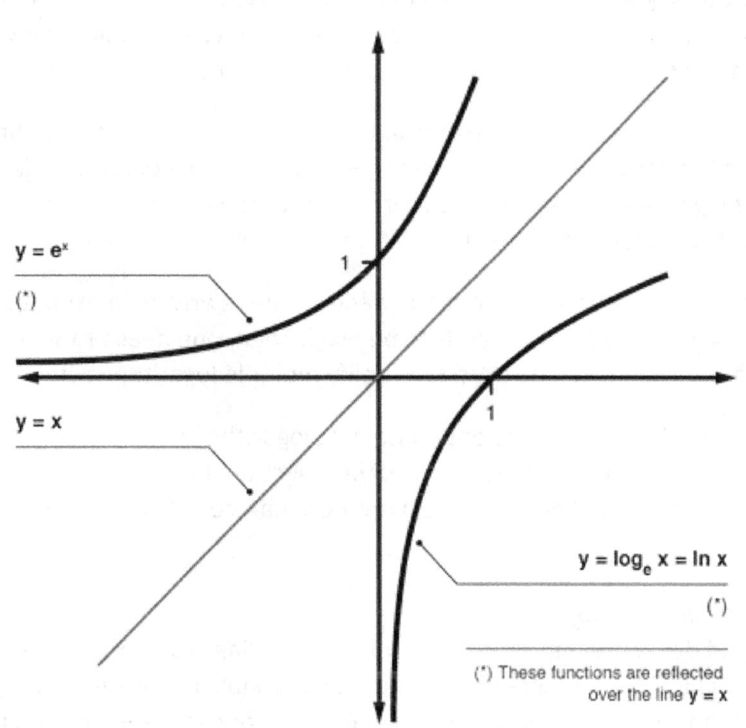

The x-intercept of the logarithmic function $y = \log_b x$ with any base is always the ordered pair $(1, 0)$. By the definition of inverse, the point $(0, 1)$ always lies on the exponential function $y = b^x$. This is true because any real number raised to the power of 0 equals 1. Therefore, the exponential function only has a y-intercept. The exponential function also has a horizontal asymptote of the x-axis as x approaches negative infinity. Because the graph is reflected over the line $y = x$, to obtain the graph of the logarithmic function, the asymptote is also reflected. Therefore, the logarithmic function has a one-sided vertical asymptote at $y = 0$. These asymptotes can be seen in the above graphs of $y = e^x$ and $y = \ln x$.

Logarithms

When working with logarithms and exponential expressions, it is important to remember the relationship between the two. In general, the logarithmic form is $y = log_b x$ for an exponential form $b^y = x$. Logarithms and exponential functions are inverses of each other.

A logarithmic scale is a scale of measurement that uses the logarithm of the given units instead of the actual given units. Each tick mark on such a scale is the product of the previous tick mark multiplied by a number. The advantage of using such a scale is that if one is working with large measurements, this technique reduces the scale into manageable quantities that are easier to read. The Richter magnitude scale is the famous logarithmic scale used to measure the intensity of earthquakes, and the decibel scale is commonly used to measure sound level in electronics.

Solving Problems Related to Exponential and Logarithmic Functions

To solve an equation involving exponential expressions, the goal is to isolate the exponential expression. Once this process is completed, the logarithm—with the base equaling the base of the exponent of both sides—needs to be taken to get an expression for the variable. If the base is e, the natural log of both sides needs to be taken.

To solve an equation with logarithms, the given equation needs to be written in exponential form, using the fact that $\log_b y = x$ means $b^x = y$, and then solved for the given variable. Lastly, properties of logarithms can be used to simplify more than one logarithmic expression into one.

Some equations involving exponential and logarithmic functions can be solved algebraically, or analytically. To solve an equation involving exponential functions, the goal is to isolate the exponential expression. Then, the logarithm of both sides is found in order to yield an expression for the variable. Laws of Logarithms will be helpful at this point.

To solve an equation with logarithms, the equation needs to be rewritten in exponential form. The definition that $\log_b x = y$ means $b^y = x$ needs to be used. Then, one needs to solve for the given variable. Properties of logarithms can be used to simplify multiple logarithmic expressions into one.

Other methods can be used to solve equations containing logarithmic and exponential functions. Graphs and graphing calculators can be used to see points of intersection. In a similar manner, tables can be used to find points of intersection. Also, numerical methods can be utilized to find approximate solutions.

Exponential Growth and Decay

Exponential growth and decay are important concepts in modeling real-world phenomena. The growth and decay formula is $A(t) = Pe^{rt}$, where the independent variable t represents temperature, P represents an initial quantity, r represents the rate of increase or decrease, and $A(t)$ represents the amount of the quantity at time t. If $r > 0$, the equation models exponential growth and a common application is population growth. If $r < 0$, the equation models exponential decay and a common application is radioactive decay. Exponential and logarithmic solving techniques are necessary to work with the growth and decay formula.

Using Exponential and Logarithmic Functions in Finance Problems

Modeling within finance also involves exponential and logarithmic functions. Compound interest results when the bank pays interest on the original amount of money – the principal – and the interest that has accrued. The compound interest equation is:

$$A(t) = P\left(1 + \frac{r}{n}\right)^{nt}$$

where P is the principal, r is the interest rate, n is the number of times per year the interest is compounded, and t is the time in years. The result, $A(t)$, is the final amount after t years. Mathematical problems of this type that are frequently encountered involve receiving all but one of these quantities and solving for the missing quantity. The solving process then involves employing properties of logarithmic and exponential functions. Interest can also be compounded continuously. This formula is given as $A(t) = Pe^{rt}$. If $1,000 was compounded continuously at a rate of 2% for 4 years, the result would be:

$$A(4) = 1000e^{0.02 \cdot 4} = \$1{,}083$$

Rate of Change Proportional to the Current Quantity

Many quantities grow or decay as fast as exponential functions. Specifically, if such a quantity grows or decays at a rate proportional to the quantity itself, it shows exponential behavior. If a data set is given with such specific characteristics, the initial amount and an amount at a specific time, t, can be plugged into the exponential function $A(t) = Pe^{rt}$ for A and P. Using properties of exponents and logarithms, one can then solve for the rate, r. This solution yields enough information to have the entire model, which can allow for an estimation of the quantity at any time, t, and the ability to solve various problems using that model.

Graphing and Identifying Domains, Ranges, Intercepts, Zeros, and Inverses of the Circular Functions

From the unit circle, the trigonometric ratios were found for the special right triangle with a hypotenuse of 1.

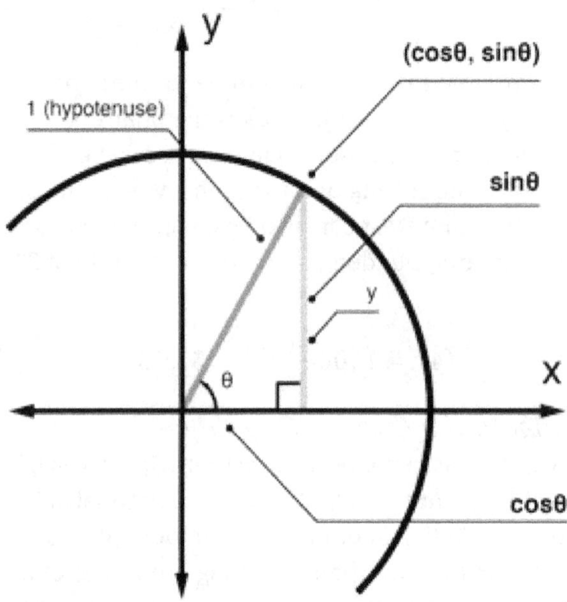

From this triangle, the following Pythagorean identities are formed

$$\sin^2\theta + \cos^2\theta = 1$$

$$\tan^2\theta + 1 = \sec^2\theta$$

$$1 + \cot^2\theta = \csc^2\theta$$

The second two identities are formed by manipulating the first identity. Since identities are statements that are true for any value of the variable, then they may be used to manipulate equations. For example, a problem may ask for simplification of the expression $\cos^2 x + \cos^2 x \tan^2 x$. Using the fact that

$$\tan(x) = \frac{\sin x}{\cos x}, \frac{\sin^2 x}{\cos^2 x}$$

can then be substituted in for $\tan^2 x$, making the expression

$$\cos^2 x + \cos^2 x \frac{\sin^2 x}{\cos^2 x}$$

Then the two $\cos^2 x$ terms on top and bottom cancel each other out, simplifying the expression to $\cos^2 x + \sin^2 x$. By the first Pythagorean identity stated above, the expression can be turned into $\cos^2 x + \sin^2 x = 1$.

Another set of trigonometric identities are the double-angle formulas:

$$\sin 2\alpha = 2 \sin \alpha \ \cos \alpha$$

$$\cos 2\alpha = \begin{cases} \cos^2\alpha - \sin^2\alpha \\ 2\cos^2\alpha - 1 \\ 1 - 2\sin^2\alpha \end{cases}$$

Using these formulas, the following identity can be proved:

$$\sin 2x = \frac{2 \tan x}{1 + \tan^2 x}$$

By using one of the Pythagorean identities, the denominator can be rewritten as:

$$1 + \tan^2 x = \sec^2 x$$

By knowing the reciprocals of the trigonometric identities, the secant term can be rewritten to form the equation:

$$\sin 2x = \frac{2 \tan x}{1} * \cos^2 x$$

Replacing $\tan(x)$, the equation becomes:

$$\sin 2x = \frac{2 \sin x}{\cos x} * \cos^2 x$$

where the $\cos x$ can cancel out. The new equation is $\sin 2x = 2 \sin x * \cos x$. This final equation is one of the double-angle formulas.

Other trigonometric identities such as half-angle formulas, sum and difference formulas, and difference of angles formulas can be used to prove and rewrite trigonometric equations. Depending on the given equation or expression, the correct identities need to be chosen to write equivalent statements.

The graph of sine is equal to the graph of cosine, shifted $\frac{\pi}{2}$ units. Therefore, the function $y = \sin x$ is equal to $y = \cos(\frac{\pi}{2} - x)$. Within functions, adding a constant to the independent variable shifts the graph either left or right. By shifting the cosine graph, the curve lies on top of the sine function. By transforming the function, the two equations give the same output for any given input.

Solving Trigonometric Functions

Solving trigonometric functions can be done with a knowledge of the unit circle and the trigonometric identities. It requires the use of opposite operations combined with trigonometric ratios for special triangles. For example, the problem may require solving the equation:

$$2\cos^2 x - \sqrt{3}\cos x = 0$$

for the values of x between 0 and 180 degrees. The first step is to factor out the $\cos x$ term, resulting in:

$$\cos x\,(2\cos x - \sqrt{3}) = 0$$

By the factoring method of solving, each factor can be set equal to zero:

$$\cos x = 0 \text{ and } (2\cos x - \sqrt{3}) = 0$$

The second equation can be solved to yield the following equation: $\cos x = \frac{\sqrt{3}}{2}$. Now that the value of x is found, the trigonometric ratios can be used to find the solutions of $x = 30 \text{ and } 90 \text{ degrees}$.

Solving trigonometric functions requires the use of algebra to isolate the variable and a knowledge of trigonometric ratios to find the value of the variable. The unit circle can be used to find answers for special triangles. Beyond those triangles, a calculator can be used to solve for variables within the trigonometric functions.

Performing Algebraic Operations on Functions

When two functions are added together, the result is known as a sum function. The domain of a sum function is the intersection of the two domains of the original functions. If the functions are $f(x)$ and $g(x)$, then it is possible to compute an expression for $(f+g)(x)$ by adding together those functions. For example, suppose that:

$$f(x) = 4x - 2 \text{ and } g(x) = x^2 - 2x$$

Then the expression for:

$$(f+g)(x) = (4x-2) + (x^2 - 2x) = x^2 + 2x - 2$$

In this example, the domain of both f and g is all real numbers, so the domain of the sum function listed above is all real numbers.

When one function is subtracted from another, the result is known as a difference function. Like the sum function, the domain of a difference function is also the intersection of the two domains of the original functions. With the functions from the previous paragraph, the subtraction is:

$$(f-g)(x) = (4x-2) - (x^2 - 2x) = -x^2 + 6x - 2$$

The domain of the difference function listed above is also all real numbers. When finding an expression for such subtraction of functions, it is very important to make sure to subtract the *entire* second function from the first function.

The result of the multiplication of two functions is known as a product function. Like sum and difference formulas, the domain of the product function is the intersection of the two domains of the original functions. In this example, the domain of $f \times g$, also written as fg, is all real numbers.

Finally, the quotient function is found by the division of two functions. By definition:

$$(f/g)(x) = f(x)/g(x)$$

With the above examples:

$$(f/g)(x) = \frac{(4x-2)}{(x^2 - 2x)}$$

Note that the denominator cannot be zero in a fraction, so:

$$\left(\frac{f}{g}\right)(x) = \frac{f(x)}{g(x)}$$

provided that $g(x) \neq 0$. Therefore, that the domain of $\frac{f}{g}$ is the intersection of the domains of both f and g, excluding any x-values that cause $g(x) = 0$. In the example discussed previously, both 2 and 0 would create a 0 denominator when plugged in for x in the function. Therefore, the domain of the quotient function in interval notation is:

$$(-\infty, 0) \cup (0,2) \cup (2, \infty)$$

The difference quotient is an important calculation and it involves performing algebraic operations on functions. For a function $f(x)$, the difference quotient is defined as:

$$\frac{f(x+h) - f(x)}{h}$$

Therefore, for the function $f(x) = 4x + 3$, its difference quotient is:

$$\frac{4(x+h) + 3 - (4x+3)}{h} = \frac{4x + 4h + 3 - 4x - 3}{h} = 4$$

Identifying and Using Composite Functions

In many scenarios, it is common for the output of one function to depend on an output of another function. Therefore, the output of the second function would be the input of the first function. A real-life situation can be seen with taxes. If you work hourly, your paycheck is based on the number of hours worked, and the taxes are based on the total paycheck. This involves what is called a *composite function.*

Given two functions *f* and *g*, the composition of *g* with *f* is written $g°f$, and it is defined by the equation:

$$(g°f)(x) = g(f(x))$$

In other words, first apply the function *f* to x, and then apply *g* to the result.

The domain of such a function is some subset of the domain of *f*. Specifically, it is those values in the domain of *f*, such that the result when *f* yields something in the domain of *g*.

Another way to think about a composite function $g°f$ is that the function $f(x)$ gets plugged into $g(x)$ whenever there is an x. Note that x is in the domain of $f(x)$ and $f(x)$ is in the domain of $g(x)$. Also, the domain of a composite function can be thought of the intersection of the domain of the input function and the domain of the composite function.

More than two functions can be involved when building composite functions as well. Consider:

$$f(x) = 2x, g(x) = x^2 + 1, \text{and } h(x) = \sqrt{x}$$

The composite function:

$$h\left(g(f(x))\right) = \sqrt{(2x)^2 + 1} = \sqrt{4x^2 + 1}$$

Its domain is the intersection of the two input functions and the composite function, which is all real numbers.

Complex Numbers

Given a complex number $a + bi$, its *complex conjugate* is $a - bi$. For example, the complex conjugate of $4 + 3i$ is $4 - 3i$. It is the number with equal real part and opposite imaginary part. The absolute value of a complex number $a + bi$, also known as its *magnitude* or *modulus* is $\sqrt{a^2 + b^2}$. It is equal to the distance from the origin to the corresponding point in the complex plane. A multiplicative inverse of any number is what one multiplies by to obtain a product of 1. In other words, it is the reciprocal. For a complex number $a + bi$, its *multiplicative inverse* is $\frac{1}{a+bi}$, which can be rewritten once rationalized as:

$$\frac{a}{a^2 + b^2} - \frac{b}{a^2 + b^2}i.$$

The complex numbers form a field, which means that two complex numbers can be added together and multiplied times one another and either result is still a complex number. Also, for any complex number $a + bi$, its additive inverse $-a - bi$ is also a complex number. Finally, every nonzero complex number has a multiplicative inverse that is a complex number. Addition can be performed using the same process as vector addition. In this case, addition is done component-wise. In component form:

$$(a + bi) + (c + di) = (a + c) + (b + d)i$$

in which the real part and imaginary part are considered separate components.

Representing Complex Numbers

Given the situation, the format in which a complex number is used is important. When given as $a + bi$, it is written in its algebraic, rectangular, or Cartesian form, and it relates to an ordered pair (a, b) in the complex plane with a real (horizontal) and imaginary (vertical) axis. A complex number that is completely imaginary lies on the vertical axis. Its vector form is found similarly by writing its real and imaginary parts into vector form $< a, b >$. Polar form of a complex number is necessary if there is desire to use complex numbers in the real number system by using polar coordinates. In this case:

$$z = a + bi = r(\cos\theta + i\sin\theta),$$

where r represents the absolute value of z and $\theta = \tan^{-1}\left(\frac{b}{a}\right)$. The ordered pair $(r,\ \theta)$ represent the polar coordinates. Finally, a complex number can be represented in exponential form, and Euler's formula $e^{i\theta} = \cos\theta + i\sin\theta$ is necessary. With this formula, the complex number's exponential form is $z = re^{i\theta}$. Also, it is true that $a = r\cos\theta$ and $b = r\sin\theta$.

Complex Number Operations

Complex number operations can be performed using geometric representations of the numbers themselves. In terms of addition, two complex numbers can be added by adding the real parts together separately from the imaginary parts. This operation can be performed within the ordered pairs. Multiplication can be thought of using polar coordinates. Its magnitude r, which is the distance from the point to the origin in the complex plane, and its argument θ, which is the angle from the horizontal axis to the line segment connecting the origin and the point itself, can be used. Two complex numbers can be multiplied by one another by multiplying their magnitudes together and adding their arguments together. Therefore, the product of the complex number with magnitude r_1 and argument θ_1 with the complex number with magnitude r_2 and argument θ_2 is the complex number with magnitude $r_1 r_2$ and argument $\theta_1 + \theta_2$.

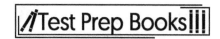

Complex Numbers as Solutions

Complex numbers may result from solving polynomial equations using the quadratic equation. Since complex numbers result from taking the square root of a negative number, the number found under the radical in the quadratic formula—called the *determinant*—tells whether or not the answer will be real or complex. If the determinant is negative, the roots are complex. Even though the coefficients of the polynomial may be real numbers, the roots are complex.

Solving polynomials by factoring is an alternative to using the quadratic formula. For example, in order to solve $x^2 - b^2 = 0$ for x, it needs to be factored. It factors into $(x + b)(x - b) = 0$. The solution set can be found by setting each factor equal to zero, resulting in $x = \pm b$. When b^2 is negative, the factors are complex numbers. For example, $x^2 + 64 = 0$ can be factored into $(x + 8i)(x - 8i) = 0$. The two roots are then found to be $x = \pm 8i$.

When dealing with polynomials and solving polynomial equations, it is important to remember the fundamental theorem of algebra. When given a polynomial with a degree of n, the theorem states that there will be n roots. These roots may or may not be complex. For example, the following polynomial equation of degree 2 has two complex roots: $x^2 + 1 = 0$. The factors of this polynomial are $(x + i)$ and $(x - i)$, resulting in the roots $x = i, -i$. As seen on the graph below, imaginary roots occur when the graph does not touch the x-axis.

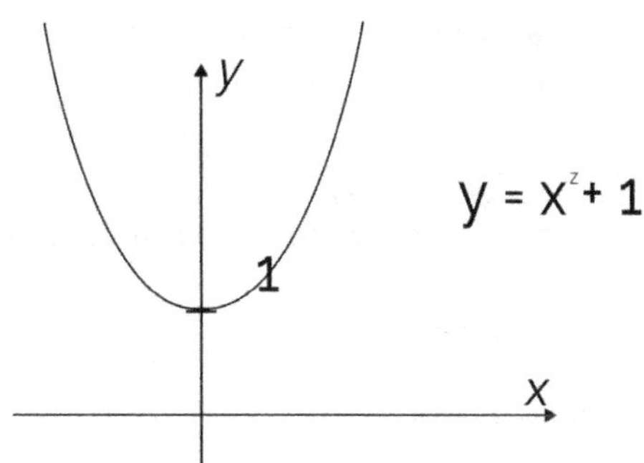

When a graphing calculator is permitted, the graph can always confirm the number and types of roots of the polynomial.

A polynomial identity is a true equation involving polynomials. For example,

$$x^2 - 5x + 6 = (x - 3)(x - 2)$$

which can be proved through multiplication by the FOIL method and factoring. This idea can be extended to involve complex numbers. Because

$$i^2 = -1, x^3 + 9x = x(x^2 + 9) = x(x + 3i)(x - 3i)$$

This identity can also be proven through FOIL and factoring.

Polar Representations of Complex Numbers

A complex number in the form $z = a + bi$ can be written in its polar form if there is necessity to use it amongst real numbers in the Cartesian coordinate system. In this case

$$z = r(\cos\theta + i\sin\theta)$$

where r represents the absolute value of z, the distance from the point to the origin, and

$$\theta = \tan^{-1}\left(\frac{b}{a}\right)$$

represents the angle, in radians, from the positive x-axis to the ray that connects the origin to the point. The ordered pair (r, θ) represents the polar coordinates. Given the polar representation,

$$z = r(\cos\theta + i\sin\theta),$$

a proof by induction can be used to obtain DeMoivre's Theorem, which says that if *n* is a natural number, $z^n = r^n(\cos n\theta + i\sin n\theta)$.

Vectors

A vector can be thought of as a list of numbers. These can be thought of as an abstract list of numbers, or else as giving a location in a space. For example, the coordinates (x, y) for points in the Cartesian plane are vectors. Each entry in a vector can be referred to by its location in the list: first, second, and so on. The total length of the list is the *dimension* of the vector. A vector is often denoted as such by putting an arrow on top of it, e.g. $\vec{v} = (v_1, v_2, v_3)$

Adding Vectors Graphically and Algebraically

There are two basic operations for vectors. First, two vectors can be added together. Let:

$$\vec{v} = (v_1, v_2, v_3), \vec{w} = (w_1, w_2, w_3)$$

The the sum of the two vectors is defined to be:

$$\vec{v} + \vec{w} = (v_1 + w_1, v_2 + w_2, v_3 + w_3)$$

Subtraction of vectors can be defined similarly.

Vector addition can be visualized in the following manner. First, visualize each vector as an arrow. Then place the base of one arrow at the tip of the other arrow. The tip of this first arrow now hits some point in the space, and there will be an arrow from the origin to this point. This new arrow corresponds to the new vector. In subtraction, we reverse the direction of the arrow being subtracted.

For example, consider adding together the vectors (-2, 3) and (4, 1). The new vector will be (-2+4, 3+1), or (2, 4). Graphically, this may be pictured in the following manner.

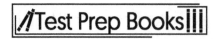

Performing Scalar Multiplications

The second basic operation for vectors is called *scalar multiplication*. Scalar multiplication allows us to multiply any vector by any real number, which is denoted here as a scalar. Let:

$$\vec{v} = (v_1, v_2, v_3)$$

and let a be an arbitrary real number. Then the scalar multiple

$$a\vec{v} = (av_1, av_2, av_3)$$

Graphically, this corresponds to changing the length of the arrow corresponding to the vector by a factor, or scale, of a. That is why the real number is called a scalar in this instance.

As an example, let:

$$\vec{v} = \left(2, -1, \frac{1}{3}\right)$$

Then:

$$3\vec{v} = \left(3 \cdot 2, 3(-1), 3 \cdot \frac{1}{3}\right) = (6, -3, 1)$$

Note that scalar multiplication is *distributive* over vector addition, meaning that:

$$a(\vec{v} + \vec{w}) = a\vec{v} + a\vec{w}$$

Representing Vectors Equations of Lines and Planes

Since vectors can be thought of as giving directions, and since lines continue on in a single direction, it is possible to represent any line by using vectors. To do so requires two things: a vector $\vec{p}$ that goes to a point on the line, and a vector $\vec{r}$ which gives the direction of a line. The equation for the line will then be all vectors of the form $\vec{v} = \vec{p} + s\vec{r}$, where s can take the value of any real number.

Suppose we know two points on the line, *A* and *B*. Then we can take $\vec{p}$ to be the vector pointing to *A*, and take $\vec{r}$ to be the vector that goes from *A* to *B*. This will be the vector going to *B* minus the vector going to *A*. Of course, there will be many different vector equations corresponding to the same line, since any two points on the line may be used.

Consider a line in the Cartesian plane which passes through the points (1, -2) and (2, 3). Call the first point *A* and the second point *B*. Then we can take

$$\vec{p} = (-1, 2), \text{and } \vec{r} = (2, 3) - (-1,2) = (3, 1)$$

Then the vector equation for the line will be $\vec{v} = (-1, 2) + s(3,1)$.

A plane in three dimensions can similarly be represented by using vectors. In this case, three vectors are needed: first, a vector $\vec{p}$ pointing to some point on the plane, and then two vectors $\vec{q}$ and $\vec{r}$ corresponding to the two directions in which the plane goes. If three points on the plane are given, *A*, *B*, and *C*, then one can take $\vec{p}$ to be the vector pointing to *A*, $\vec{q}$ to be the vector from *A* to *B*, and $\vec{r}$ to be the vector from *A* to *C*. The vector equation for the plane is then:

$$\vec{v} = \vec{p} + s\vec{q} + t\vec{r}$$

Note, however, that this requires the three given points to not all lie on the same line. If they all lie upon a single line, then they do not define a unique plane.

Suppose, then, that the points $(0, 3, 3), (-2, 2, 2), (-1, 1, 0)$ lie on a plane. We can take:

$$\vec{p} = (0, 3, 3)$$

$$\vec{q} = (-2, 2, 2) - (0, 3, 3) = (-2, -1, -1)$$

$$\vec{r} = (-1, 1, 0) - (0, 3, 3) = (-1, -2, -3)$$

The vector equation for the plane will now be:

$$\vec{v} = (0, 3, 3) + s(-2, -1, -1) + t(-1, -2, -3)$$

Two vectors are equal if, and only if, their individual components are equal. For example:

$$< 1, 2 >=< 1, 2 > \text{ but } < 1, 2 >\neq< 2, 1 >$$

Also, vector addition is performed component-wise. Such an example is:

$$< 1, 2 > +< 2, 3 >=< 3, 5 >$$

The zero vector is defined to be the vector containing only components equal to 0, and any vector plus a zero vector equals itself. Hence, the zero vector is the additive identity. Scalar multiplication is performed by multiplying each component by the scalar. For example:

$$3 \cdot< 1, 2 >=< 3, 6 >$$

Scalar multiplication and addition can be used to prove that the distributive property holds within vector addition and scalar addition. Vector multiplication is defined using the dot product, which is also known as the scalar product. The result of a dot product is a scalar. Each corresponding component is multiplied, and then the sum of all products is found. For example:

$$< 1, 2 >\cdot< 2, 3 >= 1 \cdot 2 + 2 \cdot 3 = 2 + 6 = 8$$

Alternatively, the dot product is defined to be the product of the magnitudes of each vector and the cosine of the angle between the two vectors. Therefore, if two vectors are perpendicular, their dot product is equal to zero. Finally, two vectors are parallel if they are scalar multiples of each other.

Calculus

Limits

The *limit of a function* can be described as the output that is approached as the input approaches a certain value. Written in function notation, the limit of $f(x)$ as x approaches a is:

$$\lim_{x \to a} f(x) = B$$

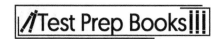

As x draws near to some value a, represented by $x \to a$, then $f(x)$ approaches some number B. In the graph of the function:

$$f(x) = \frac{x+2}{x+2}$$

the line is continuous except where $x = -2$. Because $x = -2$ yields an undefined output and a hole in the graph, the function does not exist at this value. The limit, however, does exist. As the value $x = -2$ is approached from the left side, the output is getting very close to 1. From the right side, as the x-value approaches -2, the output also gets close to 1. Since the function value from both sides approaches 1, then:

$$\lim_{x \to -2} \frac{x+2}{x+2} = 1$$

One special type of function, the *step function* $f(x) = [x]$, can be used to define right and left-hand limits. The graph is shown below. The left-hand limit as x approaches 1 is $\lim_{x \to 1^-} [x]$. From the graph, as x approaches 1 from the left side, the function approaches 0. For the right-hand limit, the expression is $\lim_{x \to 1^+} [x]$. The value for this limit is one. Since the function does not have the same limit for the left and right side, then the limit does not exist at $x = 1$. From that same reasoning, the limit does not exist for any integer for this function.

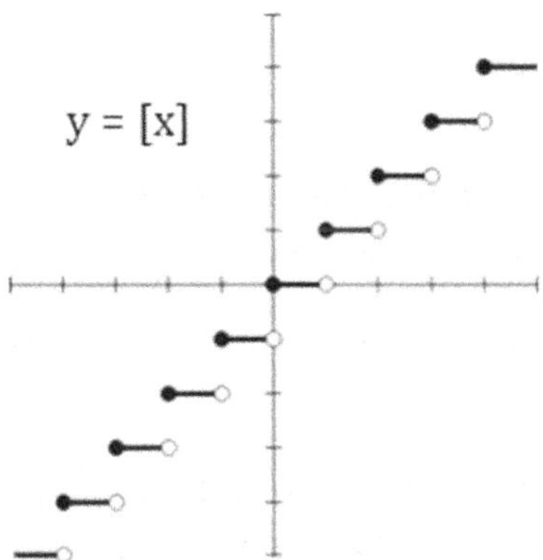

Sometimes, a function approaches infinity as it draws near to a certain x-value. For example, the following graph shows the function:

$$f(x) = \frac{2x}{x-3}$$

There is an asymptote at $x = 3$. The limit as x approaches 3, $\lim_{x \to 3} \frac{2x}{x-3}$, does not exist. The right and left-hand side limits at 3 do not approach the same output value. One approaches positive infinity, and the other approaches negative infinity. Infinite limits do not satisfy the definition of a limit. The limit of the function as x approaches a number must be equal to a finite value.

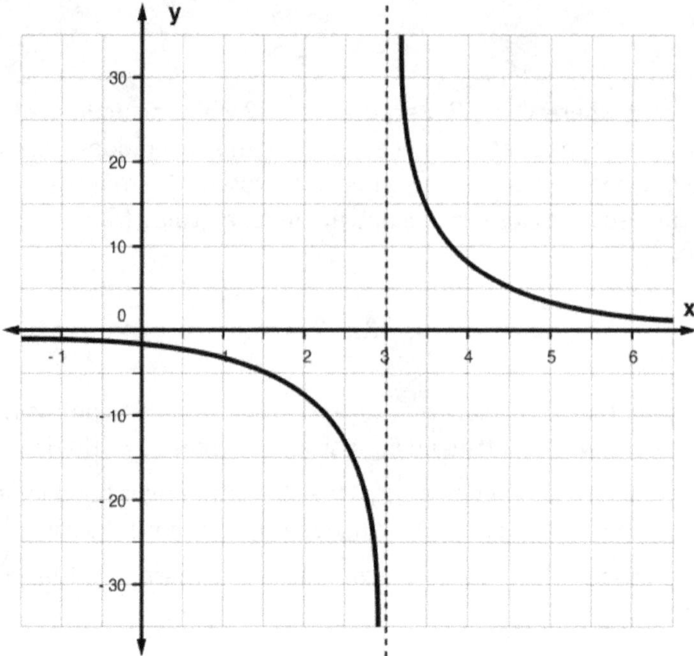

Horizontal asymptotes can be found using limits. Horizontal asymptotes are limits as x approaches either ∞ or $-\infty$. For example, to find $\lim_{x\to\infty} \frac{2x}{x-3}$, the graph can be used to see the value of the function as x grows larger and larger. For this example, the limit is 2, so it has a horizontal asymptote of $y = 2$. In considering $\lim_{x\to-\infty} \frac{2x}{x-3} = 2$, the limits can also be seen on a graphing calculator by plotting the equation $y = \frac{2x}{x-3}$. Then, the table can be brought up. By scrolling up and down, the limit can be found as x approaches any value.

Limit laws exist that assist in finding limits of functions. These properties include multiplying by a constant, $\lim kf(x) = k \lim\ f(x)$, and the addition property:

$$\lim[f(x) + g(x)] = \lim f(x) + \lim\ g(x)$$

Two other properties are the multiplication property:

$$\lim f(x)g(x) = (\lim\ f(x))(\lim g(x))$$

and the division property:

$$\lim \frac{f(x)}{g(x)} = \frac{\lim\ f(x)}{\lim\ g(x)}\ (if \lim g(x) \neq 0)$$

These properties are helpful in finding limits of polynomial functions algebraically:

In $\lim_{x\to2} 4x^2 - 3x + 8$

the constant and multiplication properties can be used together, and the problem can be rewritten as:

$$4\lim_{x\to 2} x^2 - \lim_{x\to 2} 3x + \lim_{x\to 2} 8$$

Since this is a continuous function, direct substitution can be used. The value of 2 is substituted in for x and evaluated as:

$$4(2^2) - 3(2) + 8$$

which yields a limit of 18. These properties allow functions to be rewritten so that limits can be calculated.

Continuity

To find if a function is continuous, the definition consists of three steps. These three steps include finding $f(a)$, finding $\lim_{x\to a} f(x)$, and finding:

$$\lim_{x\to a} f(x) = f(a)$$

If the limit of a function equals the function value at that point, then the function is continuous at $x = a$. For example, the function $f(x) = \frac{1}{x}$ is continuous everywhere except $x = 0$. $f(0) = \frac{1}{0}$ is undefined; therefore, the function is discontinuous at 0. Secondly, to determine if the function $f(x) = \frac{1}{x-1}$ is continuous at 2, its function value must equal its limit at 2. First:

$$f(2) = \frac{1}{2-1} = 1$$

Then the limit can be found by direct substitution:

$$\lim_{x\to 2} \frac{1}{x-1} = 1$$

Since these two values are equal, then the function is continuous at $x = 2$.

Differentiability and continuity are related in that if the derivative can be found at $x = c$, then the function is continuous at $x = c$. If the slope of the tangent line can be found at a certain point, then there is no hole or jump in the graph at that point. Some functions, however, can be continuous while not differentiable at a given point. An example is the graph of the function $f(x) = |x|$. At the origin, the derivative does not exist, but the function is still continuous. Points where a function is discontinuous are where a vertical tangent exists and where there is a cusp or corner at a given x-value.

Derivatives

Finding Derivatives of Algebraic Functions by Means of the Sum and Product, Power Rule, and Applying the Mean Value Theorem

The derivative of a function is found using the limit of the difference quotient:

$$\lim_{\Delta x\to 0} \frac{f(x+\Delta x) - f(x)}{\Delta x}$$

This finds the slope of the tangent line of the given function at a given point. It is the slope, $\frac{\Delta y}{\Delta x}$, as $\Delta x \to 0$. The derivative can be denoted in many ways, such as $f'(x)$, y', or $\frac{dy}{dx}$.

The following graph plots a function in black. The gray line represents a secant line, formed between two chosen points on the graph. The slope of this line can be found using rise over run. As these two points get closer to zero, meaning Δx approaches 0, the tangent line is found. The slope of the tangent line is equal to the limit of the slopes of the secant lines as $\Delta x \to 0$.

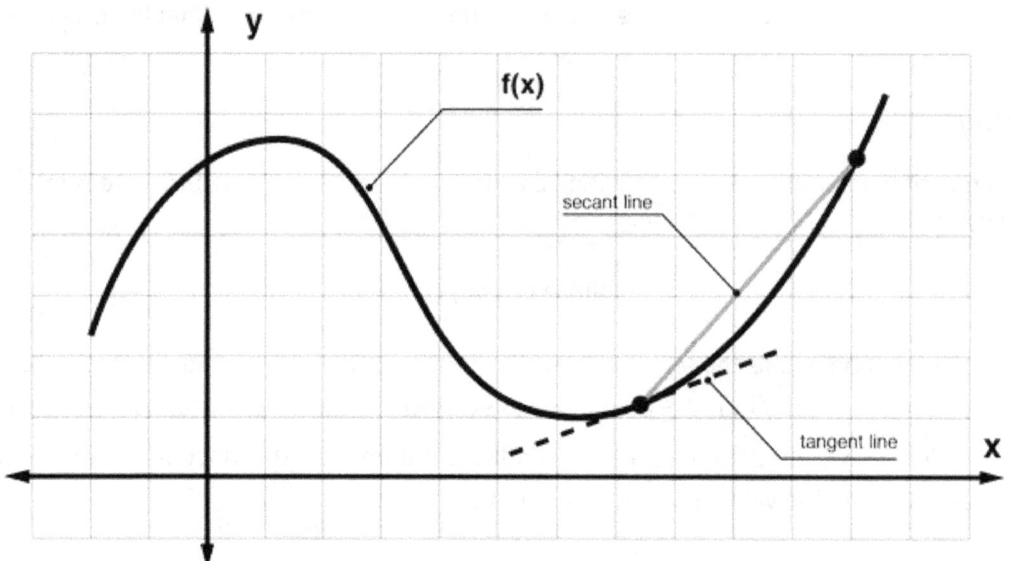

The derivative of a function can be found algebraically using the limit definition. Here is the process for finding the derivative of $f(x) = x^2 - 2$:

$$f'(x) = \lim_{h \to 0} \frac{f(x+h) - f(x)}{h}$$

$$= \lim_{h \to 0} \frac{(x+h)^2 - 2 - (x^2 - 2)}{h}$$

$$= \lim_{h \to 0} \frac{(x+h)(x+h) - 2 - x^2 + 2}{h}$$

$$= \lim_{h \to 0} \frac{x^2 + xh + xh + h^2 - 2 - x^2 + 2}{h}$$

$$= \lim_{h \to 0} \frac{x^2 + 2xh + h^2 - 2 - x^2 + 2}{h}$$

$$= \lim_{h \to 0} \frac{2xh + h^2}{h}$$

$$= \lim_{h \to 0} \frac{h(2x+h)}{h} = \lim_{h \to 0} 2x + h = 2x + 0 = 2x$$

Once the derivative function is found, it can be evaluated at any point by substituting that value in for x. Therefore, in this example, $f'(2)$=4.

Using the Chain Rule to Find Derivatives of Composite Functions

Consider the following functions:

$$y = 4u \text{ and } u = 5x - 6$$

The composite function:

$$y = 4(5x - 6)$$

can be built from the two functions as $y = f(u)$. Consider the following derivatives:

$$\frac{dy}{du} = 4, \frac{du}{dx} = 5, \text{and } \frac{dy}{dx} = 20$$

Therefore, it is true that:

$$\frac{dy}{dx} = \frac{dy}{du} \times \frac{du}{dx} = 4 \times 5 = 20.$$

This example is the foundation of the Chain Rule, which allows for the differentiation of composite functions. Basically, if $f(u)$ is differentiable at u, and u is differentiable at x, then the composite function $y = f(u)$ is differentiable at x and:

$$\frac{dy}{dx} = \frac{dy}{du} \times \frac{du}{dx}.$$

In other words, within a composite function, there is an "outside" function and an "inside" function. In the example above, the outside function is *y* and the inside function is *u*. To find the derivative of the composite function, take the derivative of the outside function and evaluate it in terms of the inside function. Then, multiply times the derivative of the inside function. In the above example, the derivative of the outside function was 4 and the derivative of the inside function was 5, so their product, 20, was the derivative.

The Chain Rule is helpful when taking derivatives that would otherwise require complicated algebra steps. Consider the following function:

$$y = (x^2 + x + 1)^2$$

Its derivative could be taken by squaring out the polynomial, collecting like terms, and then applying the Power Rule to each term. However, this is complicated and involves too many steps. The Chain Rule could be applied easily. The outside function is x^2 and the inside function is $x^2 + x + 1$. Therefore, the derivative of the composite function is the derivative of the outside function, evaluated in terms of the inside function, multiplied by the derivative of the inside function. This results in:

$$y = 2(x^2 + x + 1)(2x + 1)$$

$$(4x + 2)(x^2 + x + 1)$$

Solving Problems by Differentiation

Derivatives can be used to find the behavior of different functions such as the extrema, concavity, and symmetry. Given a function:

$$f(x) = 3x^2$$

the first derivative is $f'(x) = 6x$. This equation describes the slope of the line. Setting the derivative equal to zero means finding where the slope is zero, and these are potential points in which the function has extreme values. If the first derivative is positive over an interval, the function is increasing over that interval. If the first derivative is negative over an interval, the function is decreasing over that interval. Therefore, if the derivative is equal to zero at a point and the function changes from increasing to decreasing, then the function has a minimum at that point. If the function changes from decreasing to increasing at that point, it is a maximum. The second derivative can be used to define concavity. If it is positive over an interval, the graph resembles a U and is concave up over that interval. If the second derivative is negative, the graph is concave down. For this equation, solving:

$$f'(x) = 6x = 0 \text{ gets } x = 0, f(0) = 0$$

Also, the second derivative is 6, which is positive. The graph is concave up and, therefore, has a minimum value at (0,0).

Finding the derivative of a function can be done using the definition as described above, but rules proved via the different quotient can also be used. A few are listed below. These rules apply for functions that take the form inside the parenthesis. For example, the function $f(x) = 3x^4$ would use the Power Rule and Constant Multiple Rule. To find the derivative, the exponent is brought down to be multiplied by the coefficient, and the new exponent is one less than the original. As an equation, the derivative is:

$$f'(x) = 12x^3$$

$$\frac{d}{dx}(a^b) = 0$$

$$\frac{d}{dx}(x^n) = nx^{n-1}$$

$$\frac{d}{dx}(a^x) = a^x \ln a$$

$$\frac{d}{dx}(x^x) = x^x(1 + \ln x)$$

In relation to real-life problems, the position of a ball that is thrown into the area may be given by the equation:

$$p = 7 + 25t - 16t^2$$

The position, p, can be found for any time, t, after the ball is thrown. To find the initial position, $t = 0$ can be substituted into the equation to find p. That position would be 7ft above the ground, which is equal to the constant at the end of the equation.

Finding the derivative of the function would use the Power Rule. The derivative is:

$$p' = 25 - 32t$$

The derivative of a position function represents the velocity function. To find the initial velocity, the time $t = 0$ can be substituted into the equation. The initial velocity is found to be 25ft/s – the same as the coefficient of t in the position equation. Taking the derivative of the velocity equation yields the acceleration equation $p'' = -32$. This value is the acceleration at which a ball is pulled by gravity to the ground in feet per second squared.

Using Derivative Tests to Find Extrema, Points of Inflection, and Intervals

Rectilinear motion problems involve an object moving in a straight line. Given a position function $s = f(t)$, which outputs the position of an object given a specific time t, the object's velocity can be found by taking the derivative of the position function. Therefore, $v = f'(t)$. Its speed is equal to the absolute value of the velocity function:

$$s = |v| = |f'(t)|$$

Also, the acceleration of the object can be found by taking the second derivative of the position function. Therefore:

$$a = v' = f''(t).$$

Optimization problems also make use of derivatives. These problems involve finding either the smallest or largest value of a given function. The *Closed Interval Method* can be used to find absolute extrema of a function on a closed interval. First, the critical values need to be found on the given interval. They are found by setting the derivative equal to zero and solving, and they can also exist where the derivative is undefined. Then, the function is evaluated at those points and at the endpoints of the interval. The largest value is the absolute maximum within that interval, and the smallest value is the absolute minimum within that interval.

Interpreting the Derivatives of Circular Functions and their Inverses

Circular functions are part of the set of trigonometric functions. They have domains that are angles and ranges that are real numbers. The most widely used circular (trigonometric) functions are sine, cosine, tangent, cosecant, secant, and cotangent. Here are the derivatives of the six trigonometric functions:

The Derivatives of the Six Trigonometric Functions

$$\frac{d}{dx}(\sin(x)) = \cos(x)$$

$$\frac{d}{dx}(\cos(x)) = -\sin(x)$$

$$\frac{d}{dx}(\tan(x)) = \sec^2(x)$$

$$\frac{d}{dx}(\cot(x)) = -\csc^2(x)$$

$$\frac{d}{dx}(\sec(x)) = \sec(x)\tan(x)$$

$$\frac{d}{dx}(\csc(x)) = -\csc(x)\cot(x)$$

The functions are differentiable at every x-value in which they are defined. For example, tangent is not differentiable at $\frac{\pi}{2}$. If tangent is evaluated at $\frac{\pi}{2}$, the result is undefined because $cos\left(\frac{\pi}{2}\right) = 0$. There is actually an asymptote there on the graph of tangent. Therefore, $\frac{\pi}{2}$ is not in the domain of tangent, and therefore the function is not differentiable there.

The derivatives of tangent, cotangent, secant, and cosecant can all be derived using the Quotient Rule and the following identities:

$$\text{Pythagorean identity: } \cos^2 x + \sin^2 x = 1$$

$$\text{Reciprocal identities: } \sec x = \frac{1}{\cos x},\ \csc x = \frac{1}{\sin x},\ \tan x = \frac{\sin x}{\cos x},\ \text{and } \cot x = \frac{1}{\tan x}.$$

For example:

$$\frac{d}{dx}\tan x = \frac{d}{dx}\frac{\sin x}{\cos x}$$

$$\frac{\frac{d}{dx}\sin x \cdot \cos x - \frac{d}{dx}\cos x \cdot \sin x}{(\cos x)^2} = \frac{\cos^2 x + \sin^2 x}{\cos^2 x}$$

$$\frac{1}{\cos^2 x} = \sec^2 x$$

Also, the inverse trigonometric functions can be differentiated. Note that the domain of these six functions are real numbers and their outputs are angles. Here are the derivatives of the six inverse trigonometric functions:

The Derivatives of the Six Inverse Trigonometric Functions

$$\frac{d}{dx}(\sin^{-1}(x)) = \frac{1}{\sqrt{1 - x^2}}$$

$$\frac{d}{dx}(\cos^{-1}(x)) = -\frac{1}{\sqrt{1 - x^2}}$$

$$\frac{d}{dx}(\tan^{-1}(x)) = \frac{1}{1 + x^2}$$

$$\frac{d}{dx}(\sec^{-1}(x)) = \frac{1}{|x| \cdot \sqrt{x^2 - 1}}$$

$$\frac{d}{dx}(\csc^{-1}(x)) = -\frac{1}{|x| \cdot \sqrt{x^2 - 1}}$$

$$\frac{d}{dx}(\cot^{-1}(x)) = -\frac{1}{1 + x^2}$$

The derivatives of both the trigonometric functions and the inverse trigonometric functions can be used alone or inside rules such as the Product Rule and Quotient Rule. For instance, consider the following function:

$$y = x\sin^{-1}x + \frac{x}{\sin x}$$

The Product Rule would have to be used on the first half of the function and the Quotient Rule would have to be used on the second half. Therefore, the derivative is:

$$y = \sin^{-1}x + \frac{x}{\sqrt{1 - x^2}} + \frac{\sin x - x\cos x}{\sin^2 x}.$$

Trigonometric functions can be used to model simple harmonic motion. For instance, the position of a body hanging from a spring that is stretched 4 feet from its resting position can be described by the function $s = 4\cos t$, where t represents time in seconds. Note that at time $t = 0, s = 4$, and 4 is known as its amplitude. Its velocity, v, can be found by taking the first derivative of the position function and its acceleration, a, can be found by taking the second derivative of the position function. Therefore:

$$v = -4\sin t \text{ and } a = -4\cos t.$$

Interpreting the Derivatives of Transcendental Functions

Transcendental functions are functions that basically "transcend" algebra. In other words, they cannot be expressed in terms of algebraic functions. These functions include exponential functions, logarithmic functions, and their inverses. Consider the natural logarithmic function $y = \ln x$ and its inverse function, the exponential function $y = e^x$. The derivative of the exponential function is actually the function itself. It is the only function that holds this property. Therefore:

$$\frac{d}{dx}e^x = e^x$$

The derivative of its inverse function, $y = \ln x$, is derived using implicit differentiation. The rule is that:

$$\frac{d}{dx}\ln x = \frac{1}{x}, \text{ for } x > 0.$$

Other rules exist for exponential functions and logarithmic functions with bases other than e. Consider the exponential function with base $a, y = a^x$. Its derivative can be derived using the Chain Rule and it can be seen in the rule:

$$\frac{d}{dx}a^x = a^x \ln a, a > 0, a \neq 1.$$

This rule is applied when finding that the derivative of $y = 5^x$ is $y' = 5^x \ln 5$.

Finally, the logarithmic function with base a, which is $y = \log_a x$, can be derived using the Change of Base formula for logarithms and the derivative of the natural logarithmic function. The process is shown here:

$$\frac{d}{dx}\log_a x = \frac{d}{dx}\frac{\ln x}{\ln a} = \frac{1}{\ln a}\frac{d}{dx}\ln x = \frac{1}{\ln a} \times \frac{1}{x} = \frac{1}{x\ln a} \text{ for } a > 0, a \neq 1.$$

This rule is applied when finding that the derivative of $y = \log_2 x$ is $y' = \frac{1}{x\ln 2}$.

Determining the Derivatives of Composite Functions

Composite functions are often built from trigonometric, logarithmic, and exponential functions. In this case, in order to take the derivative, the Chain Rule must be used.

Consider the example of a composite function

$$y = \sin(4x^2)$$

It is a composite function with an outside function of $\sin x$ and an inside function of $4x^2$. The derivative of the outside function is $\cos x$, but evaluating it in terms of the inside function results in $\cos(4x^2)$. The derivative of the inside function is $8x$. Therefore, the derivative of the composite function is the product of these two expressions:

$$\frac{dy}{dx} = 8x\cos(4x^2)$$

The following function also requires the Chain Rule to find its derivative:

$$y = \log_4(1 + \ln x).$$

Note that the inside function is a transcendental function $1 + \ln x$, and the outside function is a transcendental function $\log_4 x$. Therefore, its derivative is:

$$y' = \frac{1}{(1 + \ln x)\ln 4} \times \frac{1}{x} = \frac{1}{x\ln 4(1 + \ln x)}.$$

The Chain Rule can be used as many times as necessary, depending on how many inside functions exist within a composite function. Consider the following composite function based on the circular function cosine:

$$y = (\cos(5x))^2$$

It has an outside function of x^2, a middle function of $\cos x$, and an inside function of $5x$. Its derivative involves using the Chain Rule twice, and is:

$$y' = 2(\cos(5x)) \times (-\sin(5x)) \times 5$$

$$-10\cos(5x)\sin(5x)$$

Using Implicit Differentiation

If an equation is not placed into the form $y = f(x)$, in order to be differentiated, implicit differentiation must be used. Basically, if the equation is not solved for y as a function of x, the normal rules for taking derivatives do not apply. These equations are known as implicitly defined functions. Some examples of implicitly defined functions are:

$$x^3y^2 + xy + 3 = 0 \text{ and } x^2y^2 + xy + 3 = 0$$

Solving for y as a function of x in both examples is very difficult; therefore, in order to differentiate each function, a new technique must be used.

In this case, the process is called implicit differentiation, and it involves taking the derivative of both sides of the equation with respect to x. The variable y must be treated as a function of x, so when taking the derivative of y term, the chain rule must be used. For instance:

$$\frac{d}{dx}(y^2) = 2y\frac{dy}{dx}$$

Once the derivative of both sides are taken, the equation is then solved for $\frac{dy}{dx}$ in terms of both y and x. This end result gives a formula for the slope of the tangent line at any point on the original curve.

A common function that highlights the use of implicit differentiation is one that represents a circle. Consider the equation:

$$x^2 + y^2 = 9$$

a circle centered at the origin with radius 3. Its derivative can be found by using implicit differentiation. First, take the derivative of both sides with respect to x. Remember, that whenever there is a y, the chain rule must be used because y is a function of x. This results in:

$$2x + 2y\frac{dy}{dx} = 0$$

Then, solve for $\frac{dy}{dx}$ using algebra. This results in $\frac{dy}{dx} = -\frac{x}{y'}$, which is the formula for the slope of the tangent line at any point (x, y) on the original circle. This example also could have been done using normal differentiation by first solving for y to obtain:

$$y = \pm\sqrt{9 - x^2}$$

The chain rule would be used to obtain the same result.

Knowing the derivative of the natural logarithmic function and how to differentiate implicitly are helpful tools when differentiating functions in which other rules cannot be applied. The process is known as Logarithmic Differentiation. Consider the function $y = x^x, x > 0$. There is no known rule that allows the derivative to be taken. Therefore, take the natural logarithm of both sides and use properties of logarithms to rewrite it as $\ln y = x \ln x$. Differentiating implicitly on both sides with respect to x results in:

$$\frac{1}{y}\frac{dy}{dx} = \ln x + 1.$$

Therefore:

$$\frac{dy}{dx} = y(\ln x + 1) = x^x(\ln x + 1)$$

Determining Related Rates

Related rate problems also involve derivatives. Each problem involves both an unknown quantity and known quantities that involve derivatives. The key is to relate the unknown quantity or its rate of change to the known quantities or their rates of change through a known formula or equation. The equation must be differentiated with respect to the independent variable. The functions usually have time as their independent variables, so most derivatives are with respect to time and implicit differentiation needs to be used. Consider an object moving along the path $y = x^3$, and at some time t, its x-coordinate is 8 and the x-coordinate is moving at a rate of 4 units per measurement of time. To find how fast the y-coordinate is moving, a related rates problem must be solved. Using implicit differentiation:

$$\frac{dy}{dt} = 3x^2\frac{dx}{dt}$$

The problem gives that:

$$x = 8 \text{ and } \frac{dx}{dt} = 4$$

so this equation can be used to find that the y-coordinate is moving at a rate of 768 units per measurement of time.

Integrals

Finding Antiderivatives and Interpreting C

Per the fundamental theorem of calculus, on a closed interval [a, b], the following represents the definite integral:

$$f(x): \int_a^b f(x)dx = F(b) - F(a)$$

$F(x)$ represents the antiderivative of the function $f(x)$. Other theorems allow constants to be moved to the front of the integral, negatives to be moved to the outside of the integral, and integrals to be split into two parts that make up a whole. An example of using these theorems can be seen in the following problem:

$$\int_{-1}^{3} (4x^3 - 2x)dx = (108 - 6) - (-4 + 2) = 104$$

The antiderivative of:

$$4x^3 - 2x \text{ is } x^4 - x^2$$

Within the fundamental theorem of calculus, the antiderivative $F(x)$ exists. It is true that:

$$F'(x) = f(x)$$

Therefore, it is important to know how the graph of a function and a derivative relate. Because the derivative function represents the slope of the tangent of a function, where a function is horizontal, the derivative function has zeros. On intervals where the function is decreasing, the derivative function lies below the x-axis, and on intervals where the function is increasing, the derivative function lies above the y-axis.

Slope is defined in algebra to be a rate of change; therefore, the derivative function is a rate of change. The definite integral in the fundamental theorem of calculus can also be used to represent a rate of change. If one were to calculate the definite integral of a function $f(x)$ over the interval $[a, b]$ as $F(b) - F(a)$, where $F'(x) = f(x)$, the result is the net rate of change of $F(x)$ over the same interval.

Understanding and Using Sigma Notation for Simplifying Sums

Sigma notation can be used to simplify writing down long sums. Suppose that there is a list of numbers, which can be labeled by the numbers 1, 2, 3, and so on. This label is called an *index*, and it is generally written at the lower right of the symbol representing the numbers in the list: x_i. Thus, x_1 will indicate the first number in the list, x_2 will indicate the second number, and x_i represents the *i*-th number in the list.

Suppose that for a given problem, it is necessary to plug each number in the list into some formula, *f*, then add up the results for every number. The resulting sum would be quite long and difficult to write out, since it would look like $f(x_1) + f(x_2) + f(x_3) + \cdots$ and so on. In addition, it is sometimes necessary to write down formulas that work for different lists that may have a different length. Sigma notation is a way of writing down such sums that solves this problem elegantly.

Therefore, suppose the list of numbers runs from x_1 to x_n, where *n* is an arbitrary natural number. To indicate the sum of all *n* quantities $f(x_i)$, one may use sigma notation as follows:

$$\sum_{i=1}^{n} f(x_i).$$

The large symbol is a capital Greek letter *sigma*. Below it, write the index label (in this case *i*) and the number at which to start. At the top, write the number at which the sum is to stop. Then, to the right of the sigma symbol itself, write the expression that is to be added up.

It is not necessary to always start the sum at the first value of the index. By writing some other number instead of 1, sigma notation can be used to indicate that the sum is to start at some other point in the list. So, for example:

$$\sum_{i=3}^{5} f(x_i) = f(x_3) + f(x_4) + f(x_5)$$

While:

$$\sum_{i=0}^{2} f(x_i) = f(x_0) + f(x_1) + f(x_2)$$

Approximating Areas Bounded by Curves

In calculus, the area problem involves finding the area under a positive function $y = f(x)$ from $x = a$ to $x = b$, above the x-axis. Such a region Ω is shown here:

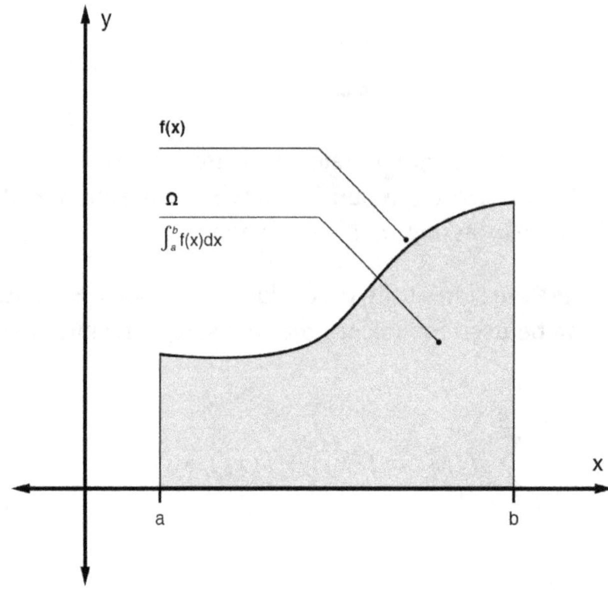

The area is defined as the definite integral of

$$y = f(x) \text{ from } x = a \text{ to } x = b$$

and is denoted as

$$\int_a^b f(x)dx.$$

In a similar manner, the area between two curves is

$$y = f(x) \text{ and } y = g(x)$$

from $x = a$ to $x = b$ where

$$f(x) \geq g(x)$$

over that same interval is given as

$$\int_a^b (f(x) - g(x))dx.$$

Arc length can also be calculated using an integral. Consider the same function $y = f(x)$ from $x = a$ to $x = b$. The length of the curve over that interval, also known as arc length, is defined as:

$$L = \int_a^b \sqrt{1 + \left(\frac{dy}{dx}\right)^2}\, dx$$

All three of these integral definitions are based on proofs based on limits.

The average value of a function can be found by the following integral:

$$\frac{1}{b-a}\int_a^b f(x)dx$$

The integral finds the area of the region bounded by the function and the x-axis, while the fraction divides the area to find the average value of the integral. An example of this is shown in the graph below. The function $f(x)$ is the black line. The light gray shading represents the area under the curve, while the rectangle drawn on top with added darker shading represents the same amount of area as the region under the graph of the given function over the interval of a to b. This rectangle has the base [a, b] and height f(c).

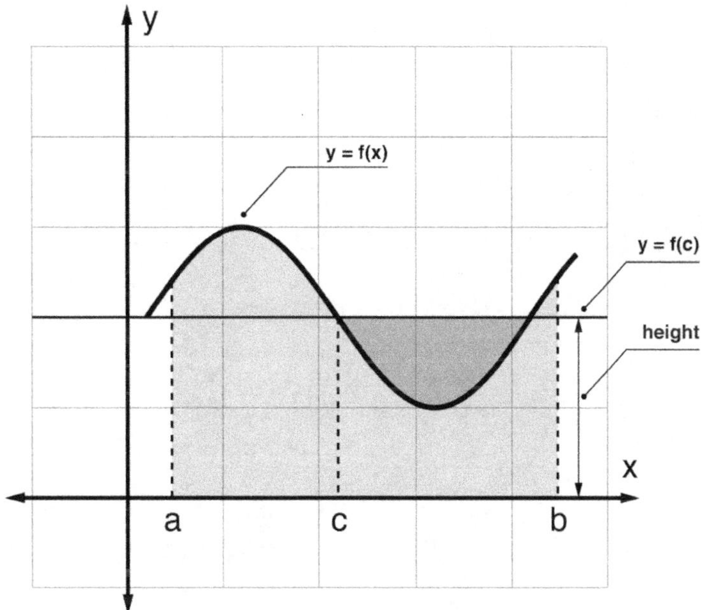

The *Mean Value Theorem* states that if f is a continuous function on interval [a, b], and f' is differentiable on (a, b), then there exists at least one number, c, in which the derivative at that point equals the slope of the secant line connecting the endpoints of the interval. This number can be found by the equation:

$$f'(c) = \frac{f(b) - f(a)}{b - a}$$

Integration

Since integration is the inverse operation of finding the derivative, the integral is found by going backwards from the derivative. In relation to the ball problem, an acceleration function can be integrated to find the velocity function. That function can then be integrated to find the position function. From velocity, integration finds the position function:

$$p = -16t^2 + 25t + c$$

where c is an unknown constant. More information would need to be given in the original problem to integrate and find the value of c.

Practice Questions

1. The mixed number $3\frac{3}{4}$ can be expressed as which improper fraction?

   a. $\frac{14}{3}$
   b. $\frac{17}{4}$
   c. $\frac{15}{4}$
   d. $\frac{11}{3}$

2. $\frac{13}{3} - \frac{4}{5} =$

   a. $\frac{53}{15}$
   b. $\frac{7}{5}$
   c. $\frac{73}{15}$
   d. $\frac{4}{5}$

3. In a room of 40 students, 25 are girls. What percentage of the students are girls?

   a. 55%
   b. 62.5%
   c. 70%
   d. 73.5%

4. A group of five friends take a test. The scores of the first four were 75, 80, 90, and 95. If the average for all five scores is 85, what must the score of the fifth student have been?

   a. 75
   b. 80
   c. 85
   d. 90

5. $3.2 \times 4.1 =$

   a. 14.2
   b. 11.33
   c. 15.6
   d. 13.12

6. $\frac{5.2 \cdot 10^2}{2.6 \cdot 10^4} =$

   a. 4×10^2
   b. 2×10^{-2}
   c. 2×10^2
   d. 4×10^{-2}

7. How should 0.042 be expressed in scientific notation?
a. 4.2×10^2
b. 4.2×10^3
c. 4.2×10^{-3}
d. 4.2×10^{-2}

8. The ratio of people who prefer Coke to people who prefer Pepsi in a company is 4:3. If there are a total of 140 people in the company, how many like Coke better than Pepsi?
a. 60
b. 70
c. 75
d. 80

9. $\frac{4x^3y^2z}{2x^2y^3z} =$

a. $2xy$
b. $\frac{2x}{y}$
c. $\frac{2y}{x}$
d. $\frac{1}{2xyz}$

10. Solve for x: $\frac{2x+3}{4x-4} = 1$.
a. 3
b. 3.5
c. 4
d. 4.5

11. What are the polynomial roots of $x^2 - x - 12$?
a. 4, -3
b. 3, -4
c. 3, -3
d. 4, -4

12. Solve for x and y, given that $2x + 3y = 8, -x + y = 1$.
a. (3, 3)
b. (2, -2)
c. (1, 2)
d. (4, 1)

13. $3^3 \times 3^2 \times 9^{-1} =$
a. 9
b. 27
c. 81
d. 243

14. Find the sum of the following polynomials: $(-3xy + x^2 - 1), (2x + 2xy), (5x - y)$.

a. $x^2 - xy + 7x - y - 1$
b. $-3x^2 + 2xy - 2x + 2$
c. $-3x^2y^2 + 4xy - 2x \pm 2y + 4$
d. $5xy - 2y$

15. What are the polynomial roots of $\frac{1}{2}x^2 - 4x - 2$?

a. $4 \pm 2\sqrt{5}$
b. $2 \pm 4\sqrt{5}$
c. $1 \pm \sqrt{5}$
d. $4 \pm 2\sqrt{15}$

16. Solve for x in terms of y, if $\sqrt[3]{x} = y^3$.

a. $x = y^{16}$
b. $x = y^9$
c. $x = y^6$
d. $x = y^4$

17. A bag contains 5 red marbles, 10 blue marbles, and 15 green marbles. What is the probability of picking a green marble out of the bag in a single try?

a. $\frac{1}{6}$
b. $\frac{1}{3}$
c. $\frac{1}{2}$
d. $\frac{2}{5}$

18. What is the probability of selecting an ace or a red card out of a standard pack of cards?

a. $\frac{1}{2}$
b. $\frac{1}{13}$
c. $\frac{7}{13}$
d. $\frac{15}{26}$

19. If 2 fair 4-sided dice are rolled, what is the probability that the results add up to 4?

a. $\frac{1}{16}$
b. $\frac{1}{12}$
c. $\frac{5}{16}$
d. $\frac{3}{16}$

For questions 20-23, students taking a test got the following scores: {93, 85, 90, 75, 70, 75, 80, 85, 85}.

20. What is the mean score?
    a. 82
    b. 83
    c. 84.5
    d. 85

21. What is the median of the data set?
    a. 75
    b. 80
    c. 85
    d. 93

22. What is the difference between the mode of the data set and the mean?
    a. 1
    b. 2
    c. 3
    d. 5

23. Suppose that a tenth and eleventh student took the test. What would their average score need to be in order for the class average to be 80?
    a. 80
    b. 70
    c. 71
    d. 74

24. Solve for x: $x^3 - 16x = 0$.
    a. 0, 2, -2
    b. 0, 4, -4
    c. 0, 8, -8
    d. 0, 16, -16

25. Solve for x: $\sqrt{x-1} = \sqrt{x+1} - 1$.
    a. $\frac{3}{4}$
    b. $\frac{6}{5}$
    c. $\frac{2}{5}$
    d. $\frac{5}{4}$

26. Solve for x: $x^2 - 8x = -16$.
    a. 1
    b. 2
    c. 3
    d. 4

27. What is the slope of a line passing through the points (1, 4) and (3, 10)?
    a. 2
    b. 3
    c. 4
    d. 5

28. What is the slope of a line described by the equation $x + 2y + 4 = 0$?
    a. $\frac{1}{2}$
    b. 1
    c. $-\frac{1}{2}$
    d. -1

29. What is the equation of a line that passes through the point (2, 3) with a slope of 4?
    a. $y = 4x - 5$
    b. $y = 3x - 8$
    c. $y = \frac{1}{2}x + 3$
    d. $y = \frac{3}{2}x + 4$

30. Recall that there are 2.54 centimeters (cm) to every inch (in). The factor for converting distances between D_{cm}, the distance in centimeters, and D_{in}, the distance in inches, is $2.54\frac{cm}{in}$. How would one obtain the distance in inches, given the distance in centimeters?
    a. $D_{in} = 2.54D_{cm}$
    b. $D_{in} = \frac{D_{cm}}{2.54}$
    c. $D_{in} = D_{cm}^{2.54}$
    d. $D_{in} = D_{cm} + 2.54$

31. What is the formula relating an area A_{cm} in centimeters to an area A_{in} in inches?
    a. $A_{cm} = 6.4516A_{in}$
    b. $A_{cm} = 5A_{in}$
    c. $A_{cm} = 3.46A_{in}$
    d. $A_{cm} = 8.16A_{in}$

32. Find $\frac{d}{dx}\frac{(x^2+4)}{x}$.
    a. $\frac{x^2-4}{x^2}$
    b. $\frac{x^2+4}{x^2}$
    c. $\frac{x^2-4}{x}$
    d. $\frac{x^2+4}{x}$

33. Find $\frac{d}{dx}2x^3$.
   a. $8x^2$
   b. $5x$
   c. $6x^2$
   d. $\frac{x^4}{2}$

34. Find $\frac{d}{dx}xe^x$.
   a. $(x+1)e^x$
   b. e^x
   c. $x+e^x$
   d. e^x-2x

35. Evaluate the derivative of $6x^2+4x-64$ at $x=2$.
   a. -32
   b. 4
   c. 28
   d. 29

36. Find $\frac{d}{dx}\tan(2x)$.
   a. $\csc^2 4x$
   b. $\sec^2 4x$
   c. $2\csc^2 2x$
   d. $2\sec^2 2x$

37. Suppose that $2y^2+x^2=3$. What is the slope of the tangent line to this curve at the point (1, 1)?
   a. 1
   b. -1
   c. $\frac{1}{2}$
   d. $-\frac{1}{2}$

38. Find $\frac{d}{dx}(\frac{1}{2}x^2-4x-2)$.
   a. $4x+1$
   b. $x-4$
   c. x^2+2x
   d. $\frac{1}{x}$

39. Find $\int e^{\frac{3x}{2}} dx$.
a. $3e^{\frac{3x}{2}} + C$
b. $2e^{\frac{3x}{2}} + C$
c. $\frac{2}{3}e^{\frac{3x}{2}} + C$
d. $\frac{3}{2}e^{\frac{3x}{2}} + C$

40. Find $\int \frac{4}{x} dx$.
a. $-\frac{2}{x^2} + C$
b. $4x + C$
c. $\frac{4}{\ln|x|} + C$
d. $4\ln|x| + C$

41. Find $\int 3\cos x\, dx$.
a. $3\sin x + C$
b. $-3\sin x + C$
c. $\frac{1}{3}\csc x + C$
d. $3\tan x + C$

42. Find $\int_{-1}^{1} x^3\, dx$.
a. $\frac{1}{8}$
b. 0
c. $-\frac{1}{4}$
d. $\frac{1}{2}$

43. Find $\int_2^4 3x dx$.
a. 18
b. 19
c. 20
d. 24

44. Find the area between the curves $y = x$ and $y = x^2$, between the points $x = 0, x = 1$.
a. $\frac{1}{16}$
b. $\frac{1}{6}$
c. $\frac{1}{4}$
d. $\frac{1}{3}$

45. In feet per second, the velocity of an object dropped off a building is $v(t) = -32t - 8$. If the object was dropped from 500 feet, what equation describes its height in feet as a function of time in seconds?

a. $h(t) = -32t - 8 - 500$
b. $h(t) = -32t^2 - 8t + 500$
c. $h(t) = -16t + 500$
d. $h(t) = -16t^2 - 8t + 500$

46. Approximate the area under $2x^2 + 1$ from $x = -1$ to $x = 2$ using left endpoints and 3 intervals.

a. 13
b. 9.5
c. 7
d. 17

47. Solve for x: $x^2 + 2x + 5 = 0$.

a. $-1 \pm 2i$
b. $1 \pm i$
c. $1 \pm 2i$
d. $-1 \pm i$

48. What is $\vec{v} - \vec{w}$, if $\vec{v} = (3, -2, 1), \vec{w} = (2, 1, -4)$?

a. $(1, 4, 2)$
b. $(-3, 5, 1)$
c. $(2, 2, 2)$
d. $(1, -3, 5)$

Answer Explanations

1. C: Convert the whole number 3 to a fraction with a denominator of 4:

$$\frac{3}{1} \times \frac{4}{4} = \frac{12}{4}$$

Add this to the fractional part of the mixed number:

$$\frac{12}{4} + \frac{3}{4} = \frac{15}{4}$$

2. A: Convert the fractions to a common denominator of 15:

$$\frac{13}{3} \times \frac{5}{5} - \frac{4}{5} \times \frac{3}{3} = \frac{65}{15} - \frac{12}{15} = \frac{53}{15}$$

3. B: The fraction of students who are girls is $\frac{25}{40}$. To convert this to a fraction over 100, multiply the numerator and denominator by 2.5

$$\frac{25}{40} \times \frac{2.5}{2.5} = \frac{62.5}{100}$$

The percentage is the numerator of a fraction with a denominator of 100, so it is 62.5%.

4. C: Let the fifth student's score be x. Then

$$\frac{1}{5}(75 + 80 + 90 + 95 + x) = 85$$

This equation simplifies to:

$$\frac{1}{5}(340 + x) = 85, 340 + x = 425, x = 85$$

5. D: Consider this as:

$$32 \times 10^{-1} \times 41 \times 10^{-1}$$

$$32 \times 41 \cdot 10^{-2} = 1312 \times 10^{-2} = 13.12$$

6. B: First, $\frac{5.2}{2.6} = 2$. Next:

$$\frac{10^2}{10^4} = 10^2 \times 10^{-4} = 10^{-2}$$

So, the answer is 2×10^{-2}.

7. D: Scientific notation requires that the non-decimal portion of the number lie between 1 and 10, which requires moving the decimal point to the right 2 places, or multiplying by 10^2, to get 4.2. Therefore, the original number is 4.2×10^{-2} to move the decimal point back to the left 2 places.

8. D: If the ratio is 4:3, then the fraction of people who prefer Coke is $\frac{4}{7}$. Multiplying $\frac{4}{7} \times 140 = 80$.

9. B:

$$\frac{4x^3y^2z}{2x^2y^3z} = 2x^3x^{-2}y^2y^{-3}zz^{-1}$$

$$2x^{3-2}y^{2-3}z^{1-1} = 2xy^{-1}z^0 = \frac{2x}{y}$$

10. B: Multiply both sides by $4x - 4$

$$\frac{2x+3}{4x-4}(4x-4) = 1(4x-4)$$

The equation becomes:

$$2x + 3 = 4x - 4$$

Subtract $4x$ from both sides and subtract 3 from both sides to get $-2x = -7$. Now, divide both sides by:

-2. $x = \frac{7}{2} = 3.5$

11. A: The divisors of 12 are 1, 2, 3, 4, 6, and 12. Since the outcome is negative, one factor must be positive and one negative. The only pair from this list that will multiply to -12 and add to -1 is 3 with -4. Therefore, this polynomial factors into $(x-4)(x+3)$. The roots of this can be immediately read to be 4 and -3.

12. C: Multiply the second equation by 2 to obtain

$$-2x + 2y = 2$$

Add this result to the first equation to eliminate the x term

$$(2x + 3y) + (-2x + 2y) = 8 + 2$$

becomes $5y = 10$, so $y = 2$. Substituting this into the second equation gives $-x + 2 = 1$, which simplifies to $x = 1$. So, the solution is (1, 2).

13. B: Rewrite this as:

$$3^3 \times 3^2 \times (3^2)^{-1}$$

$$3^5 \times 3^{-2} = 3^3 = 27$$

14. A: The sum is:

$$-3xy + x^2 - 1 + 2x + 2xy + 5x - y$$

Gathering terms with the same monomials gives:

$$x^2 + (-3 + 2)xy + (2 + 5)x - y - 1$$

$$x^2 - xy + 7x - y - 1$$

15. A: Apply the quadratic formula with $a = \frac{1}{2}, b = -4, c = -2$. This gives:

$$\frac{4 \pm \sqrt{(-4)^2 - 4 \cdot \frac{1}{2}(-2)}}{2 \cdot \frac{1}{2}}$$

$$4 \pm \sqrt{16 + 4} = 4 \pm \sqrt{20}$$

$$4 \pm 2\sqrt{5}$$

16. B: Raise both sides to the third power:

$$(\sqrt[3]{x})^3 = (y^3)^3, x = y^9$$

17. C: The total number of marbles is 5 + 10 + 15 = 30. Of these, 15 are green. All marbles have an equal probability of getting picked, so the probability is $\frac{15}{30} = \frac{1}{2}$.

18. C: A standard pack of cards has 52 cards and 4 of those are aces. There are also 26 red cards in a deck. However, there is an overlap of the 2 red aces. The probability of getting one of these cards is

$$\frac{4}{52} + \frac{26}{52} - \frac{2}{52} = \frac{28}{52} = \frac{7}{13}$$

19. D: There is a total of 16 possible ways to roll the dice, corresponding to each possible pairing of numbers 1 through 4. To get results that add to 4, there are 3 ways: the rolls could be 1 and 3, 2 and 2, or 3 and 1. Therefore the probability is $\frac{3}{16}$.

20. A: There is a total of 9 tests, so the mean is given by

$$\frac{1}{9}(70 + 75 + 75 + 80 + 85 + 85 + 85 + 90 + 93) = \frac{738}{9} = 82$$

21. C: There are 9 entries, so the median is $\frac{9+1}{2} = 5$, therefore it is the fifth entry, when the entries are ordered from lowest to highest. Reordering gives {70, 75, 75, 80, 85, 85, 85, 90, 93}. The fifth entry is 85.

22. C: The mode is the most frequent number to appear. Reading through the list shows that 85 appears 3 times, and all other numbers appear at most twice. So, the mode is 85. The difference between 85 and 82 (the mean) is 3.

23. C: The new average would be

$$\frac{1}{11}(70 + 75 + 75 + 80 + 85 + 85 + 85 + 90 + 93 + 2x)$$

where x is the average of these 2 additional students. Set this equal to 80

$$\frac{1}{11}(738 + 2x) = 80, 738 + 2x = 880, 2x = 142, x = 71$$

Be careful to note here, in the formula for the average, the need to add in *twice* the average because there are *2* students whose average comes out to x.

24. B: An x can be factored out to turn this equation into $x(x^2 - 16) = 0$. Therefore, one of the solutions is zero. Solving $x^2 - 16 = 0$ gives $x^2 = 16$, or $x = \pm 4$.

25. D: Square both sides of the equation:

$$(\sqrt{x-1})^2 = (\sqrt{x+1} - 1)^2$$

Becomes:

$$x - 1 = x + 1 - 2\sqrt{x+1} + 1$$

Isolate the remaining square root on one side to get:

$$-3 = -2\sqrt{x+1}$$

Square both sides again:

$$(-3)^2 = (-2\sqrt{x+1})^2$$

Becomes:

$$9 = 4(x+1), 9 = 4x + 4, 5 = 4x, x = \frac{5}{4}.$$

26. D: This equation becomes:

$$x^2 - 8x + 16 = 0$$

-4 and -4 will add to get -8 and multiply to give 16, so this factors into $(x - 4)^2 = 0$, which has the solution of 4.

27. B: The slope is given by the formula $\frac{y_2 - y_1}{x_2 - x_1}$, which in this case becomes:

$$\frac{10-4}{3-1} = \frac{6}{2} = 3$$

28. C: There are several ways to approach this problem. One way is to solve for *y*, getting:

$$2y = -x - 4, y = -\frac{1}{2}x - 2$$

which is in slope-intercept form. In this form the slope is the coefficient of *x*, or $-\frac{1}{2}$.

29. A: Begin by writing the equation in point-slope form:

$$y - y_0 = m(x - x_0)$$

In this case, this gives the equation:

$$y - 3 = 4(x - 2)$$

Solving for y, the slope-intercept form is the result, $y = 4x - 5$.

30. B: The formula to convert from inches to centimeters is $D_{cm} = 2.54D_{in}$. From the formula $D_{cm} = 2.54D_{in}$ divide both sides by 2.54 to solve for D_{in}, to get:

$$D_{in} = \frac{D_{cm}}{2.54}$$

31. A: There are $2.54\frac{cm}{in}$. Area is in in^2, so to eliminate the inches, one needs to multiply by this conversion twice

$$2.54\frac{cm}{in} \times 2.54\frac{cm}{in} in^2$$

cancels the inches and results in cm^2. So, the formula is

$$A_{cm} = 2.54^2 A_{in} = 6.4516A_{in}$$

32. A: The derivative can be found by using the quotient rule

$$\frac{x\frac{d}{dx}(x^2+4) - [(x^2+4)\frac{d}{dx}x]}{x^2} = \frac{x(2x) - (x^2+4)(1)}{x^2}$$

The derivative simplifies to $\frac{x^2-4}{x^2}$.

33. C: Apply the power rule, to get:

$$2 \times 3x^{3-1} = 6x^2$$

34. A: Apply the product rule with:

$$f(x) = x, g(x) = e^x$$

The derivatives are:

$$f'(x) = 1, g'(x) = e^x$$

Therefore:

$$\frac{d}{dx}xe^x = 1 \times e^x + xe^x = (x+1)e^x$$

Note: Avoid the temptation to simply use the product of the derivatives of each term for the answer. The full product rule must be applied to get the correct answer.

35. C: Using the power rule and the rule for derivatives of constants, the derivative of this expression is $12x + 4$. Evaluating this at $x = 2$ gives:

$$12 \times 2 + 4 = 24 + 4 = 28$$

36. D: This requires the chain rule, with:

$$f(x) = \tan x \,, g(x) = 2x$$

Then:

$$f'(x) = \sec^2 x \,, g'(x) = 2$$

Plugging this into the chain rule formula gives :

$$(\sec^2 2x) \times 2 = 2\sec^2 2x$$

Make sure to use the entire formula for the chain rule here.

37. D: Using implicit differentiation, begin with:

$$\frac{d}{dx}(2y^2 + x^2) = \frac{d}{dx}3$$

which gives:

$$4yy' + 2x = 0$$

Solving for y' gives $y' = -\frac{x}{2y}$. Plugging in the point (1, 1) gives $y' = -\frac{1}{2}$.

38. B: Applying the power rule and the rule for constants gives:

$$\frac{1}{2} \cdot 2x^{2-1} - 4 \cdot 1x^{1-1} + 0 = x - 4$$

39. C: To find $\int e^{\frac{3x}{2}} dx$, apply the substitution rule first where:

$$u = \frac{3}{2}x, \frac{2}{3}du = dx$$

Then, substitute the known values $\frac{2}{3}\int e^u dx$, and apply the integration rule. Then back substitute to get the solution:

$$\frac{2}{3}e^{\frac{3x}{2}} + C$$

40. D:

$$\int \frac{4}{x} dx = 4 \int \frac{1}{x} dx = 4\ln|x| + C$$

Note that 1/x is the exceptional case to which the power rule for integration does not apply.

41. A: $\int 3\cos x\,dx = 3\int \cos x\,dx = 3\sin x + C$.

42. B: Begin by finding an antiderivative of x^3, which is $\frac{x^4}{4}$. The constant of integration can be assumed to be zero, since this is a definite integral. Therefore:

$$\int_{-1}^{1} x^3\,dx = \frac{x^4}{4}\bigg|_{-1}^{1}$$

$$\frac{1^4}{4} - \frac{(-1)^4}{4} = \frac{1}{4} - \frac{1}{4} = 0$$

43. A: Begin by finding an antiderivative of $3x$, which is $\frac{3x^2}{2}$. Again, the constant of integration can be taken to be zero, since this is a definite integral. Then:

$$\int_{2}^{4} 3xdx = \frac{3x^2}{2}\bigg|_{2}^{4} = \frac{3\cdot 4^2}{2} - \frac{3\cdot 2^2}{2} = \frac{3\cdot 16}{2} - 6$$

$$24 - 6 = 18$$

44. B: On this interval, $y = x$ is the curve on top, and $y = x^2$ is the curve on the bottom. So the area is given by the definite integral:

$$\int_{0}^{1} (x - x^2)dx = \left(\frac{x^2}{2} - \frac{x^3}{3}\right)\bigg|_{0}^{1}$$

$$\left(\frac{1^2}{2} - \frac{1^3}{3}\right) - \left(\frac{0^2}{2} - \frac{0^3}{3}\right) = \frac{1}{2} - \frac{1}{3} = \frac{1}{6}$$

45. D: Position is an antiderivative of velocity, so it must have the form:

$$h(t) = -16t^2 - 8t + C$$

At the starting time of $t = 0$, this should equal 500, so setting:

$$500 = -16\cdot 0^2 - 8\cdot 0 + C$$

gives $C = 500$, or:

$$h(t) = -16t^2 - 8t + 500$$

46. C: Break up the interval from -1 to 2 into 3 intervals. Each interval has a width of 1. The left endpoints of these intervals are -1, 0, and 1. Evaluate $2x^2 + 1$ at each of these points. This evaluation gives 3, 1, and 3, respectively. Therefore, the 3 rectangles have areas of:

$$3 \times 1 = 3, 1 \times 1 = 1, 3 \times 1 = 3$$

Add these areas to obtain $3 + 1 + 3 = 7$.

47. A: Apply the quadratic formula with $a = 1, b = 2, c = 5$. This gives

$$\frac{-2 \pm \sqrt{2^2 - 4 \cdot 1 \cdot 5}}{2 \cdot 1} = -1 \pm \frac{1}{2}\sqrt{4 - 20}$$

$$-1 \pm \frac{1}{2}\sqrt{-16} = -1 \pm \frac{1}{2}i\sqrt{16}$$

$$-1 \pm \frac{i}{2} \cdot 4 = -1 \pm 2i$$

48. D: To perform this operation, subtract the vectors component by component:

$$(3 - 2, -2 - 1, 1 - (-4)) = (1, -3, 5)$$

Dear PCAT Test Taker,

We would like to start by thanking you for purchasing this study guide for your PCAT exam. We hope that we exceeded your expectations.

Our goal in creating this study guide was to cover all of the topics that you will see on the test. We also strove to make our practice questions as similar as possible to what you will encounter on test day. With that being said, if you found something that you feel was not up to your standards, please send us an email and let us know.

We would also like to let you know about other books in our catalog that may interest you.

PTCB

This can be found on Amazon: amazon.com/dp/162845833X

We have study guides in a wide variety of fields. If the one you are looking for isn't listed above, then try searching for it on Amazon or send us an email.

Thanks Again and Happy Testing!
Product Development Team
info@studyguideteam.com

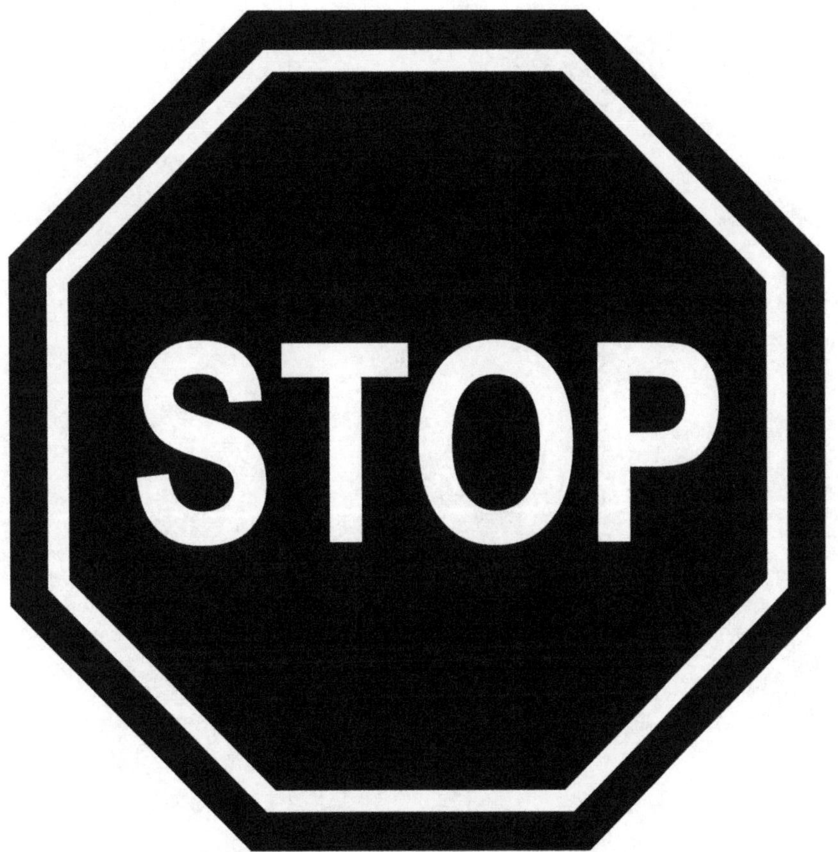

FREE Test Taking Tips DVD Offer

To help us better serve you, we have developed a Test Taking Tips DVD that we would like to give you for FREE. **This DVD covers world-class test taking tips that you can use to be even more successful when you are taking your test.**

All that we ask is that you email us your feedback about your study guide. Please let us know what you thought about it – whether that is good, bad or indifferent.

To get your **FREE Test Taking Tips DVD**, email freedvd@studyguideteam.com with "FREE DVD" in the subject line and the following information in the body of the email:

a. The title of your study guide.

b. Your product rating on a scale of 1-5, with 5 being the highest rating.

c. Your feedback about the study guide. What did you think of it?

d. Your full name and shipping address to send your free DVD.

If you have any questions or concerns, please don't hesitate to contact us at freedvd@studyguideteam.com.

Thanks again!

CPSIA information can be obtained
at www.ICGtesting.com
Printed in the USA
BVHW011335150820
586534BV00012B/174

9 781628 458480